LASSEN VOLCANIC
National Park

A COMPLETE
HIKER'S GUIDE

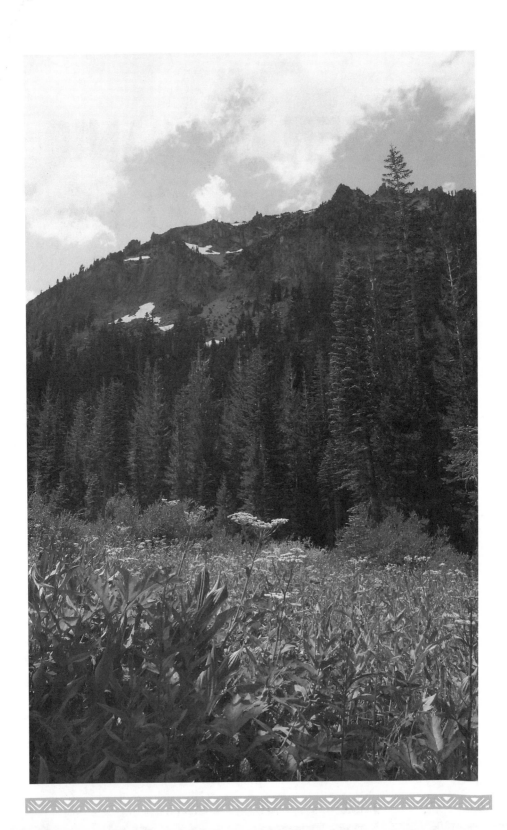

LASSEN VOLCANIC
National Park

A COMPLETE
HIKER'S GUIDE

MIKE WHITE

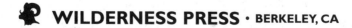 **WILDERNESS PRESS** · BERKELEY, CA

Lassen Volanic National Park: A Complete Hiker's Guide

1st EDITION 1981
2nd EDITION 1986
3rd EDITION 2003
4th EDITION March 2008

Copyright © 2008 by Mike White

Front cover photo copyright © 2008 by Laurence Parent Photography
Back cover photo copyright © 2008 by Mike White
Interior photos, except where noted, by Mike White
Cover and book design: Larry B. Van Dyke
Book editor: Eva Dienel

ISBN 978-0-89997-470-5
UPC 7-19609-97470-3

Manufactured in Canada

Published by: **Wilderness Press**
               1200 5th Street
               Berkeley, CA 94710
               (800) 443-7227; FAX (510) 558-1696
               info@wildernesspress.com
               www.wildernesspress.com

Visit our website for a complete listing of our books and for ordering information.

Cover photos: Hat Lake below Reading Peak *(front)*;
                    View from Lassen Peak *(back)*
Frontispiece: Loomis Peak from Manzanita Creek

SAFETY NOTICE: Although Wilderness Press and the author have made every attempt to ensure that the information in this book is accurate at press time, they are not responsible for any loss, damage, injury, or inconvenience that may occur to anyone while using this book. You are responsible for your own safety and health while in the wilderness. The fact that a trail is described in this book does not mean that it will be safe for you. Be aware that trail conditions can change from day to day. Always check local conditions and know your own limitations.

Dedication

To Darrin, Randy, and John, for helping me to see things from a grander perspective and for their visible examples of walking by faith.

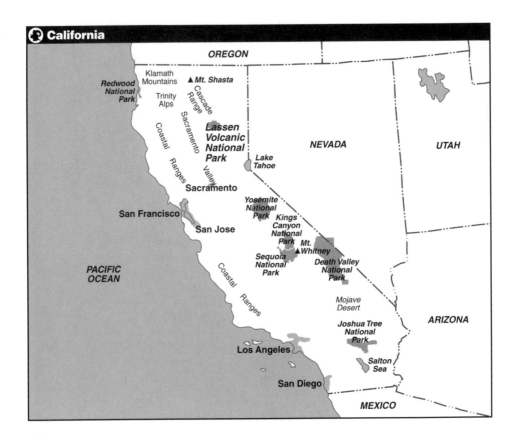

California

OREGON

Redwood National Park

Klamath Mountains ▲ Mt. Shasta

Trinity Alps

Coastal Ranges

Sacramento

Cascade Range

Lassen Volcanic National Park

Lake Tahoe

NEVADA

UTAH

Sacramento Valley

San Francisco

San Jose

Yosemite National Park

Kings Canyon National Park

Mt. ▲ Whitney

Sequoia National Park

Death Valley National Park

PACIFIC OCEAN

Coastal Ranges

Mojave Desert

Joshua Tree National Park

ARIZONA

Los Angeles

San Diego

Salton Sea

MEXICO

Contents

Acknowledgments   *xiii*

Preface   *xiii*

Chapter **1**   **Introduction** **1**
Human History   2
Flora and Fauna   8
Geology   14
Climate   18
Locator Map   20

Chapter **2**   **Traveling the Backcountry** **21**
Fees   21
About Lassen and Surrounding Lands   22
Wilderness Ethics and Trail Courtesy   25
Maps   27
Wilderness Permits   27
Wilderness Use Regulations for Lassen Volcanic National Park   28
Backpacking Equipment Checklist   29
Winter in the Lassen Area   29

Chapter **3**   **About This Guide** **31**
Symbols   31
Trip Information   32
Map Legend   33

Chapter **4**   **Lassen Scenic Byway Road Log** **35**
Segment 1: Main Park Road Through Lassen Volcanic
National Park   36
Segment 2: Highway 44 from Crossroads Junction to
Old Station   47
Segment 3: Highway 44 from Old Station to Highway 36
Junction   48
Segment 4: Highway 44 Junction to Highway 89 Junction
West of Mineral   49

Segment 5: Highway 89 from Old Station through Hat Creek Valley   50

Chapter 5 Lassen Scenic Byway Trips 53

Introduction to the Main Park Road 53

SOUTHWEST ENTRANCE TRAILHEADS:
1 Brokeoff Mountain   56
2 Mill Creek Falls   58
3 Ridge Lakes   60
4 Sulphur Works   61

ROAD SUMMIT TRAILHEADS:
5 Bumpass Hell to Kings Creek Picnic Area   62
6 Lassen Peak   65
7 Paradise Meadow   70
8 Terrace, Shadow, and Cliff Lakes   72

KINGS CREEK MEADOWS TRAILHEADS:
9 Cold Boiling Lake and Crumbaugh Lake   73
10 Kings Creek to Southwest Campground   74
11 Twin Meadows   76
12 Upper Kings Creek   77
13 Sifford Lakes   78
14 Kings Creek Falls   80
15 Kings Creek Falls and Bench Lake Loop   81

SUMMIT LAKE TRAILHEADS:
16 Summit Lake   83
17 Corral Meadow   84
18 Corral Meadow-Swan Lake Loop   85
19 Echo and Twin Lakes   87
20 Cluster and Twin Lakes Loop   89
21 Dersch Meadows to Cliff Lake   92

EMIGRANT PASS TRAILHEADS:
22 Nobles Trail to Badger Flat   94
23 Hat Lake to Paradise Meadow   96
24 Devastated Area Interpretive Trail   97

MANZANITA LAKE TRAILHEADS:
25 Crags Lake   98
26 Manzanita Creek   100
27 Manzanita Lake   102
28 Lily Pond Nature Trail   104
29 Nobles Trail to Lost Creek   105

*Introduction to the Hat Creek Recreation Area
and Thousand Lakes Wilderness* 106

BUNCHGRASS TRAILHEAD:
30 Durbin and Barrett Lakes 109

HAT CREEK TRAILHEADS:
31 Spattercone Nature Trail 111
32 Subway Cave 112
33 Pacific Crest Trail: Subway Cave to Hat Creek Rim 114
34 Hat Creek Trail 116

FOREST ROAD 22 TRAILHEAD:
35 Pacific Crest Trail to Hat Creek Rim Lookout 119

MUD LAKE TRAILHEAD:
36 Pacific Crest Trail: Hat Creek Rim 121

TAMARACK TRAILHEAD:
37 Barrett Lake-Lake Eiler Loop 123

CYPRESS TRAILHEAD:
38 Upper Twin, Everett, and Magee Lakes, and Magee Peak 125

MAGEE TRAILHEAD:
39 Magee Peak 128

Introduction to Butte Lake and Caribou Wilderness 130

BUTTE LAKE TRAILHEADS:
40 Bathtub Lake Loop 132
41 Prospect Peak 134
42 Cinder Cone Nature Trail 136
43 Lower Twin-Horseshoe-Snag Lakes Loop 138
44 Widow-Jakey-Snag Lakes Loop 143

CONE LAKE TRAILHEAD:
45 Widow Lake 147
46 Triangle, Twin, and Turnaround Lakes 149

CARIBOU LAKE TRAILHEAD:
47 Middle Caribou Lakes Loop 151
48 Emerald, Rim, and Cypress Lakes 154

SILVER LAKE TRAILHEAD:
49 Trail Lake from Silver Lake 155

ECHO LAKE TRAILHEAD:
50 Trail Lake from Echo Lake 157

HAY MEADOW TRAILHEAD:
51 Beauty, Evelyn, Long, and Hidden Lakes Loop 158

Introduction to the Greater Susanville-Chester Area *160*

EAGLE LAKE TRAILHEADS:
52 Eagle Lake Recreation Trail 162
53 Osprey Overlook Trail 164

SUSANVILLE TRAILHEAD:
54 Bizz Johnson Trail 166

LAKE ALMANOR TRAILHEAD:
55 Lake Almanor Recreation Trail 167

Introduction to Juniper Lake *168*

JUNIPER LAKE TRAILHEADS:
56 Mount Harkness 171
57 Juniper Lake Loop 174
58 Crystal Lake 176
59 Inspiration Point 177
60 Horseshoe and Indian Lakes Loop 179
61 Horseshoe, Snag, and Swan Lakes Loop 181
62 Cameron Meadow-Grassy Creek Loop 185
63 Jakey Lake 187
64 Jakey Lake-Widow Lake Loop 189

Introduction to Warner Valley and Drakesbad *193*

WARNER VALLEY TRAILHEAD:
65 Warner Valley to Mount Harkness 194
66 Lower Kings Creek to Corral Meadow 197

DRAKESBAD TRAILHEADS:
67 Boiling Springs Lake 199
68 Terminal Geyser and Little Willow Lake 201
69 Drake Lake 204
70 Dream Lake and Devils Kitchen 207
71 Sifford Lakes 209
72 Kings Creek Falls 211
73 Corral Meadow Loop 213

Introduction to the Southern Borderlands *216*

WILLOW LAKE TRAILHEAD:
74 Willow Lake to Terminal Geyser 218

DOMINGO SPRINGS TRAILHEAD:
75 Pacific Crest Trail: Northbound to Drakesbad   220

HIGHWAY 36 TRAILHEAD:
76 Pacific Crest Trail: Highway 36 to Domingo Springs   223

SPENCER MEADOW TRAILHEAD:
77 Spencer Meadow Loop   226
78 Blue Lake   229

MARTIN CREEK TRAILHEAD:
79 Heart Lake via Glassburner Meadow   231

SOUTH FORK DIGGER CREEK TRAILHEAD:
80 Heart Lake via South Fork Digger Creek   233

MILL CREEK TRAILHEAD:
81 Mill Creek Trail   234

DEER CREEK TRAILHEAD:
82 Deer Creek Trail   237

BLACK ROCK TRAILHEAD:
83 Mill Creek Trail-Ishi Wilderness   239

Chapter 6 Bucks Lake Wilderness Trips. 243

Introduction to Bucks Lake Wilderness   243

HIGHWAY 70 TRAILHEAD:
84 Pacific Crest Trail to Three Lakes   245

SILVER LAKE TRAILHEAD:
85 Gold Lake   247
86 Silver Lake to Spanish Peak   248

BUCKS SUMMIT TRAILHEAD:
87 Bucks Summit to Spanish Peak   250

BUCKS CREEK TRAILHEAD:
88 Bucks Creek Loop   252
89 Bucks Creek to Mill Creek Campground   253

MILL CREEK CAMPGROUND TRAILHEAD:
90 Bucks Lake Wilderness Loop   255

MILL CREEK TRAILHEAD:
91 Three Lakes   259

Chapter 7 McArthur-Burney Falls Trips

Introduction to McArthur-Burney Falls Memorial State Park   263

BURNEY FALLS TRAILHEAD:

92 Falls Loop   264
93 Headwaters Pool-Pacific Crest Trail Loop   265
94 Burney Creek-Rim Trail Loop   266

PIONEER TRAILHEAD:

95 Pioneer Cemetery Trail   267

Appendices 269

   I Backpacks and Dayhikes Features Chart   269
  II The Bear Facts and Other Animal Concerns   273
 III Minimum-Impact Stock Regulations   276
 IV Nonprofit Organizations   277
  V Quick Guide to Frequently Used Numbers and Websites   278
 VI Suggested Reading   280

Index 281
About the Author 285

Acknowledgments

Without the love, support, and encouragement of my wife, Robin, none of my projects would ever come to fruition—by far and away, she deserves the highest praise for assisting me in this particular endeavor. Roslyn Bullas and her team at Wilderness Press were also instrumental in the process of retooling this guide into a new book and deserve much praise as well. While hiking many of the trails in the greater Lassen region was a solitary affair, a few willing souls did tag along with me for some of my adventures, including Jered Singleton, Chris Taylor, Keith Catlin, Chaise Correa, Eric Millette, and a group of kids from RCF's junior high camp. Officials from both the National Park Service and Forest Service were very helpful when called upon, especially Nancy Bailey from Lassen Volcanic. Lastly, I would like to thank Jeff Schaffer, who authored the previous editions of the Lassen guide, leaving a fine foundation to build upon.

Preface

Prior to working on this guide, I did what most people do when taking a summer foray to Lassen Volcanic National Park: I drove along the scenic main park road, made a quick visit to view the historic photographs of Lassen's eruptions at the Loomis Museum, and took dayhikes along the park's two most popular trails—to Lassen Peak, the park's highest summit and the site of the most recent eruptions, and to Bumpass Hell, the park's most active hydrothermal area. My most significant discovery during a season of fieldwork for this project was the abundance of spectacular scenery that lay beyond these popular destinations.

The Lassen area is truly a dayhiker's paradise, with a plethora of paths that lead to wildflower-carpeted meadows, forest-rimmed lakes, crystalline streams, interesting hydrothermal features, and view-packed summits. Although the vast majority of trails are well-suited for one-day adventures, backpackers also will find plenty of backcountry campsites for solitude and breathtaking scenery.

Although hundreds of thousands of people visit the park every year, the highest concentration of visitation occurs along the main park road, leaving a huge tract of untamed land available for those willing to venture away from the asphalt. The good news is that Lassen is likely to stay wild. Somewhat isolated in the mountains of northern California, far from major population centers, the Lassen area maintains a sense of remoteness and serenity that should remain for generations to come.

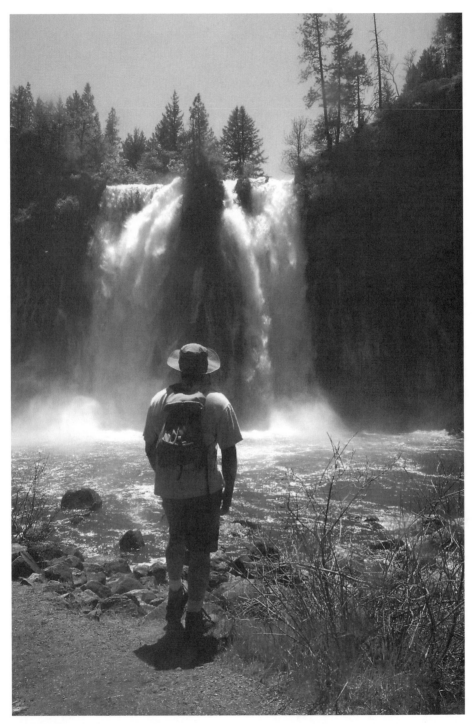

Burney Falls

Chapter 1

Introduction

Majestic Lassen Peak, a 10,457-foot lava dome towering over its mostly forested surroundings, is the centerpiece of Lassen Volcanic National Park. Until the 1980 eruption of Mt. Saint Helens in Washington state, Lassen Peak was the most recent volcano to blow in the continental US, when a series of events occurred from 1914 to 1917. These dramatic eruptions, along with several active hydrothermal areas and plenty of visible evidence of past volcanic activity, have created an extremely scenic and interesting landscape. In recognition of the region's numerous volcanic domes, cinder cones, mud pots, geysers, fumaroles, and hot springs, as well as its pristine lakes and wildflower-carpeted meadows, a groundswell of public support eventually compelled the federal government to approve the creation of Lassen Volcanic National Park in 1916.

The park is certainly more than dormant volcanoes and active fumaroles, hot springs, and mud pots, however. Meadows carpeted with brilliant wildflowers adorn numerous forest clearings, and a bounty of beautiful and placid lakes dot the backcountry. In the high country, a number of delightful streams spill down, creating significant waterfalls and picturesque cascades as the water makes its way to the Sacramento River in the western valley below.

As happens in many national parks, most of the nearly 383,000 average annual visitors to Lassen Volcanic congregate in one area: the main park road, which winds 33 miles from the southwest border to the northwest border, climbing over an 8500-foot pass along the way. Of those visitors, only about 10 to 15 percent stay overnight in one of the five campgrounds located along the main park road (the park has three other campgrounds, located near Butte and Juniper lakes and in Warner Valley). Of that percentage, only 15 percent backpack in the park's wilderness. Although the park contains about 150 miles of trail, most visitors head to two trails: the Lassen Peak and Bumpass Hell trails, which together represent only about 4 percent of the total trail mileage.

All of this means that in the backcountry, there is approximately one square mile for every backpacker (although reality dictates that backpackers tend to congregate around the park's major lakes). The potential for solitude for those willing to step away from the main park road is high, and you don't have to be a hardy backpacker to enjoy the trails of Lassen Volcanic. Indeed, the park is a dayhiker's paradise, with just about any destination accessible in one day or less. Solitude is also a reasonable expectation in the surrounding Lassen National Forest, including in the Thousand Lakes and Caribou wildernesses. Farther south, Bucks Lake Wilderness in Plumas National Forest is similarly uncrowded.

The majority of visitors to Lassen Volcanic come not for backcountry solitude, but rather for the scenic attractions, namely Lassen Peak and the hydrothermal areas. Families flock to the park to relax in a campground, hike a short trail, or swim or fish in one of the park's numerous lakes.

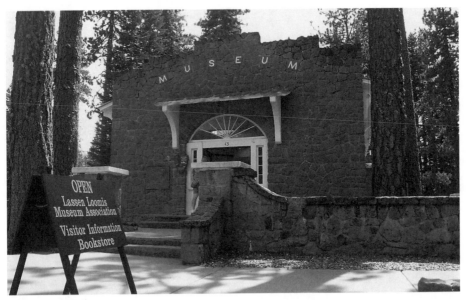

Loomis Museum

The scenery almost always pleases, and the warm and sunny summer weather is usually cooperative. Camping can be quite pleasant, although competition for available sites at campgrounds along the main park road can be high, especially during weekends (reservations are recommended at Manzanita Lake, Summit Lake North, and Summit Lake South campgrounds).

Despite the fact that fishing is better outside the park, plying the waters for that elusive trout remains a popular pastime within Lassen Volcanic, especially at lakes with adjacent campgrounds, including Manzanita, Summit, and Butte. The Park Service quit stocking park lakes in the 1980s, and of the 23 lakes with fish, only 9 have self-sustaining populations. Manzanita Lake is catch-and-release only, and fishing there is not allowed near the boat launch and inlet. Manzanita Creek, above the lake, is also off-limits to anglers. In addition, fishing is prohibited around the boat launches of Butte and Juniper lakes. A valid California fishing license is required for fishing in any waterway within the park.

The national forest areas outside the park offer many fine fishing opportunities,

including at Hat Creek, Deer Creek, Eagle Lake, Bucks Lake, and Lake Almanor. Unlike the national park, many of the waterways in the national forest are regularly stocked with fish. Backcountry fishing is perhaps best in Caribou Wilderness, where the numerous lakes and lack of use combine to provide good conditions for anglers. Special restrictions apply to some of the streams and lakes; check with the California Department of Fish and Game (www.dfg.ca.gov) for more information.

Human History

Native Americans and Early Settlement

Prior to the arrival of Europeans, Native Americans routinely traveled to the Lassen area in search of fish and game and to gather of a variety of nuts, seeds, and berries to supplement their diets. They also gathered roots and grasses for making baskets. Archaeological surveys within the park indicate that Native Americans regularly used these lands for habitation and work sites. Unfortunately, as happened in much of the rest of North America, the Native Americans who occupied the greater Lassen region were systematically destroyed by disease, destruction of habitat, and outright extermination. Lassen Peak was near the nexus of the territory of four distinct groups of Native Americans: the Yahi, Yana, Atsugewi, and Maidu. Both the Yahi and Yana lived primarily in the western foothills near the east edge of the Sacramento Valley. The Atsugewi inhabited an area to the north and northeast of Lassen Peak, while the Maidu lived to the south in the drainages of the north and middle forks of the Feather River. Although no permanent settlement was ever established within the future boundary of Lassen Volcanic, Native Americans from these tribes would often migrate to the area during the summer months and set up temporary camps. Euro-American fur trappers introduced diseases that devastated the population of the tribes, and settlers upset migratory wildlife patterns and reduced the animals' numbers.

By the late 1800s, with westward expansion in full swing, the conflicts between Native Americans and Euro-Americans increased, which inevitably led to the downfall of the four tribes. A band of four Yahi survived into the early 1900s in the rugged Deer Creek area until only one remained. Ishi, dubbed "the last wild Indian in North America," walked out of the mountains in 1911, and lived nearly five more years in the white man's civilization until his death from tuberculosis in 1916. Ishi has been immortalized in *Ishi in Two Worlds* (University of California Press, 1961), an excellent book by Theodora Kroeber, and by the small wilderness area that bears his name and contains some of the wild foothills terrain that provided him refuge for so many years.

Europeans arrived in the area in the early 1800s, when some of the first settlers were fur trappers exploring the streams of the upper Sacramento Valley but avoiding the lands around Lassen Peak. Instead, they generally came into the valley from the north or south, leaving the Lassen area

to the east virtually untrammeled by Euro-Americans until the last half of the 19th century.

Settlement of the Lassen area increased dramatically after the construction of two emigrant trails that brought people north from an area near the current site of Rye Patch Reservoir in Nevada. The first trail was built by Peter Lassen, who arrived from San Francisco in 1844, when he obtained an extensive tract of land in the upper valley (near present-day Marysville) from the Mexican government, which controlled California at that time.

After the discovery of gold in California, Lassen sought support to develop a route for emigrants that ran directly to his holdings in northern California, instead of over Donner and Carson passes, where the previously established pioneer routes traveled. To establish his claim in 1848, Lassen and a small party of 12 wagons followed part of the previously established Applegate Trail to Goose Lake in southern Oregon. Just beyond the lake, Lassen's party broke away from the Applegate Trail and forged a new route along the Pit River. Difficult terrain produced long detours resulting in delays that ultimately placed them in peril of starvation. Fortunately, a group of miners from Oregon followed their tracks and quickly caught up with the struggling group, sharing food and breaking trail the rest of the way to Lassen's ranch.

Although several thousand travelers ultimately used the route, the long and arduous Lassen Trail was deemed a less desirable way to reach northern California and was soon discarded for the standard routes farther south. Peter Lassen eventually lost his ranch, and resettled near present-day Greenville and then Honey Lake before being shot to death in 1859. As the first settler to establish a permanent residence within the region, and as one of California's oldest and most respected pioneers, Peter Lassen is honored today with his name attached to several geographic features.

The second route, the Nobles Emigrant Trail, was established by William H. Nobles in the early 1850s. Nobles discovered his new emigrant route while on the way back from a prospecting expedition in 1851, and by the following year, the first emigrants made the journey, which passed near Cinder Cone and over what is now known as Nobles Pass in the vicinity of Manzanita Lake. Although it ultimately carried four to five times as many emigrants as did the Lassen Trail—and it received praise as a far superior route—the Nobles Trail failed to lure a high percentage of westward traffic away from the more noteworthy Donner Pass and Carson Pass routes. As a result, it was not chosen as the best route for the construction of the Transcontinental Railroad (which ultimately was built over Donner Pass, with a subsequent route through Feather River Canyon), and eventually Nobles Trail was doomed to obscurity. The Tehama County Wagon Road, built in the early 1860s between Red Bluff and Susanville, met a similar fate with the expansion of the railroad in 1867.

Early Explorations

As towns in the Sacramento Valley became settled, exploration of the vast, undeveloped lands of the southern Cascades increased—and that exploration included pioneering routes up Lassen Peak itself. In the beginning, Lassen Peak was called San Jose, Mt. Joseph, and Mt. Saint Joseph, but in 1851, a miner named Grover K. Godfrey, after a chance meeting with Peter Lassen, christened the mountain Lassen Peak, crediting Peter Lassen as the first Euro-American to set foot on the summit. However, evidence of Lassen's first ascent is inconclusive, as no one saw him on the summit, nor was any evidence found of his presence. The first documented climb of Lassen Peak was made by Godfrey himself in 1851.

By the mid-1850s, others set their sights on the peak as well. In 1863, the California State Geological Survey, under the direction of Josiah Dwight Whitney, sent a team led by William H. Brewer into the Lassen wilderness, exploring hot springs and climbing Lassen Peak a couple of times. Clarence

King, famed geologist, mountaineer, and the first director of the US Geological Survey, was the most notable in attendance. After a week of exploration, the survey laid important groundwork for understanding the volcanic origins of the landscape. In August of 1863, Helen Brodt became the first non-native female to reach the summit. Her first name was later bestowed upon the attractive lake at the peak's base.

In the last part of the 19th century, several explorers contributed to more knowledge of the area. In 1874, Harvey W. Harkness, a mycologist and natural historian, headed into the area near Snag and Juniper lakes to check out false reports of recent volcanic activity, and, in the process, he became the first to climb Cinder Cone. In 1878, Lieutenant Samuel E. Tillman led a small band of men from the George Wheeler Survey (which Congress had approved to map the American West), from Chico to Susanville across the southern part of the future parklands. The Wheeler Survey laid important groundwork for future surveys conducted by the soon-to-be formed US Geological Survey. In 1883, Joseph Silas Diller, a veteran US Geological Survey geologist, led a broad exploration into the southern Cascades. Diller returned two years later to more closely inspect the lands around Lassen Peak, and he continued his investigations of the area for four decades. Among other notable achievements, including authoring several books of natural history, Diller was credited as the first to identify Lassen Peak as part of the Cascade Range and not the Sierra Nevada.

Seeds of Preservation

Fortunately for the long-term protection of the area's resources, mining proved to be largely unprofitable, and small-scale logging did only reasonably better. However, grazing was another story, as the lush grasses found in the numerous meadows provided an excellent food source for both sheep and cattle. In the latter half of the 19th century, ranchers herded their stock into the higher elevations as the snow melted in summer and the rich forage appeared shortly afterward. As a result, settlements took hold along the Tehama County Wagon Road in Battle Creek and Mill Creek meadows, and a small village developed at Mineral Springs. A few Sacramento Valley residents started to visit these areas in the summer to escape the oppressive heat, and they developed a fledgling resort community there by the mid-1860s. About a decade later, an even smaller development was taking place at Manzanita Lake along the old Nobles route.

The first stirrings for protecting land in the Lassen area were the result of numerous fires that consumed substantial tracts of forest land. Some of these fires were set by natural causes, but stockmen attempting to expand grazing areas started the majority of them. In part, the resulting destruction the fires posed to watersheds spurred the Department of the Interior to propose the idea of forest preserves. In 1905, jurisdiction of these preserves was transferred to the Department of Agriculture, which renamed them national forests shortly thereafter. Despite a lack of staff and resources, the small group of rangers, under the supervision of chief ranger Louis A. Barrett, was so effective in regulating the stockmen that most of them eventually left the Lassen area. The creation of the Forest Service in 1905 had both positive and negative impacts on the health of Lassen National Forest. Grazing was curtailed, but other parts of the forest fell victim to logging, railroad, and power companies. Perhaps the most visible example occurred when Big Meadow was inundated by Lake Almanor in 1914 upon completion of the first dam by the Great Western Power Company (which was later absorbed into the Pacific Gas and Electric Company).

In 1906, Barrett and a group of citizens reacted to these threats by petitioning the federal government to protect the hot springs and volcanic features surrounding Lassen Peak. The Forest Service commissioned the well-traveled Barrett to make recommendations on which lands were worthy of national park status. Instead of a park, which required time-consuming congressional approval and administration by the Department of Interior, Barrett proposed two national monuments overseen by the Forest Service that could easily be established by presidential proclamation. In May of 1907, President Theodore Roosevelt created Cinder Cone National Monument and Lassen Peak National Monument.

The Creation of Lassen Volcanic National Park

For the next seven years, the Forest Service administered the two national monuments and surrounding national forest. Although Congressman John H. Raker, who represented northeastern California and was frequently a guest at Drakesbad Guest Ranch in Warner Valley, had submitted two proposals, the creation of a national park may never have happened without the eventual eruptions of Lassen Peak. Raker's efforts generated little national interest but raised significant opposition from sheep and cattle interests that continued to use the proposed parklands for grazing. The first minor eruption of Lassen Peak, on May 30, 1914, prompted a flock of sightseers, reporters, photographers, and scientists to visit the mountain. Benjamin F. Loomis was among this group of interested observers, and his photographic documentation, some of which can be viewed at the Loomis Museum, provides an excellent record of the subsequent volcanic events. A series of minor eruptions took place over the next year, until the first major event occurred on May 19, 1915, when lava spilled over the crater rim, initiating a substantial mudflow down Hat and Lost creeks. Three days later, a gradual buildup culminated in Lassen Peak's biggest eruption, which sent a dark cloud billowing 4 miles into the atmosphere and a hot blast of air down the course of the previous mudflow, devastating a much wider swath of timber. Volcanic ash from the eruption was carried as far as Reno, about 100 miles away. Volcanic activity tapered off after that eruption, with the last cited activity in 1921.

Seizing the opportunity presented by a renewed interest in an active volcano, local residents and civic groups, spearheaded by journalist Michael E. Dittmar and business-man Arthur L. Conard, convinced Raker to resubmit his bill. Despite opposition from the Forest Service, which was reluctant to relinquish control of its lands to the Inte-rior Department, the Senate and House overwhelmingly passed the bill. On August 9, 1916, President Woodrow Wilson signed the bill into law, setting aside 79,561 acres as Lassen Volcanic National Park. A little over two weeks later, the president signed a separate bill creating the National Park Service, with the dual mission of preserving natural resources and promoting human enjoyment of these public lands.

Just like other national parks at the time, Lassen Volcanic was initially under-funded and understaffed and had to fend off attempts by angry stockmen to abolish the park. Early visitation to Lassen Volcanic was minimal, with roads going only as far as Sulphur Works and Drakesbad in the south and Manzanita Lake in the north. In 1925, Benjamin Loomis organized a crew to extend the road from Manzanita Lake to Crescent Meadow, from which point a trail was built to the top of Lassen Peak (the current Manzanita Creek Trail follows part of this old road). Soon after that, the park received additional funding for the construction of both state and park roads that eventually made Lassen Volcanic much more accessible to the public.

Recent History

In the mid-1920s, Lassen Volcanic National Park took two major strides forward when Walker Collins became the first permanent park ranger, and the town of Mineral was selected as the site for park headquarters. Thanks to legislation sponsored by Con-gressman Harry Englebright, in 1929 Las-sen Volcanic was expanded by just over 25,000 acres, to a configuration represen-tative of the current boundary. Around the same time, Benjamin Loomis, having built the Mae Loomis Memorial Museum in 1927 in honor of his daughter, donated his 40-acre tract of land near Reflection Lake to the Park Service. Shortly afterward, PG&E also agreed to deed 280 acres nearby that included Manzanita Lake. Despite these two significant donations, the sizable tracts of private land that remained within the park boundaries proved to be much more difficult to obtain. Significant inholdings included Sulphur Works and a large tract in Hot Springs Valley, Drakesbad, Juniper Lake, and Terminal Geyser. These acquisi-tions proved to be so difficult that the last of these issues was not to be completely resolved until 1997.

By 1931, the road across the park was complete, paving the way for Manzanita Lake in the north and Sulphur Works in the south to replace Drakesbad as the primary entry points to the park. That same year, the current Lassen Peak Trail was opened, providing hikers a route to the summit that was shorter and had less elevation gain than the previous route from Manzanita Creek. The Park Service responded to the greater influx of visitors by hiring seasonal rang-ers and naturalists, printing publications, and developing a variety of programs that enhanced enjoyment of the park. During the 1930s, the Civilian Conservation Corps made invaluable contributions to the park's infrastructure, including the construction of campgrounds at Manzanita Lake, Summit Lake, Warner Valley, and Butte Lake.

A long and contentious battle with the Supan family over acquisition of their property at Sulphur Works and Hot Springs Valley ended in 1952 when a condemnation suit was settled with a jury award of just under $50,000 for their 260 acres. Modern-day visitors may be amazed to learn that a restaurant, gas station, souvenir shop, bath-house, four cabins, and a ski tow had once occupied the relatively pristine site, and that homesites in Hot Springs Valley had at one time been offered for sale.

After decades of valuable stewardship by the Sifford family, 400 acres surrounding Drakesbad were sold to the Park Service during the same time period as the Sulfur Works acquisition. Efforts to purchase private land around Juniper Lake in 1957 were largely successful, although a number of rustic cabins blight the northwest shore to this day. The Snell family had purchased the land around the lake in 1914 with the intention of building a road, store, and cafe; stocking the lake with trout; and subdividing the land into cabin sites.

A more recent difficulty arose in the extreme southern part of the park when an oil company bulldozed a road to Terminal Geyser in 1962. Sixteen years later, without contacting the Park Service, Phillips Petroleum Corporation cleared a 1.5-acre site and sunk a test well immediately below Terminal Geyser and within a stone's throw of the Pacific Crest Trail. A year later, Phillips returned to the site, without notifying the Park Service, but this time the Interior Department condemned the property and then issued a "declaration of taking" in 1980. After years of litigation, Phillips Petroleum Corporation and its trustees were awarded more than $11 million for damages. The Park Service had the well plugged in 1997 and began restoration of the site the next year. None of these developments is visible today. With the conclusion of the Phillips Petroleum debacle, almost all of the park's private inholdings had been obtained.

With better access, visitors to Lassen Volcanic steadily increased during the decades leading up to World War II. Winter use of the area reached a crescendo during the mid-1930s, prompting a private concessionaire to install a rope tow below Sulphur Works for downhill skiing enthusiasts. Summer visitors to Drakesbad were so numerous that many groups had to be turned away for lack of lodging facilities and space for campsites. The number of visitors topped out at 108,000 in 1941 before dropping precipitously during the war years.

The park received a huge increase in visitation following World War II, which severely taxed both the neglected infrastructure and the insufficient number of staff. After the war, winter users benefited from improvements to the ski area and the eventual construction of the Lassen Chalet in 1966. By the mid-1950s, visitation had tripled the previous high set in 1941, and by 1972, it reached a half million visitors, with the park's infrastructure still in need of major upgrades. Although improvements were slow in coming, Congress accepted a recommendation from the Park Service to classify 78,982 acres of the park as wilderness in 1972, ensuring that Lassen Volcanic's backcountry would remain wild and undeveloped.

In 1974, after a USGS report identified potential hazards from seismic activity, the Park Service decided, for public safety reasons, to close commercial facilities at Manzanita Lake, including the lodge and cabins, general store, gas station, gift shop, and camper services. Park facilities such as Manzanita Lake Campground, its picnic area, the Loomis Museum, and employee housing also were shut down. The closures, which were located in the path of a potential rockslide from Chaos Crags, sparked considerable controversy. A portion of the campground outside the projected avalanche path was reopened after two years, but the rest of the facilities remained closed until 1981, when a new park master plan was approved. Under this plan, day-use activities would be permitted at Manzanita Lake and Chaos Crags. Further scientific study minimized the extent of the risk from a potential rockfall avalanche, prompting the Park Service in 1987 to preserve the historic buildings in the area and allow day use of the nature trails. However, the ban on overnight accommodations and closure of campground loops A and B remained in effect.

In the early 1980s, an effort to alleviate overcrowding on winter weekends included the installation of a triple chairlift at the ski area near the park's southwest entrance. However, by the mid-80s, the ski area proved to be commercially unviable, due in part to the opening of a competing ski area on Mt. Shasta and successive years of drought that produced very poor snow conditions. Since downhill skiing didn't fit philosophically with the national park mission, coupled with the fact that the Lassen ski area was originally seen as only a short-term priority until a full-scale operation could be built on Forest Service land nearby, the Park Service allowed the concessionaire to pull out of its contract and the chairlift was subsequently removed.

Increased visitor use steadily continued through the 1980s and 1990s. The 21st century dawned with old and new challenges to the park's dual mission of protecting the cultural and natural resources while allowing the public to enjoy those resources. In July of 2003, a general management plan was released to chart the course of the Park Service within Lassen Volcanic National Park for the next 10 to 15 years. Along with expanded protection of plants and animals and a desire for increased environmental awareness by visitors, a number of specific improvements were proposed. The Park Service is planning to decide whether to expand wilderness designation by nearly 25,000 acres, as well as whether to increase ranger patrols in the backcountry, improve the Lassen Peak and Bumpass Hell trails, and implement better maintenance of all trails in general. New trail projects include relocation of the Warner Valley Trailhead to a less environmentally sensitive area, construction of a trail from the Warner Valley Campground to Drakesbad, consolidation of the Juniper Lake trailheads to a single area, and an upgrade of pedestrian and bike trails in the Manzanita Lake area. Perhaps the most noticeable improvement will be the construction of the Kohm Yah-mah-nee visitor center near the site of the old Lassen Chalet by the southwest entrance. Slated to open in October 2008, the visitor center will provide year-round services, including an information desk, interpretive exhibits and displays, an auditorium where a new park film will be shown, a bookstore, gift shop, restaurant, restrooms, drinking fountains, first-aid services, after-hours backcountry registration vestibule, and an amphitheater. Road projects will include better cultural and interpretive facilities and improved pullouts along the main park road, and upgrades to the Warner Valley Road. Several of the park's campgrounds and picnic areas will be improved or relocated to less environmentally sensitive areas.

In the 21st century, the rise in gas prices has affected visitation to Lassen Volcanic National Park, where getting to the park relies almost exclusively on the private automobile. In 2001, just over 372,000 people visited the park. After peaking at nearly 407,000 in 2003, visitation dropped to 381,611 in 2006. As visitor use remains high and resulting challenges to the ecosystem continue, the Park Service will continue to be stretched to uphold the dual mission of protection and enjoyment of Lassen Volcanic. With federal resources being funneled to other priorities, the challenges become even more daunting. Without the additional support of private individuals and nonprofit organizations, the challenge for the future will be monumental (see Appendix IV for organizations that support Lassen Volcanic).

Flora and Fauna

Lassen Volcanic National Park and the surrounding national forest lands contain a rich diversity of both animals and plants. The park is home to almost 300 species of mammals, birds, reptiles, amphibians, and fish. Mammals comprise approximately 57 of those species, and range from common predators like black bears and mountain lions to smaller rodents like mice and chipmunks. Birds make up the lion's share of species, with approximately 216 species in the park. Some of the more intriguing birds include bald eagles, peregrine falcons, and spotted owls. Fish occupy a spot at the other end of the numeric scale, with only nine species present—five are native to California, and the rest are introduced species.

Amphibians and reptiles each have six representative species within the park.

Forests and wildflowers are the predominant plants that characterize the backcountry of Lassen Volcanic National Park and the surrounding forest lands. The park hosts around 700 species of vascular plants—ferns, herbs, shrubs, and trees—grouped into about 75 plant families. In comparison, the Mt. Shasta area and Crater Lake National Park host about 485 and 570 species, respectively, in approximately 60 families each. All three of these areas are nearly equal in size, have a volcanic origin, and span a similarly wide range of elevation. Additionally, ponderosa pines are found at the lower elevations and alpine flowers are at the highest in all three areas.

Lassen exceeds the Mt. Shasta and Crater Lake areas in plant diversity because of its location and geologic history. Lassen Volcanic and the surrounding lands lie near the north end of the Sierra Nevada, the south end of the Cascade Range, the west edge of the Great Basin, and the east edge of the Sacramento Valley floral provinces. This region is a virtual melting pot for plants, receiving immigrants from these four major plant areas. The greater Lassen area is also one of active, though sporadic, volcanism, where geologically recent volcanoes and lava flows bury older volcanic rocks, resulting in a variable collage of soils that range from fresh lava, pumice, and ash to deep, weathered, organically rich sediments. Just like around Mt. Shasta and Crater Lake, glaciers flowed through the area, creating canyons and meadows. However, unlike those two areas, glaciers in Lassen left behind a plethora of lakes of all sizes and depths, thereby creating additional environments for plant succession. With a wider range of environments, plants from very diverse communities have successfully migrated to Lassen Volcanic. Consequently, every Lassen environment, no matter how seemingly extreme and uninviting, has found some willing takers.

Today, each plant growing in the greater Lassen area has specific water, tem-

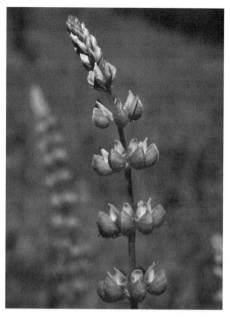

Lupine

perature, and mineral requirements, which limit distribution. Certainly, global warming has already had a minor impact on the distribution of plant species and a much more dramatic impact should be anticipated for the future. Plants may migrate into higher elevations searching for cooler temperatures and more abundant water supplies, and conifers may start to invade some of the meadows for which the park is famous. While glaciers have long been absent from the Lassen landscape, the permanent snowfields on the namesake peak will diminish and eventually disappear altogether, providing additional ground for plants to take root. Wildflowers such as sulfur flower and sticky cinquefoil have wide tolerances and consequently enjoy above average distribution.

Overspecialization leads to extinction, yet non-specialization leads to the loss of habitat to more specialized, better-adapted species. Similar to animals, plants must adapt along a careful path if their lines are to survive through the ages. Generally, plants tend to prefer fairly specific environments, called habitats, with plants of similar habitats collectively forming a group referred to as a plant community.

The following major plant communities represent those that you are likely to encounter on a visit to the Lassen region, if you were to travel by car from the Burney Falls area south along Highway 89 and the main park road to the base of Lassen Peak, and from there by foot up the Lassen Peak Trail to the 10,457-foot summit. Also mentioned are some of the more common animals found within these communities.

Mixed Conifer Forest (Part 1)

Plants: Lowest in elevation (about 3000 feet, near Burney Falls), this community has the longest growing season, roughly nine months. Winters tend to be mild, with ample rain and snow. Winter snow usually disappears by early or mid-spring, and the landscape can be fairly dry by early summer, with wildflowers going to seed usually before the hot summer drought. As the dominant conifer of this community, the ponderosa pine is one of two three-needled pines in the southern Cascades (Jeffrey pine is the other). Similar in appearance, ponderosa pines can be distinguished from Jeffrey pines by their smaller cones (3 to 6 inches) with scales that curve out rather than in. Douglas firs, sugar pines, white firs, and incense cedars may be found intermixed in the ponderosa pine forest. Common shrubs include currant, gooseberry, squawcarpet, and snowberry.

In lower elevations along the western part of Lassen National Forest, Douglas firs are often the dominant conifers, with a substantial mixture of oaks in the forests farther west, toward the foothills. In the drier, open areas, chaparral is quite common in this zone as well.

Animals: The mild climate of this community provides a good home for a wide range of wildlife. Small mammals include skunks and a host of rodents. Great horned and pygmy owls are common birds, along with the white- and red-breasted nuthatch,

brown creeper, olive-sided flycatcher, common flicker, and pileated woodpecker.

Sagebrush-Juniper Woodland

Plants: Heading south up Hat Creek Valley, Highway 89 stays close to Hat Creek, oftentimes within the ponderosa pine forest. The mountains to the west, which increase in height farther to the south, intercept most of the Pacific storms, depriving lands to the east of life-giving moisture. Consequently, a sagebrush and juniper community thrives on the hot and dry Hat Creek Rim above the east side of the valley. Pockets in the valley itself have even more extreme conditions, where former creeks and wet meadows were buried beneath geologically recent lava flows. Only the hardiest of species can take hold in the young and sterile lava. Along with the western juniper, mountain mahogany is a familiar tree/shrub. Rabbitbrush and bitterbrush are associates of the sagebrush. Drought-tolerant wildflowers, such as mule ears and sulfur flower are common wildflowers.

Animals: Animals common to the mixed conifer forest, such as the golden-mantled ground squirrel and coyote, are found in the sagebrush-juniper woodland, as well as some animals from the Great Basin environment, such as the sagebrush lizard and black-tailed jackrabbit.

Mountain Chaparral

Plants: Where soils are thin and dry, extensive tracts of brush, especially greenleaf manzanita, cover the landscape. Lesser associates include pinemat manzanita, chinquapin, tobacco brush, snowbrush, huckleberry oak, and bitterbrush. These tracts begin around 4000 feet along the east base of Sugarloaf Peak in Hat Creek Valley, but see the greatest development between 5000 and 6000 feet just outside Lassen Volcanic's northwest corner. Large fires are usually the instruments responsible for converting open forests into pure brushland, although extensive logging has a similar impact. These areas provide browsing deer with plenty of forage and excellent fawning sites. So dense are some of these tracts that reforestation can be delayed for a century or more.

Animals: With abundant food and plenty of cover for protection against predators, the mountain chaparral community is teeming with birds and animals. Scurrying lizards are more than likely the most common animals, but other notable species include cottontail rabbit, deer mouse, dusky-footed wood rat, mountain quail, and fox sparrow.

Mixed Conifer Forest (Part 2)

Plants: At higher elevations than the Mixed Conifer Forest (Part 1), somewhere between 5000 and 6000 feet, ponderosa pines intermix with and then yield to Jeffrey pines. Characteristic stands of Jeffrey pine forest can be found within Lassen Volcanic around Manzanita Lake. These conifers and their associated vegetation, which varies considerably from place to place, grow in areas of elevation up to 8000 feet on slopes with gravelly, well-drained soils. Cones of the Jeffrey pines are 6 to 8 inches long with scales that generally curve in. Jeffrey pine bark is said to emit a vanilla or pineapple scent when scratched. Associates include white fir and western juniper. Tobacco brush, greenleaf manzanita, and sagebrush are common shrubs found within this environment. Drought-tolerant wildflowers grace the forest floor in early to midsummer.

South of Manzanita Lake, Highway 89 ascends into a white fir forest belt, where soils are deep but well-drained and slopes vary from gentle to moderate. Common associates of this zone include sugar pine and incense cedar. The white fir forest is generally cool and shady, causing snow on the forest floor to linger through June, about a month or so longer than the drier slopes beneath a Jeffrey pine forest at the same elevation. These shady conditions inhibit the development of much groundcover, although root parasites like snow plant and pinedrops do well in the low-light environment. Where the forest is more open, pinemat manzanita and bush chinquapin are the most common shrubs, and lupine, paintbrush, and penstemon are the most frequently seen wildflowers.

Animals: Lodgepole chipmunks, red fox, and Steller's jays are just a few of the many species of animals living in the mixed conifer forest.

Upper Montane Forest

Plants: Three types of conifers make up the majority of trees found in the upper montane forest. Lodgepole pine, the most widely distributed pine in the western US, is common around lakes and meadows, and along stream banks. Red fir blankets the upper end of this zone, often in pure stands, but also in mixed stands with lodgepole pine and lesser amounts of western white pine. This mixed forest of lodgepole pine, red fir, and western white pine is the trademark forest within Lassen Volcanic National Park.

The lodgepole pine forest is found between 5500 feet and 7500 feet where sufficient groundwater is present. These two-needled conifers are first seen near the Lost Creek bridge, becoming more common on the way to the Devastated Area. This stretch of terrain appears to be dry, but an abundant supply of groundwater lies a mere 5 to 10 feet below the surface. Lodgepole pines thrive along mountain streams and around meadows, and just about every lake in the Lassen area is surrounded by these trademark trees. Streamside environments are also well-suited for a number of shrubs in this community, including thinleaf alder, creek dogwood, Labrador tea, red mountain heather, serviceberry, mountain spirea, currant, and a few varieties of willow. Receiving much more light than their white fir forest counterparts, wildflowers can be

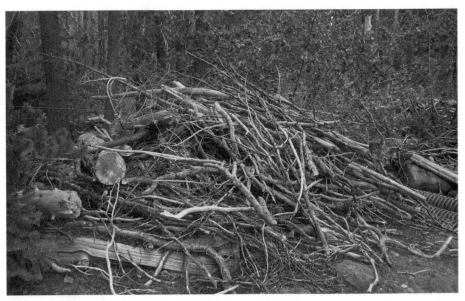

Beaver activity

quite abundant in a lodgepole pine forest, especially along streams, where varieties include monkeyflower, fireweed, leopard lily, monkshood, lupine, gentian, saxifrage, and buttercup. Where the groundwater is much farther below the surface, the groundcover shifts to drought-tolerant species such as spreading phlox.

The other form of upper montane forest, the red fir forest, clothes almost half of Lassen Volcanic. In neighboring Caribou Wilderness, red firs mingle extensively with lodgepole pines, and together these two species blanket at least three-quarters of the terrain. With a general range between 6000 to 8000 feet, the red fir forest is cooler and hangs onto snow long into the summer, with some patches remaining well into July. Due to the harsher environment, red firs and their occasional associate, the western white pine, don't grow nearly as tall as their counterparts in the white fir forest. At the lower-elevation end of the range, red firs intermix regularly with white firs, which are very similar in appearance, especially as young trees, when they both resemble Christmas trees with silver trunks full of resin blisters. As the trees mature, the trunks

of red firs take on a reddish-brown hue, while the trunks of white firs appear grayish. The red and white fir are distinguished by their needles: Red fir needles are angled and bend up at the base, and the tips have sharp points, while white fir needles appear flat, twist at the base, and have blunt tips. Waist-high shrubs at the lower elevations have been supplanted almost exclusively by foot-high pinemat manzanita, although the forest floor is virtually barren where red firs form dense, nearly pure stands.

Animals: Animals in the upper montane forest tend to be reclusive and are therefore rarely seen. Black bear, mule deer, coyote, mountain lion, and bobcat are large mammals that range through but are not limited to the upper montane forest. Small mammals include the long-tailed weasel, snowshoe hare, red fox, golden-mantled ground squirrel, and pine marten. Bats can often be seen patrolling the skies above lakes after dusk. Birds may be somewhat easier to spot and birdwatchers should watch for the black-backed woodpecker, Williamson sapsucker, and hermit thrush.

Mountain Meadows

Plants: Continuing toward Lassen Peak, the road passes through two fine sets of meadows around 6600 and 7300 feet: Dersch Meadows, between the Devastated Area and Summit Lake, and Kings Creek Meadows, higher up, between Summit Lake and Lassen Peak. Although they can be quite dry by late summer, mountain meadows are usually boggy enough in early and midsummer to resist invasion from threatening lodgepole pines. More water-tolerant than lodgepole pines, willows and alders often are found in and around these types of meadows, where grasses, sedges, and rushes are the most dominant members of the community. Moist meadows offer excellent conditions for water-loving wildflowers such as cinquefoil, monkeyflower, paintbrush, larkspur, aster, stickseed, Mariposa lily, penstemon, gentian, corn lily, yampah, and yarrow.

Animals: Mule deer often browse on the rich plant life in mountain meadows, particularly around dawn and dusk. Black bears like to dine on the berries that typically grow on shrubs around the fringe of these meadows, but they are seen by humans much less often than the deer. Badgers tend to be even more reclusive than the bears. More common to the meadows are a host of rodents, including golden-mantled ground squirrels, shrews, voles, moles, pocket gophers, and meadow mice. The skies above mountain meadows feature a number of bird species, including killdeer and sparrow. Western toads are common amphibians.

Subalpine Zone

Plants: As the main park road climbs to an 8500-foot pass, a much harsher climate is evident. At these elevations, the winter snowpack averages around 15 feet, with snowdrifts of 25 feet or more that can last into August following stormy winters. Winter winds can be extremely fierce, allowing only the hardiest of plants to survive. Plant survival is further complicated by a growing season that lasts only three to four months. Two conifers, mountain hemlock and whitebark pine, are able to withstand this harsh environment. Mountain hemlocks grow at elevations of around 9200 feet in areas of deep snow, which provides the trees with a blanket of insulation during the cold winters. Whitebark pines tend to be hardier, but at elevations with progressively more severe conditions, these trees take on a dwarfed, prostrate form, called krummholtz (crooked wood). Near timberline (approximately 10,000 feet), those trees grow no taller than a low bush. Both mountain hemlocks and whitebark pines tend to grow in clusters or small groves, as conditions are generally too severe to support a dense forest. This leaves plenty of rocky and gravelly open space with a thin cover of perennial wildflowers, grasses, and sedges with very few shrubs. Common wildflowers of the subalpine zone include silverleaf lupine, sulfur flower, pussypaws, paintbrush, mountain pride, and Davis' knotweed.

Animals: Although summers are short in this community, the rich and varied flora found in the subalpine zone provides a fine home for a number of animals. Chipmunks or golden-mantled ground squirrels are probably the most often seen mammals in this community, along with the smaller pika. Common birds include mountain bluebird, Clark's nutcracker, mountain chickadee, and Cassin's finch.

Alpine Zone

Plants: Hikers climbing up the Lassen Peak Trail pass through the subalpine zone on the way to the first alpine plant species near 9000 feet. Near 10,000 feet, the last of the trees, grasses, and sedges disappear, and alpine wildflowers are the only plants that remain from there to the summit. Fierce winter winds across these open slopes blow away the protective snow and expose alpine plants to wind-chill temperatures of −50°F. Therefore wildflowers develop a ground-hugging aspect, rarely growing higher than a couple of inches above the soil. During the one- to two-month period of frost-free temperatures, alpine wildflowers shoot out of the ground and dot the otherwise bleak environment with color. Common alpine wildflowers include Davidson's penstemon, beautiful polemonium, Tolmie's saxifrage, Shasta knotweed, and golden draba. At least one alpine wildflower, Lassen Peak smelowskia, is found only within Lassen Volcanic, on Lassen Peak itself, and in a saddle between the peak and Chaos Crags.

Animals: The harsh elements of the alpine zone limit the animal species to a small number of rodents and birds that typically pass through the area rather than take up permanent residence. Watch for pikas on the ground, and Clark's nutcrackers and gray-crowned rosy finches in the sky.

Geology

Lassen Volcanic and the surrounding forest lands contain some of the most interesting geology in northern California. Lassen Peak itself erupted around 100 years ago, and the area is a veritable classroom for the study of volcanism, as well as a living laboratory for how nature recovers from such devastating events. Along with Lassen Peak's plug dome, the region holds many geologic wonders, including cinder cones, lava flows, lava tubes, and spattercones. Glaciation has also been a major influence on the area, and the effects of it can be observed in many parts of the park.

The oldest rocks in the Lassen area, which date back several million years or more, are similar to those in the Sierra Nevada and Klamath Mountains, and geologists speculate that they were deposited on a marine shelf just west of the shore of an ancient continent. No trace of these rocks exists in the Lassen area, for younger rocks have buried them hundreds or even thousands of feet deep. However, old marine sedimentary rocks are abundantly exposed east and south of Lake Almanor, and it's

safe to infer that they extend northwest under the Lassen area.

But one can't infer that Lake Almanor's igneous granitic rocks extend northwest under the Lassen area. Although geologic maps tend to imply that granitic rocks underlie the area, some geologists believe these rocks have been faulted about 100 miles to the west, lying today in the Klamath Mountains. These rocks began as molten material—magma—rising through the earth's crust and solidifying into plutons near the surface. Some of the magma probably reached the surface and erupted, creating volcanoes and lava flows similar to those seen today.

During the extensive period when plutons were forming, geologists theorize that the Lassen landscape lay very close to sea level. Part of this area may have been under a shallow sea, while another part may have been a lowland swamp. By 35 million to 40 million years ago, geologists believe, the land was raised farther above sea level, though swamps still prevailed locally. Vegetation flourished in the subtropical climate, with the swamps accumulating deposits that later turned to coal. When additional uplifting occurred and the climate became subtropical, the area experienced the first major eruptions of volcanic rock, mostly fluid lava flows of basalt and basaltic andesite. Such flows gradually buried the older landscape under hundreds of feet of lava. Although extensive, these flows probably erupted at a rate no grater than that occurring in the Cascade Range today. However, over great periods of time, such eruptions can significantly alter the landscape.

Due to continuing eruptions in the Lassen area, evidence of Pliocene age volcanoes remains mostly buried, with well-studied Mt. Maidu a notable exception. Battle Creek—with the assistance of glaciers—eroded much of the overlying rocks, exposing the volcano's innards. Mt. Maidu's eruptions, which likely began 2.25 million years ago, slowly built up a large volcano that may have towered over the town site of Mineral by a vertical mile or more.

About 1.2 million to 800,000 years ago, great quantities of rhyolite and dacite lava erupted on the volcano's flanks—more than 8 cubic miles of volcanic rock, including erupted ash.

Considerable time elapsed before the next known volcano began to form. Mt. Tehama, which originated about 600,000 years ago, slowly grew to a sizable mountain of perhaps 11,000 feet, standing about 10 miles northeast of eroded Mt. Maidu. More so than Mt. Maidu, this volcano was a child of the ice age, with glaciers that repeatedly developed on its flanks, gnawing deeper and deeper into the peak. The northeast flank became the site of several eruptions that oozed large amounts of dacite over the landscape and created Bumpass Mountain as well as the domes of Reading Peak, Flatiron Ridge above Warner Valley, Ski Heil Peak northwest of Lake Helen, and an unnamed dome immediately east of Lake Helen.

Both during and after periods of Mt. Tehama's flank eruptions, glaciers continued to eat away at the volcano, and by 100,000 years ago, they may have eaten back to the very core. By this time, Mill Creek canyon, through which the main park road climbs, had already formed, for glaciers that followed certainly flowed down the canyon. Today, only the flanks of Mt. Tehama remain, and Brokeoff Mountain is the largest and highest remnant. To the north, Mt. Diller, along with Pilot Peak, Diamond Peak, and Mt. Conard, also are remnants of this large volcano. Mt. Conard once stood 4000 feet above today's Sulphur Works.

While Mt. Tehama was dominating the scene in the area of Lassen Volcanic, another volcano was dominating the Hat Creek Valley area. Thousand Lakes Volcano stood about 17 miles north-northwest of Mt. Tehama and may have risen to a height of 9000 to 10,000 feet. Similar to Tehama, this volcano was gutted through repeated episodes of glaciation, almost entirely on the northeast slopes. Today, only the southern and western flanks remain, crowned by Crater, Magee, and Fredonyer peaks.

What's left of the volcano occupies all but the eastern third of Thousand Lakes Wilderness.

Although Mt. Tehama and the Thousand Lakes volcano may have stolen the show with impressive "fireworks" from their lofty summits, they weren't the only eruptive sites. The region as a whole experienced considerable volcanism throughout the ice age, burying most of the pre-ice age rocks. Perhaps during or after the middle of the ice age, roughly 1 million years ago or less, the vast lava plateau north of Lassen Volcanic began to rift, and a large complex block gradually dropped, forming Hat Creek Valley. Faulting had been occurring for millions of years, with uplifted blocks subjected to more aggressive erosion and down-dropped blocks subjected to burial by incoming sediments and lava flows. Volcanic activity took place at the head of Hat Creek Valley, where two vents spilled lava of andesite and basalt, which, over time, created the twin volcanoes of Table Mountain and Badger Mountain.

By the time Mt. Tehama's dacite domes erupted about 250,000 years ago, the area outside the future park boundaries had largely taken on the appearance of today's landscape. Ensuing glaciers carved the higher landforms, accentuating hills and ridges and leaving lakes behind when the glaciers disappeared. Inside the park, a significant glacial episode began, perhaps about 215,000 years ago, and lasted until about 140,000 years ago. During this time, or shortly thereafter, prominent volcanoes were born and then matured, including Mt. Harkness, Sifford Peak, Prospect Peak, and West Prospect Peak just outside the park. It's likely that during the youngest glacial period, three relatively small volcanoes formed, including Hat Mountain, Fairfield Peak, and Crater Butte, which gave rise to extensive lava flows between the main park road on the west and Horseshoe, Snag, and Butte lakes on the east.

The era following the ice age volcanism, 20,000 to 2000 years ago, could be referred to as the age of cinder cones and lava flows.

In the eastern Thousand Lakes Wilderness, about a dozen cinder cones erupted along a 7-mile-long line (perhaps a fault). Lava flows accompanied the eruptions, and several spilled over in Hat Creek Valley. Of postglacial origin, the most recent eruptions may have occurred as little as a few hundred years ago. An area of even more impressive activity occurred just beyond the north boundary of Caribou Wilderness, where a line of about two dozen cones stretches 10 miles south-southeast from Poison Lake alongside Highway 44. More than a dozen cones lie to the west. Lassen Volcanic developed fewer cones, although the plateau containing Hat Mountain, Fairfield Peak, and Crater Butte quite possibly experienced some eruptions during this period, as may have Prospect Peak. Crescent Crater, a decapitated dacite dome on the northeast flank of Lassen Peak, erupted before Lassen Peak itself.

Without Lassen Peak, the national park that bears its name probably would not exist. Geologists theorize that the monstrous dacite dome, one of the world's largest, welled up perhaps 27,000 years ago, pouring out thick, pasty lava. During that time, most of what's now the park may have been buried by an ice cap, with the peak erupting right on the ice cap's divide. This action cut off the source areas of glaciers flowing away from the divide, and consequently reduced their size severely. Glaciers soon began to form on the rubble-filled slopes of Lassen Peak, but the end of the glacial period was near, perhaps only 1000 to 2000 years away. In that time—brief by geological standards—the glaciers may have transported a quarter billion tons of Lassen Peak's loose dacite debris to a dumping ground a few miles to the east. Perhaps due to the loose nature of the slopes, and/or the short time involved, glaciers only mildly scalloped Lassen Peak.

The geologic history of Lassen Volcanic, Caribou Wilderness, and, to a lesser extent, Thousand Lakes Wilderness is a story of the interplay between volcanic eruptions building up and flowing glaciers grinding

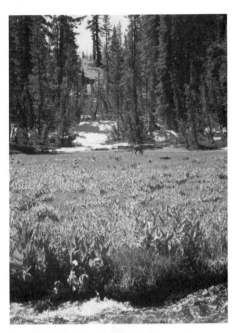

Deer in Kings Creek Meadows

down the landscape. Glaciers may have been gnawing away at Mt. Tehama even before the peak reached maximum height. The same may be true of any volcano above 8000 feet, as glaciers gradually developed and grew until they united with other glaciers to form an ice cap. These ice caps—which were hundreds of feet thick—buried most of the landscape above 6000 feet. Glaciers with large sources of ice accumulation extended beyond the general ice cap, and in the process, descended as low as 4500 feet and carved large canyons, most notably along Warner Creek. Although the creek cut down along a fault (Warner Valley is a result of the faulting), the canyon appears mostly to be the result of glacial action. Quarter-mile-thick glaciers flowed through, exerting great pressure on the valley floor. With this force, and the abundant supplies of abrasive sand and rock, the powerful glaciers cut canyons 500 to 1000 feet deeper than those in pre-glacial times.

When the last glaciers retreated in the Lassen area, about 9000 to 11,000 years ago, they left behind more than 600 basins that became ponds or lakes. Although lava flows or volcanoes formed some of these water bodies, most are the result of glacial erosion. Without these glaciers, the Lassen Volcanic-Caribou Wilderness complex would have only a dozen or so lakes. Thousand Lakes Wilderness would have only one—lava-dammed Lake Eiler.

While glaciers plucked away at mountainsides and canyon walls, creating steep and impressive slopes, they also transported loads of rock and debris downslope. Much of the debris was composed of relatively fine sediments, which became the foundation for many a fine mountain meadow. Without the glacial action, mountain meadows, with their dazzling array of wildflowers, would be almost nonexistent.

The finishing touches to the Lassen region occurred over the last 2000 years. After the ice age, Sugarloaf Peak began growing in the upper part of Hat Creek Valley, expanding to the point where the valley was almost cut in two. The landscape changed dramatically when Hat Creek Valley formed 1000 to 2000 years ago, as a result of eruptions of basalt flows that buried everything in their path. Also about this time (or perhaps several thousand years earlier), a series of eruptions at the lower end of the valley created Cinder Butte and spread lava for miles around.

In Lassen Volcanic, violent eruptions preceded the imminent eruption of Chaos Crags, a cluster of several volcanic domes. However, in those cases, the dacite lava was too thick and pasty to flow anywhere, so the lava simply piled up into domes. These massive domes lie between even more massive Lassen Peak and the Sunflower Flat domes. About 1670 A.D., part of a dome broke loose, possibly as a result of some steam explosions, and crashed down, rushing west across a gently sloped landscape at speeds well over 100 miles per hour. The 200 million cubic yards of debris came to a rest, creating a 2.5-acre area of total destruction known today as Chaos Jumbles. Manzanita Lake, Reflection Lake, and Lily Pond were later formed as a result of the altered and blocked drainage.

East of Chaos Crags, between 1630 and 1670, a rather fluid lava flow spilled across land in the Butte Lake area. Perhaps only days or weeks later, the flow was followed by the formation of a cinder cone. At least three more flows and two more cinder cone eruptions took place during that time. Today, these features are known as Fantastic Lava Beds and Cinder Cone. Some of the lava flows greatly altered the shape of Butte Lake, and one of the flows blocked a creek draining north into Butte Lake, allowing water to pool up to form Snag Lake.

The final volcanic events, which led to the eventual establishment of the park, involved a series of eruptions beginning on Memorial Day 1914. The activity reached catastrophic proportions on May 19, 1915, when a mudflow, generated by hot lava that spilled over Lassen Peak's summit crater onto an ash-laden snowfield, rumbled down the northeast side of the peak, leaving behind a several-mile-long area of desolation down both Hat and Lost creeks. On May 22, Lassen produced the fiercest eruption, the 174th recorded, with a corresponding blast of hot air that totally destroyed an area along the course of the previous mudflow. This path, about 3 miles long and 1 mile wide, is now known as the Devastated Area. After this eruption, the volcano began to calm down.

The Cascade Range consists of a series of active volcanoes, stretching from southernmost British Columbia to Lassen Volcanic. In the near future, geologically speaking, eruptions within the park may cease, and over time the area will erode to resemble the landscape to the south—an area where prior evidence of volcanism is diminished by more rolling terrain and maturing forests. This demise will be due to the northward migration the Juan de Fuca Plate, which is responsible for the previous volcanism. This chunk of the earth's crust is diving beneath northern California, Oregon, Washington, and southern British Columbia; when it reaches a certain depth, part of the plate melts, and part of that melt rises toward the surface as lava or some other product. Since the Juan de Fuca Plate is drifting north, the associated volcanism will travel northward as well. About 4 million years ago, the southern limit of activity in the Cascade Range was located well to the south, around Sonora Pass, near the northern boundary of Yosemite National Park. One million years from now, it will be around Burney Falls.

Climate

The climate of the Lassen area creates two tourist seasons: summer, primarily between the Fourth of July and Labor Day weekend, which sees the highest visitation levels, and winter, when a blanket of snow carpets the area, usually from Thanksgiving into April. Summer is the season for hiking, backpacking, fishing, camping, and sightseeing. During the winter, a much smaller number of visitors enjoy the serene landscape while cross-country skiing, snowshoeing, sledding, or backcountry snowboarding.

Late summer and early fall is the shoulder season when fewer people visit, but Lassen Volcanic generally has fair weather during this time, unless winter storms arrive early. Spring is the period of least visitation, as tourists usually avoid the area while waiting for winter's snowpack to melt.

In general, the summer season is quite mild, neither too hot nor too cold, and precipitation is uncommon. The precipitation that does occur during the summer months usually comes from a random thunderstorm. Most of Lassen Volcanic's campgrounds and lakes are located at elevations higher than the Manzanita Lake weather station, so summer temperatures are somewhat cooler than the temperatures listed in the chart on page 19. Thousand Lakes Wilderness and Caribou Wilderness experience similar deviations. Temperatures on June mornings may be near freezing, although usually temperatures register in the high 30s. By afternoon, daytime highs climb into the 60s, except when a passing cold front drops the temperature by 10 to 15 degrees. The warmest period of summer generally occurs between mid-July and mid-August,

Climate Chart

Lassen Park Headquarters, Mineral, CA (4500 feet)											
	JAN	FEB	MAR	APR	MAY	JUN	JUL	AUG	SEP	OCT	NOV	DEC
Average Max. Temp. (°F)	40	44	46	54	63	72	81	81	75	63	50	42
Average Min. Temp. (°F)	21	23	24	28	34	40	44	42	39	34	29	24
Average Snowfall (inches)	40	30	31	16	5	0.2	0	0	0.1	0.6	11	27
Manzanita Lake (5850 feet)											
	JAN	FEB	MAR	APR	MAY	JUN	JUL	AUG	SEP	OCT	NOV	DEC
Average Max. Temp. (°F)	39	42	43	50	60	70	80	78	71	60	47	41
Average Min. Temp. (°F)	19	20	22	28	35	42	46	45	41	33	27	23
Average Snowfall (inches)	40	31	37	23	9	1	0	0.1	0.6	0.3	20	34

with dawns ranging from the high 30s to low 40s, and afternoon highs in the low to mid-70s. Since the air is thinner at park elevations than at sea level, solar radiation is much greater, which makes 70 feel more like 80. As you climb higher, the radiation increases, and you can feel uncomfortably hot at an air temperature of 60°F atop 10,457-foot Lassen Peak.

By Labor Day weekend, as autumn is in the air and fall colors start appearing in the higher elevations, temperatures have dropped markedly. Daytime highs climb into the low 60s, which is still comfortable for outdoor recreation. However, mountain lakes, which were in the mid- to upper 60s just a few weeks earlier, now drop into the low 60s to high 50s, temperatures most find too chilly for enjoyable swimming. Depending on the year, the first storm of the season may appear in late September or early October, blanketing the park with a quickly melting coat of snow. Otherwise, fall is a splendid time in the mountains, as most of the tourists have departed and the days remain mild enough for one to make the most of the quiet solitude. By mid- to late October, the first significant Pacific storm usually sweeps across the area, closing the main park road and most of the area's trails.

Winter typically arrives in the Lassen area by Thanksgiving, and winter recreation begins soon after that, when a deep enough snowpack forms to provide decent conditions for snowshoeing and cross-country skiing. The winter season generally continues into late March or early April. Depending on conditions, the Park Service begins plowing sections of the main park road sometime in April, and then opens parking lots at the Devastated Area and Bumpass Hell in order to extend the season for snow sports into spring. Usually, the snowpack lasts through April up to 6000 feet, through May up to 7000 feet, and through June at 8000 feet. Lassen Peak retains a few year-round snowfields on the north side of the mountain.

Hikers can ply their craft all year at McArthur-Burney Falls Memorial State Park, although snow may sporadically dust the ground anytime between December and February. Hat Creek Valley, which is slightly higher than Burney Falls but lies in the rain shadow of the southern Cascades, usually offers snow-free hiking from early April through Thanksgiving. Lassen National Forest offers some lower-elevation trails for early- and late-season hiking, including Mill Creek Trail in Ishi Wilderness, Deer Creek Trail, Lake Almanor Trail, Eagle Creek Trail, and Bizz Johnson Trail. The lowest trails in Lassen Volcanic National Park and Caribou and Thousand Lakes wildernesses may be open as early as the first week in June, but the bulk of the trails don't shed their snow until the end of June. Higher trails, such as the ones to Bumpass Hell, Brokeoff Mountain, Magee Peak, and Lassen Peak, can hang onto substantial snowfields well into July. Nevertheless, most trails are easy to follow by mid-July. Estimates of snow-free trails may vary considerably from year to year, perfectly illustrated by the winters of 2005–2006 and 2006–2007, when an unusually late and wet winter was followed by one of the driest winters on record. During that period, some trail openings varied by as much as two months from one year to the next. Swimmers will find the warmest lake temperatures from late July to mid-August. (For current conditions, check the park website at www.nps.gov/lavo.)

Locator Map

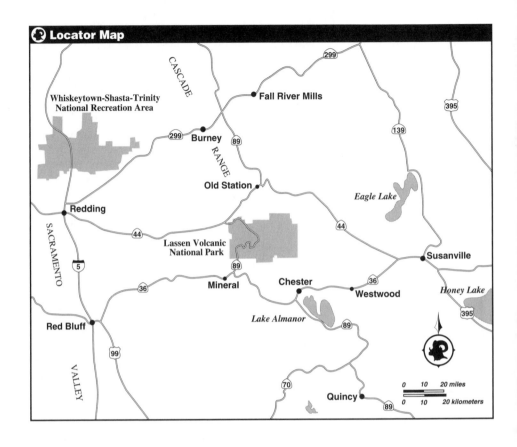

Chapter 2

Traveling the Backcountry

Fees

Rangers collect entry fees for Lassen Volcanic National Park at both the southwest entrance near the Kohm Yah-mah-nee visitor center and the northwest entrance near Manzanita Lake. When rangers staff entrance stations, payment may be made using cash, personal check, or credit card. After-hours entrance into the park requires self-registration at those locations (exact change or checks only). Entry fees (exact change or checks only) are also collected at self-registration stations at the more remote locations of the park, including Butte Lake, Juniper Lake, and Warner Valley.

Type of Pass	Fee	Duration	Terms
Vehicle Pass	$10	1 week	Access to Lassen Volcanic National Park
Annual Pass	$25	1 year	Access to Lassen Volcanic National Park and Whiskeytown National Recreation Area
Interagency Annual Pass	$80	1 year	Access to all national parks and federal recreation sites charging an admission fee
Interagency Senior Pass	$10	Lifetime	US citizens or permanent residents 62 or older. Access to all national parks and federal recreation sites charging an admission fee
Interagency Access Pass	Free	Lifetime	US citizens or permanent residents who are blind or permanently disabled. Access to all national parks and federal recreation sites charging an admission fee

About Lassen and Surrounding Lands

As has happened in many parts of the country, 9/11 and higher gas prices have taken their toll on the auto-based tourist industry within the greater Lassen area. Consequently, many tourist-related facilities outside the park have been forced to reduce their hours or to close altogether, making choices for securing such necessities as gas, food, and other supplies much more limited. Within the park itself, gasoline is available only at the Manzanita Lake Camper Store (for premium prices). A small selection of food, gifts, and supplies can be purchased from the Kohm Yah-mah-nee visitor center near the southwest entrance and the Manzanita Lake Camper Store near the northwest entrance. The Loomis Museum operates a small bookstore. Drakesbad Guest Ranch, located within the remote southern part of the park, offers lodging and meals (reservations required).

Information:
Lassen Volcanic National Park
PO Box 100
Mineral, CA 96063
(530) 595-4444
www.nps.gov/lavo

Park Service Ranger Stations and Visitor Centers:
Lassen Volcanic National Park Headquarters
Open Monday–Friday, 8 AM–4:30 PM; closed holidays
PO Box 100
Mineral, CA 96063
(530) 595-4444
(530) 595-3262 (fax)
Maps and books, park passes, restroom, wilderness permits

Kohm Yah-mah-nee Visitor Center
Near Southwest Entrance
Open October 2008

Loomis Museum
Late May to mid-June (Friday–Sunday)
9 AM–5 PM
Mid-June to early September (daily)
9 AM–5 PM
Early to late September
(Wednesday–Sunday) 9 AM–5 PM
(530) 595-4444 ext. 5180
Exhibits, books and maps, restrooms, picnic area, telephone, wilderness permits

Manzanita Lake Camper Store
Late May to mid-June (daily)
9 AM–5 PM
Mid-June to early September (daily);
8 AM–8 PM early
September to early October (daily)
9 AM–5 PM
(530) 335-7557
Restrooms, phone, showers, laundry, food, supplies, gifts, gas

USFS Headquarters:

Lassen National Forest
2550 Riverside Drive
Susanville, CA 96130
(530) 257-2151
www.r5.fs.fed.us/lassen

Plumas National Forest
159 Lawrence Street
Quincy, CA 95971
(530) 283-2050
www.r5.fs.fed.us/plumas

Forest Service District Ranger Stations:
Lassen National Forest
Almanor Ranger District
900 E. Highway 36
PO Box 767
Chester, CA 96020
(530) 258-2141

Lassen National Forest
Eagle Lake Ranger District
477-050 Eagle Lake Road
Susanville, CA 96130
(530) 257-4188

Lassen National Forest
Hat Creek Ranger District
43225 E. Highway 299
PO Box 220
Fall River Mills, CA 96028
(530) 336-5521

Plumas National Forest
Feather River Ranger District
875 Mitchell Avenue
Oroville, CA 95965-4699
(530) 534-6500

Plumas National Forest
Mt. Hough Ranger District
39696 State Highway 70
Quincy, CA 95971
(530) 283-0555

State Parks
McArthur-Burney Falls
Memorial State Park
24898 Highway 89
Burney, CA 96013
(530) 335-2777

Lodging

The only lodging option within park boundaries is the Drakesbad Guest Ranch, located at the end of the Warner Valley Road, 17 miles north of Chester. Drakesbad Guest Ranch was established in 1900 and was operated by the Sifford Family for nearly 60 years until the property was sold to the Park Service. On the National Register of Historic Places, the ranch continues to operate much as it did when it was run by the Siffords, without electricity or phone service. The 17 rooms have either a half or full bath and are lit by kerosene lamps and heated by propane. The ranch's swimming pool is heated by natural hot springs, and a certified massage therapist is on site. Meals (included in lodging fee), which are served in the dining room, include buffet breakfasts and lunches, and sumptuous dinners. A selection of beers and wines is also available.

Along with an abundance of nearby hiking opportunities, guests can enjoy a wide range of activities at the ranch, including fly-fishing, horseback riding, canoeing, volleyball, croquet, badminton, horseshoes, and ping-pong.

The ranch is usually open from early June to early October, weather permitting, and rates are based on double occupancy. Reservations are accepted beginning in mid-February. Book ahead for July and August, when occupancy rates can reach capacity. Newcomers attempting to make a reservation may feel as though they have to wait for the passing of an entire family in order to have any shot of securing a room during that period.

Outside of the park, four full-service communities—Fall River Mills, Burney, Susanville, and Chester—offer motel-style lodging. Closer to the park, a number of resorts offer more rustic accommodations.

Lassen Volcanic National Park
Drakesbad Guest Ranch
(530) 529-1512
www.drakesbad.com

Surrounding Forest Lands
Lassen Mineral Lodge
PO Box 160
Highway 36 East
Mineral, CA 96063
(530) 595-4422
www.minerallodge.com

Hat Creek Resort
12533 Highway 44/89
Old Station, CA 96071
(800) 568-0109
www.hatcreekresortrv.com

Rim Rock Ranch Resort
Highway 44/89
Old Station, CA 96071
(530) 335-7114
www.rimrockcabins.com

Rancheria RV Park
15565 Black Angus Lane
Hat Creek, CA 96040
(530) 335-7418
www.rancheriarv.com

St. Bernard Lodge
44801 Highway 36
Mill Creek, CA 96061
(530) 258-3382
www.stbernardlodge.com

Childs Meadow Resort
41500 Highway 36
Mill Creek, CA 96061
(888) 595-3383 or (530) 595-3383
www.childsmeadowresort.com

Mill Creek Resort
#1 Mill Creek Resort
Mill Creek, CA 96061
(888) 595-4449
www.millcreekresort.net

Campgrounds

Within Lassen Volcanic National Park, there are 11 campgrounds with more than 450 campsites. Campsites at Butte Lake, Butte Lake Group, Juniper Lake Group, and Lost Creek Group are available by reservation only. Sites at Manzanita Lake, Summit Lake North, and Summit Lake South campgrounds are available by reservation and on a first-come, first-served basis. Sites at Crags, Juniper Lake, Southwest Walk-In, and Warner Valley campgrounds cannot be reserved. The Forest Service offers additional campgrounds outside the park.

National Park Service Reservations
(877) 444-6777
www.recreation.gov

National Forest Service Reservations
(877) 444-6777
www.recreation.gov

Lassen Volcanic National Park

Main park road:
Southwest Walk-in
Summit Lake South
Summit Lake North
Crags
Manzanita Lake

Butte Lake Area:
Butte Lake

Juniper Lake and Warner Valley Area:
Juniper Lake
Warner Valley

Lassen National Forest

Hat Creek Area:
Big Pine
Hat Creek
Cave
Rocky
Bridge
Honn

Highway 44:
Crater Lake
Bogard
Silver Bowl
Rocky Knoll
Goumaz

Eagle Lake:
Christie
Merrill
Aspen
Eagle

Highway 36:
Roxie Peconom
Almanor
Benner Creek
High Bridge
Warner Creek
Domingo Springs
Warner Spring
Gurnsey Creek

Hole in the Ground
Battle Creek

Highway 32:
Elam Creek
Alder Creek
Potato Patch

Ishi Wilderness
Black Rock

Bucks Lake:
Queen Lily
North Fork
Gansner Bar
Silver Lake
Whitehorse
Grizzly Creek
Sundew
Hutchins
Lower Bucks
Mill Creek

California State Parks

McArthur-Burney Falls Memorial State Park:
Pioneer
Rim

Pacific Gas & Electric

Lake Almanor Area:
Rocky Point
Last Chance

Bucks Lake Area:
Haskins Valley

Wilderness Ethics and Trail Courtesy

The American wilderness evokes notions of wild and undeveloped open space where humans are merely visitors who leave no trace of their presence. The "leave only footprints, take only photographs" motto of the back-to-earth 1970s era embodies such a concept. The goal of every backcountry visitor, hiker, backpacker, and equestrian, should be to leave the wilderness the same way it was found, if not better. The following guidelines should help to keep the wild in wilderness.

Camping

- Camp a minimum of 100 feet from any water source.
- Choose campsites well away from trails.
- Never construct "improvements" (fireplaces, rock walls, drainage swales, etc.).
- Camp on exposed dirt and rock surfaces only, not on vegetation.
- Where campfires are allowed, use only downed timber—never cut trees, dead or alive.
- Use only existing fire rings for campfires, where permissible.
- Never leave a campfire unattended.
- Fully extinguish all campfires by thoroughly soaking them with water.

Sanitation

- Bury all human waste at least 6 inches deep, a minimum of 100 feet from trails, and a minimum of 500 feet from water sources.
- Pack out toilet paper, or burn it in areas where fires are permissible.
- Cook only the amount of food you can eat to avoid having to dispose of leftovers.
- Wash and rinse dishes, clothes, and yourself a minimum of 100 feet from water sources; never wash directly in lakes or streams.
- Pack out all trash—do not attempt to burn plastic or foil packaging.
- Filter, boil, or purify all drinking water.

On the Trail

- Stay on the trail—never cut switchbacks.

- Preserve the serenity of the backcountry—avoid making loud noises.
- Yield the right-of-way to uphill hikers.
- Yield the right-of-way to equestrians—step off the trail on the downhill side.
- Avoid traveling in large groups.
- Because trails can change, due to either natural or human causes, hikers should check with the appropriate agencies for trail updates prior to their hike.

Regulations for Lassen Volcanic National Park

- Group size is limited to 20 people on the trail, and 10 people per backcountry campsite (6 people are allowed in established campgrounds).
- Pets, weapons, metal detectors, wheeled vehicles, and motorized equipment are prohibited.
- No camping within 300 feet of other groups, nor within 100 feet of lakes or streams.
- Camping is prohibited within a half mile of any developed area or park road open to vehicular traffic, except in designated campgrounds.
- Camping is prohibited within a quarter mile of any hydrothermal feature.

In addition to the above restrictions, camping is prohibited within a quarter mile of the following areas: Bumpass Hell Trailhead to Bumpass Hell, Cascade Springs, Cinder Cone and Painted Dunes, Cliff Lake, Crags Lake, Crumbaugh Lake, Hat Creek Cabin, Echo Lake, Kings Creek Falls, Lassen Peak and Trail, Little Willow Lake, Mt. Harkness, Summit Trail from Summit Lake to Echo Lake, Upper and Lower Kings Creek Meadow, and Shadow Lake.

- Campfires are not allowed anywhere in the Lassen Volcanic backcountry.
- Hunting is not allowed.
- Leave all natural and cultural features undisturbed—preserve and protect them.

Maps

USGS Topographic Maps

A number of recreational maps are available for hikers and backpackers in the Lassen Volcanic area, including the maps provided in this guide. The 7.5-minute quadrangles (scale of 1:24,000), published by the United States Geological Survey, are the most accurate and usable topographic maps available. The USGS maps, $6 per sheet, are available directly from the USGS at www.store.usgs. gov, or from Forest Service ranger stations and information stations.

Today, there are computer software programs that use USGS maps as a base and usually have numerous features for customizing printable maps for personal use. The only significant disadvantage of the maps created from the software programs is the inability of most home computer printers to match the 22-by-29-inch size of the USGS maps. Some outdoor retailers, such as REI, have installed kiosks in their stores where customers can create and print comparable maps on-site.

Forest Service Maps

Lassen National Forest ($9, 1:26,720, 2002): A half inch equals 1 mile on this map of forest lands within Lassen National Forest.

Plumas National Forest ($9, 1:26,720, 2001): A half inch equals 1 mile on this map of forest lands within Plumas National Forest.

Forest Service Wilderness Maps

A Guide to the Bucks Lake Wilderness by Plumas National Forest ($9, 1:31,680, 1991): Two inches equal 1 mile on this map of the wilderness.

A Guide to the Ishi, Thousand Lakes, & Caribou Wildernesses by Lassen National Forest ($9, 1997): One inch equals 1 mile on this map of the wilderness areas.

Wilderness Press Map

Wilderness Press publishes *Lassen Volcanic National Park* ($10, 1:62,500, updated 2004), a topographic sheet map that covers the entire park as well as Caribou and Thousand Lakes wilderness areas, Hat Creek Valley, and McArthur-Burney Falls State Park.

Wilderness Permits

Dayhikers

Dayhikers are not required to have a permit for entry into Lassen Volcanic's backcountry (however, all visitors must pay an entrance fee to get into the park), Thousand

USGS Map Name	Trip Numbers
1. Burney Falls	95, 96, 97, 98
2. Murken Bench	35, 36
3. Thousand Lakes Valley	30, 37, 38, 39
4. Old Station	31, 32, 33, 34, 36
5. Manzanita Lake	25, 26, 27, 28, 29
6. West Prospect Peak	18, 19, 20, 21, 22, 23, 24
7. Prospect Peak	18, 20, 40, 41, 42, 43, 44, 45, 64, 65, 67
8. Bogard Buttes	45, 46, 47
9. Pikes Point	52, 53
10. Lassen Peak	1, 2, 3, 4, 5, 6, 10, 26, 80, 82, 83
11. Reading Peak	5, 6, 7, 8, 9, 10, 11, 12, 13, 14, 15, 16, 17, 18, 19, 20, 21, 23, 69, 70, 71, 72, 73, 74, 75, 76, 77, 78, 80, 81
12. Mt. Harkness	59, 60, 61, 62, 63, 64, 65, 66, 67, 68, 69, 77, 78
13. Red Cinder	47, 48, 49, 50, 51, 58
14. Swain Mountain	57
15. Pegleg Mountain	56, 57
16. Roop Mountain	54, 55, 56
17. Susanville	54
18. Childs Meadows	80
19. Stover Mountain	78, 79
20. Westwood West	57
21. Westwood East	57
22. Panther Spring	86
23. Barkley Mountain	86
24. Almanor	58
25. Belden	87
26. Storrie	87
27. Bucks Lake	87, 88, 89, 90, 91, 92, 93, 94

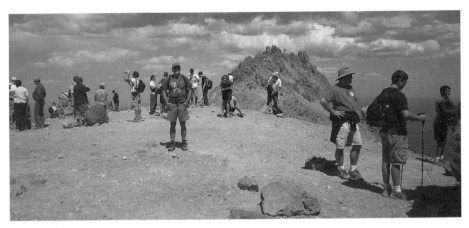

Near Lassen Summit

Lakes Wilderness, Caribou Wilderness, Ishi Wilderness, Bucks Lake Wilderness, or other areas of Lassen and Plumas national forests.

Overnight Backpackers

Currently, only Lassen Volcanic National Park requires overnight visitors in the backcountry to register for a wilderness permit, and quotas are not in effect. However, the Forest Service does require a fire permit for use of stoves or campfires in the backcountry. Wilderness permits can be obtained in person from any contact station during regular business hours. Applications may be downloaded from the park's website (www.nps.gov/lavo/planyourvisit/wilderness-permit-information.htm) and returned to the park via an email response, or faxed to: Front Desk, (530) 595-3262. Allow two weeks for processing. After business hours, backpackers may self-register at Butte Lake, Warner Valley, and Juniper Lake ranger stations; at the southwest and northwest entrance stations; and at the Kohm Yahmah-nee visitor center.

Wilderness Use Regulations for Lassen Volcanic National Park

- Ground fires are prohibited; use only camp stoves.
- Boil, treat, or filter water before drinking.
- Pets are prohibited (except on roads and roadside picnic areas).
- Wilderness permits are required for all stock day use.
- Travel is restricted to designated open trails (no cross-country travel).
- Water stock with a bucket; no grazing is permitted.
- Camp a minimum of 100 feet from any trail or high-water mark of lakes and streams.
- Group size is limited to 10 people per site. Groups must camp at least 300 feet from each other to lessen resource damage.
- Dig your hole for toileting at least 100 feet from any water and cover waste with 6 inches of soil.
- Keep wash water, soaps, detergents (even biodegradable varieties), fish entrails, and other waste out of all lakes and streams.
- Pack out all trash; don't bury or burn it.

- Use of weapons or metal detectors is prohibited.
- Motorized equipment and wheeled vehicles are prohibited.
- Do not construct *improvements* such as shelters, drainage ditches, rock walls, or bough beds.
- Leave all natural and cultural features undisturbed—preserve and protect them.

For Your Safety

- Ground around thermal areas is dangerously thin; never walk off-trail near hydrothermal areas.
- Stay on trails at all times for safety and to prevent erosion.
- Avoid higher and exposed terrain during electrical storms.
- Do not feed wildlife.
- Keep a clean camp and store food properly.
- Be aware of and prepared for changing weather conditions.

Backpacking Equipment Checklist

Gear

- ☐ Backpack (pack cover optional)
- ☐ Water bottles or hydration system
- ☐ Water purifier
- ☐ Sleeping bag (liner optional)
- ☐ Sleeping pad
- ☐ Tent (footprint optional)
- ☐ Stove, fuel, and accessories
- ☐ Cooking pots, cleaning pad, and biodegradable soap
- ☐ Bowl, cup, and utensils
- ☐ Food (bear canister)

10 Essentials (and More)

- ☐ Map of area
- ☐ Compass and GPS unit
- ☐ Sunglasses and sunblock
- ☐ Extra food
- ☐ Extra clothing
- ☐ Headlamp or flashlight (extra batteries and bulb)
- ☐ First-aid kit
- ☐ Fire starter or candle
- ☐ Matches in waterproof container
- ☐ Multi-tool knife
- ☐ Toilet paper (11th essential)
- ☐ Insect repellent
- ☐ Toiletries
- ☐ Repair kit (duct tape, cord, safety pins, etc.)
- ☐ Signaling device (whistle, mirror)
- ☐ Wilderness permit (where required)

Clothing

- ☐ Boots
- ☐ Optional footwear for stream crossings or at camp
- ☐ Socks
- ☐ Underwear (polypropylene or equivalent)
- ☐ Shirt
- ☐ Pants
- ☐ Vest (down or pile)
- ☐ Jacket (down or pile)
- ☐ Parka (Gore-Tex or equivalent)
- ☐ Rain pants (Gore-Tex or equivalent)
- ☐ Hat
- ☐ Gloves or mittens
- ☐ Bandanna
- ☐ Optional gear: camera, binoculars, book

Winter in the Lassen Area

Winter covers most of the Lassen backcountry with a thick blanket of snow. However, a few alternatives do exist for those seeking some opportunities during the winter months. The relatively low elevations around both McArthur-Burney Falls Memorial State Park (Trips 92–95) and Ishi Wilderness (Trip 83) insure that trails are snow-free in all but the coldest winters. Burney Falls, right off of Highway 89, typically has year-round access, but the dirt roads to Ishi Wilderness are not maintained from November to April and should be driven with caution (these roads are rough even in summer). Many of the trails in the Hat Creek area (Trips 31–36) are free of snow up to nine months of the year.

Visitors who embrace the coming of winter snows will find the Lassen area to be a winter wonderland for cross-country skiers and snowshoers alike. When snow closes all but a couple of miles of the main park road, the park's backcountry expands significantly, creating myriad opportunities for one-day outings and multiday adventures to ice-covered lakes, tall peaks, scenic canyons, and hydrothermal features.

The park has two winter centers, both positioned near the end of plowed sections of the main park road. The scenic Manzanita Lake area is the northern hub for winter recreation. Here, visitors can snowshoe around Manzanita Lake, or ski or snowshoe unmarked backcountry routes up Manzanita Creek or along the Nobles Emigrant Trail. At an elevation of 5800 feet, the area around Manzanita Lake usually has decent snow coverage from December through mid-March. As winter gives way to spring, the Park Service begins plowing the main park road from the Loomis Museum to a parking lot at the Devastated Area near 6500 feet. From that point, skiers, snowshoers, and mountaineers have a higher base from which to pursue their snow-related activities into the months of spring. Check the park's website (www.nps.gov/lavo) for progress of the road plowing.

The parking area near the southwest entrance is the southern hub for winter recreation. During winter, the Southwest Campground, which has vault toilets and running water, is open for snow camping. Once the Kohm Yah-mah-nee visitor center

is complete in 2008, expanded services will be available on a limited basis for winter visitors, including food service, a gift shop, and sale of interpretive and educational materials. Family snow play is a favorite activity, and the hills around the parking area, once the site of a small alpine ski area, provide excellent slopes for sledding, tubing, and snowboarding. Ranger-led, two-hour snowshoe walks are held on a first-come, first-served basis on Saturday afternoons from early January to early April, weather permitting (snowshoes are provided for a suggested $1 donation).

There are many possible backcountry routes from the southwest entrance, from short day trips to multiday outings. The 29-mile trans-park trek along the snow-covered main park road is a particularly coveted route for advanced skiers. Mountaineers can accept the challenge of a multiday trip to the summit of Lassen Peak. Skiers will find more information on possible routes in Marcus Libkind's *Ski Tours in Lassen Volcanic National Park* (Bittersweet Publishing Company, 1989), and snowshoers should consult the author's *Best Snowshoe Trails of California: 100 of the Finest Routes in the Cascades & the Sierra* (Wilderness Press, 2004), which includes 13 tours in the park.

All backcountry users should be well-versed in winter travel and avalanche awareness. Overnight camping in the backcountry requires a wilderness permit, available by self-registration at the Kohm Yah-mah-nee visitor center or at the Loomis ranger station. Permits may also be obtained in person at park headquarters, or from the park website (www.nps.gov/lavo) by fax or email. Day users of the trails can sign in and out using registers at the southwest and Loomis ranger station areas.

During spring, as plowing the main park road continues, parking becomes available at Sulphur Works (6950 feet), then the Bumpass Hell Trailhead (8200 feet), and finally at the Lassen Peak Trailhead (8500 feet), which helps to extend the park's snow sports season well into spring.

Chapter 3

About This Guide

This guide is designed for dayhikers in search of places in and around Lassen Volcanic National Park, and for backpackers interested in exploring the majesty of the southern Cascades on short weekend trips, weeklong excursions, and anything in between. Some evaluations of the trails in this book are subjective, but every effort was made to insure that the descriptions are meaningful to the average hiker and backpacker.

The 95 trips in this guide are divided into several sections corresponding to their geographical subregion. The first chapter of hikes, Chapter 4, covers a combination of state highways and the main park road through Lassen Volcanic on a loop designated as the Lassen Scenic Byway. Beginning with trips from trailheads accessible from State Highway 89, which becomes the main park road within Lassen Volcanic National Park, the loop proceeds northbound through the park to the junction of State Highway 44, just outside the northwestern park boundary. Heading east on Highway 44/89, the order of descriptions proceeds to Hat Creek Valley, where the highways divide, with Highway 89 heading north toward the Shasta area and Highway 44 heading east toward Susanville. Here, the descriptions deviate temporarily from the loop route to include trailheads accessible from Highway 89 in Hat Creek Valley, including trails into Thousand Lakes Wilderness. The Lassen Scenic Byway loop continues from the 89/44 junction, with trailheads in the Butte Lake area of Lassen Volcanic and then in the Caribou Wilderness on the way to a junction with Highway 36, about 5 miles west of Susanville. From there, the circuit continues west on 36 with access to trailheads near Susanville and trailheads emanating from the Lassen Volcanic areas of Juniper Lake and Warner Valley. Farther west, nearing the Highway 89 junction at the start of the Lassen Scenic Byway loop, Highway 36 leads to addi-

tional trailheads south of Lassen Volcanic. Trails of Bucks Lake Wilderness, south of State Highway 70 and west of Quincy are featured in Chapter 5. The final chapter of hikes, Chapter 6, describes trails within McArthur-Burney Falls Memorial State Park, north of Lassen Volcanic and easily accessible from Highway 89.

Each chapter includes a brief introduction to familiarize readers with the features of each area, with specific information about campgrounds, access, amenities, and ranger stations. Individual trail descriptions follow the information provided in the chapter introduction.

Symbols

Each description begins with a display of symbols that provides a quick and easy way to visually assess the following characteristics of each trip:

Trip Difficulty

E = Easy

M = Moderate

MS = Moderately strenuous

S = Strenuous

Type of Trip

↗ = Out and back

↗ = Point to point (shuttle required)

↻ = Loop

♫ = Semiloop

Duration

DH = dayhike (single-day outing)
BP = backpack

Trip Information

Each trip description also includes the following information:

Distance

Distances listed are in miles. Mileages for out and back, point to point, loop, and semiloop trips are listed as total mileage.

Elevation

Elevations listed are in feet. The first set of numbers represents the starting elevation, followed by significant high and low points. The second set of numbers represents the total elevation gain and loss. (To convert feet to meters, multiply by 0.3048).

Season

This entry lists the general period for when the trail should be open and mostly free from snow. However, these conditions may vary considerably from year to year.

Use

This entry gives a general idea of the trail's popularity (light, moderate, or heavy).

Map

USGS 7.5-minute maps covering the area of the trail are listed here. Occasionally, supplemental maps may be recommended.

Trip Description

The main body of the description includes an introduction of the route, directions to the trailhead, and a detailed guide to the trail.

In the margins beside the main text, readers will find quick-reference icons indicating various features found along the trip route:

⌂ = Campgrounds

≋ = Swimming holes

👁 = Noteworthy views

❀ = Seasonal wildflowers

♨ = Hydrothermal features

Additional entries concerning options and regulating information accompany the main descriptions.

Options   [O]

This entry highlights options for extending or varying the trip, including side trips, additional cross-country routes, and peaks to climb in the vicinity.

Regulatory Information   [R]

This entry concerns permits, quotas, and any specific restrictions that may apply to the trip.

🌐 Map Legend

▪▪▪▪▪▪▪▪▪▪	**Featured Trail**	▬▬▬	**National Park**
▬ ▬ ▬ ▬	**Other Trail**	▬▬▬	**National Monument; Wilderness Area**
▬▬**35**▬▬	**Trip Number**	▬▬▬	**National Forest**
T	**Trailhead**	═(**5**)═	**Interstate**
P	**Parking**	═(**89**)═	**State Highway**
A	**Campground**	(S5) (S22)	**County Road**
⌂	**Ranger Station**	**10**	**Major Forest Service Road**
?	**Information**	34N69	**Minor Forest Service Road**
$	**Fee Collection Gate**		
▲	**Mountain**		
ⅲ	**Meadow or Marsh**		
▪	**Building**		

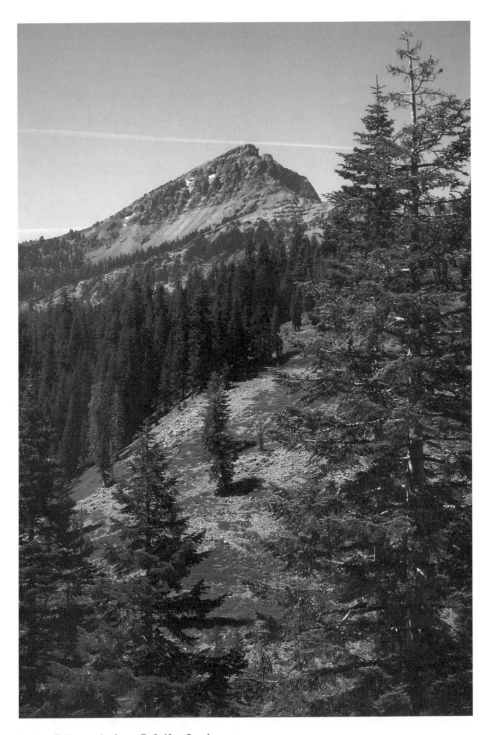

Brokeoff Mountain from E. Sulfur Creek

Chapter 4

Lassen Scenic Byway Road Log

Designated in July of 1993, the Lassen Scenic Byway comprises a combination of state highways to form a scenic, 185-mile, paved loop through and around Lassen Volcanic National Park. The following road log highlights significant points along this loop. Some of these points correspond to markers or interpretive signs within the boundary of the park, but most are unofficial landmarks that you can locate only if you pay close attention to your car's odometer. Broken into five sections, the log begins at the junction of state highways 36 and 89 near the southwest entrance to Lassen Volcanic, proceeds through the park over the high point near the Lassen Peak Trailhead, and then descends past the northwest entrance near Manzanita Lake to the Crossroads Junction between state highways 89 and 44.

Within the first segment are several of the park's most visited attractions, including the Kohm Yah-mah-nee visitor center; Southwest, Summit Lake, Lost Creek, Crags, and Manzanita Lake campgrounds; Lake Helen, Kings Creek, Summit Lake, and Manzanita Lake picnic areas; and Brokeoff Mountain, Sulphur Works, Ridge Lakes, Bumpass Hell, Lassen Peak, Terrace Lake, Summit Lake, Dersch Meadows, Hat Lake, Nobles, and Manzanita Lake trailheads.

Segment 2 continues the loop from the Crossroads Junction northeast to the small community of Old Station, near where Highway 89 turns north and Highway 44 heads southeast toward Susanville. This nearly 14-mile segment accesses three Forest Service campgrounds, two picnic areas, a vista point, the Spattercone Trailhead, the Old Station Information Center, and a few commercial establishments, as well as Forest Service roads leading to trailheads in Thousand Lakes Wilderness.

Continuing the loop, Segment 3 follows Highway 44 from the junction near Old Station around the north boundary of Lassen Volcanic and the northeast boundary of neighboring Caribou Wilderness to

the junction of state highways 44 and 36, approximately 5 miles west of Susanville. After climbing out of Hat Creek Valley, the highway passes the Hat Creek Rim Overlook, Butte Lake Road, Bogard Rest Area, and roads accessing Silver Lake, Caribou Wilderness, and a couple of Forest Service campgrounds. This segment of Highway 44 offers no commercial enterprises.

Segment 4 continues the loop on a westward journey from the 44/36 junction, passing the Devils Corral Trailhead and an access road to a Forest Service campground on the way to the tiny town of Westwood. Beyond Westwood, the highway crosses the northern arm of massive Lake Almanor before reaching the full-service community of Chester and junctions with roads to Juniper Lake, Warner Valley, and Domingo Springs, and with Highway 89 heading southeast along the west shore of Lake Almanor. From Chester, the highway continues west, past St. Bernard Inn, Deer Creek Lodge, and a trailhead for the Pacific Crest Trail on the way to a junction with Highway 32, which heads southwest toward Chico. Beyond this junction, Highway 44 continues past Gurnsey

Campground, Spencer Meadows Trailhead, and Childs Meadow Resort to the east junction of Highway 72 to Mill Creek. Another 3.5 miles leads to the close of the loop at the 44/89 junction near Morgan Summit.

Segment 5 splits away from the Lassen Scenic Byway loop near Old Station and proceeds north through Hat Creek Valley, toward McArthur-Burney Falls Memorial State Park. Along this road are a number of Forest Service campgrounds and access roads to trailheads in the Hat Creek area and Thousand Lakes Wilderness, as well as commercial campgrounds with restaurants and general stores.

Segment 1: Main Park Road Through Lassen Volcanic National Park

0.0 Highway 36 west of the 36/89 junction: Westbound from the 36/89 junction, Highway 36 descends toward Red Bluff, soon passing turnoffs to Forest Road 30N16 (providing access to Martin Creek Trailhead) and to the east junction of State Highway 172 (providing access to Mill Creek Resort, Hole in the Ground Campground, and the Mill Creek Trailhead) before reaching the town of Mineral, 5 miles from the junction. Mineral is home to the Lassen Mineral Lodge, RV campground, gas station and convenience store, post office, and LVNP headquarters at the west end of town. Battle Creek Campground is 1.2 miles west of headquarters, near the junction of Forest Road 17 (providing access to the South Fork Digger Creek Trailhead).

2.0 Road 29N22: This well-graded dirt road branches west, winding 1.25 miles to a junction with a primitive road climbing west over a low ridge to McGowan Lake. After another 1.25 miles, Road 29N22 crosses a lateral moraine and descends south along its west side, reaching a junction with Road 30N16 in 0.5 mile, which descends 2.2

miles south to Highway 36 about midway between Lassen Mineral Lodge and the 36/89 junction.

4.4 Park Boundary: The stone entrance marker, known as the Raker Memorial in honor of California Congressman John E. Raker, whose bill helped establish the park in 1906, was erected in 1931, the same year the main park road was completed.

5.0 Brokeoff Mountain Trailhead: This trail climbs to the summit of 9235-foot Brokeoff Mountain, one of the few places within the park that supports alpine vegetation.

5.3 Southwest Entrance: Just past the entrance station is the large parking area for the Southwest Walk-in Campground and the Mill Creek Falls Trailhead.

5.4 Kohm Yah-mah-nee Visitor Center: Built on the site of the old Lassen Chalet, the visitor center is slated for completion in 2008. Facilities include an information desk, interpretive exhibits and displays, auditorium with park film, bookstore, gift shop, restaurant, restrooms, first-aid services, backcountry permits, and a nearby amphitheater.

6.4 Sulphur Works and Ridge Lakes Parking Area: From this parking area, a quarter-mile, self-guided nature trail leads visitors through an active hydrothermal area. The parking lot also serves as the trailhead for the steep, 1-mile climb to Ridge Lakes. In 1866, T. M. Boardman and Dr. Mathias Supan purchased the "Sulphur Works" and started mining the sulfurous clay. Later, Supan's son, Milton, sought greater profit by abandoning the mine in favor of opening a resort. This resort remained in the Supan family until 1952, when the Park Service acquired the property through a condemnation suit. No evidence of the resort exists today.

7.1 Brokeoff Mountain Viewpoint: Brokeoff Mountain, the prominent, 9235-foot peak to the west, is the park's second highest mountain. The nearly vertical north cliff leaves many visitors with the impression that a northern part of the peak broke away. The mountain got its misleading name because everyone from early settlers to Howel Williams, a famous geologist of the late 1920s and early 1930s, believed that the northern part of the mountain had faulted downward (though Williams admitted there was no proof of such a process). Today, there is little evidence indicating any significant faulting ever occurred. The steep north face, much like the deep canyon of Mill Creek below it, can be attributed largely to the erosive action of glaciers working over a lengthy geologic period. The glaciers' task was made easier by the abundance of highly decomposed rocks seen around Sulphur Works and farther up the road north of Diamond Peak. Brokeoff Mountain, Diamond Peak, and other nearby summits were once part of a large volcano, dubbed Mt. Tehama.

The main park road continues around Diamond Peak, which is an accumulation of resistant volcanic rock lying immediately east of Mt. Tehama's principal vent. However, the rock wasn't resistant enough to resist the pull of gravity. Perhaps initiated by a large earthquake, a half-mile-wide rockslide broke loose from the south slope of the peak and crashed southeast down to East Sulphur Creek below. A smaller slide broke loose below the viewpoint, descending into West Sulphur Creek. Future slides can't be ruled out for this area.

During midsummer, this pullout and the next one (at Diamond Point) provide fine spots for viewing an assortment of wildflowers growing on the dry, sunny ridges and slopes descending below the road. One of the more interesting flowers in this area is the "unrecognized pigweed," which is a strange name for a strange wildflower, whose tiny flowers lack petals. Although it's a member of the same plant family that includes beets and spinach, the leaves of this gray-green plant are slightly poisonous. Cream bush, alpine prickly currant, California stickseed, granite gilia, Douglas wallflower, Applegate's paintbrush, giant red paintbrush, scarlet gilia, and showy penstemon are also prevalent.

7.7 Diamond Point: Sweeping views from Diamond Point include Mt. Conard, the spreading mass breaking the skyline 1.5 miles southeast that is an eastern remnant of Mt. Tehama. Once referred to as Black Butte, the name was changed in 1948 to honor Arthur L. Conard, the organizer and president of the Lassen Park Development Association, which fought for the establishment of Lassen Volcanic National Park in 1916. On the skyline to the right of Mt. Conard is the southernmost part of the Cascade Range. To the southeast, the primarily volcanic rocks of the Cascade Range gradually yield to the granitic rocks of the Sierra Nevada.

Be mindful of traffic on the main park road if you wish to examine the nearby cliff of volcanic rock. The rock occurs in layers, or beds, and these beds dip to the east toward their source from ancient Mt. Tehama. The beds are composed of tuffs, accumulations of small fragments of volcanic rock usually 4 millimeters or less in diameter, and breccias, accumulations of fragments 32 millimeters or less in diameter. Lapilli, uncommon in this cliff, are accumulations of fragments 4 to 32 millimeters in diameter. All three of these types are expelled from volcanic vents during an eruption.

8.0 Lassen Peak View: The Lassen Peak Trail switchbacks up the southeast ridge of the mountain. Eagle Peak stands just below and east of Lassen, and previously seen Mt. Conard lies to the south-southeast.

8.2 Fallen Boulders: As you can see from the nearby boulders, the summit pinnacles atop Diamond Peak are quite unstable and could break loose at any moment, or they could sit there for another thousand years. One large boulder at the head of a boggy meadow appears to be composed of a number of smaller boulders cemented together. This boulder is a remnant of an autobrecciated lava flow—a flow that was still moving slowly while hardening, resulting in the nearly solid flow breaking into countless pieces due to the motion.

But since the material was still sticky, the rocks were bonded together into a cohesive unit. The boggy meadow contains an assortment of small, water-loving plants, including dwarf plantain-leaved buttercup, three-leaved lewisia, alpine shooting star, and Baker's violet.

9.3 Scenic Turnout: This turnout provides one of the best views of Diamond Peak's pinnacle-studded summit. Lassen Peak is also clearly seen, as is severely glaciated Little Hot Springs Valley. Conifers in the immediate vicinity are primarily red firs and western white pines.

9.6 Diamond Peak View: This peak may have been named for the summit pinnacles, which can appear diamond shaped from some vantage points. Another theory is that the peak was named for quartz and calcite crystals occasionally found in the rock, although neither is diamond shaped. Diamond Peak's minerals, similar to the rest of Mt. Tehama, are about two-thirds feldspars, with the remainder evenly split between quartz (a glassy-looking mineral) and several pyroxenes (dark, heavy minerals). There is a fair amount of calcium in some of the minerals, and the calcium is carried in a solution that is sometimes deposited nearby as calcite.

This viewpoint is around 7770 feet in elevation, near the lower edge of the subalpine zone, as indicated by the appearance of droopy-topped mountain hemlocks intermixed with the many firs and pines.

Farther up the road are some hydrothermally decomposed volcanic rocks, similar in appearance to those at Sulphur Works. At present, there is no indication of significant hydrothermal activity, although there certainly must have been some here in the past. At one time, hydrothermal activity was quite widespread within the park, but nowadays such activity appears to be waning and is confined to localized pockets.

10.6 Emerald Point: Here at 8040 feet, visitors are firmly within the subalpine zone, where mountain hemlocks become common. John Muir, the famed 19th century mountaineer, naturalist, and conservationist, considered the mountain hemlock the most beautiful of all of California's conifers. Muir also felt that some of the finest groves of these droopy-tipped trees occurred on the southern slopes of Lassen Peak. Mountain hemlocks thrive in areas of heavy snow accumulation, and Muir realized the importance of a deep snowpack to the trees' survival:

When the first soft snow begins to fall, the flakes lodge in the leaves, weighing down the branches against the trunk. Then the axis bends yet lower and lower, until the slender top touches the ground, thus forming a fine ornamental arch. The snow still falls lavishly, and the whole tree is at length buried . . . It is as though this were only Nature's method of putting her darlings to sleep instead of leaving them exposed to the biting storms of winter.

Young lodgepole pines, western white pines, and red firs are also flexible enough to bend with the snow, though their trunks are often deformed because of the snow load, especially on steep slopes.

A fine view from Emerald Point includes the dark remnant peaks of Mt. Tehama. Mt. Conard, to the south, is a remnant of the volcano's east flank. Deep in Mill Creek canyon, at the foot of Mt. Conard, are some of the oldest rocks in the park. Across from Mt. Conard stands the long summit ridge of Brokeoff Mountain, ancient Mt. Tehama's highest remnant. North of that summit is Mt. Diller, on the volcano's northeast flank. Pilot Pinnacle, to the west, is the fin on the ridge northeast of Diller, and it is also part of Mt. Tehama. To the north is Ski Heil Peak, composed of a volcanic rock called dacite. This rock erupted atop a now buried vent rather than from Mt. Tehama's summit vent. Eagle Peak, to the right, and Lassen Peak are also dacite domes that erupted from local vents.

10.8 Emerald Lake: Descending glaciers scooped out basins that later filled with water and became Emerald Lake and Lake

Helen, which is on the left. It's not uncommon to see snow around these lakes, which are at approximately 8100 feet and 8164 feet respectively, until late July or early August following an average winter. Emerald Lake is a fine spot to view ankle-high fawn lilies, with their showy white and yellow flowers. Red mountain heather, a low, subalpine shrub, grows along most of the shoreline.

11.1 Glacial Erratic and the Bumpass Hell Trailhead: A 10-foot-high glacial erratic (a boulder carried by a glacier) rests on the brink of a bedrock escarpment at the south end of the Bumpass Hell parking lot. Note how the bedrock has been planed smooth by the glacier, creating a surface referred to as glacial polish. The parking area has another superb view of the same peaks seen from Emerald Point. A small knoll near the glacial erratic has dry, gravelly soils supporting sun-loving vegetation such as buckwheat, granite gilia, mountain pride, coyote mint, mariposa tulip, and cream bush. Pinemat manzanita is the low-growing shrub below the conifers.

The usually full parking lot is a testament to the popularity of the Bumpass Hell Trail. Clark's nutcrackers frequent the area in search of leftover crumbs from the hordes of tourists that embark from the trailhead. These large, gray members of the jay family are just as noisy as the Steller's jays at campgrounds and picnic areas at the lower elevations.

11.3 Lake Helen: Lake Helen, at 8162 feet, was named for Helen T. Brodt, the first white woman known to summit Lassen Peak in 1864. The lake sits in a high basin that accumulates more snow than most other areas in the park, with a spring snowpack usually 10 to 20 feet deep and occasional drifts up to 30 feet. Long-lasting snow patches are common through midsummer, and the corresponding water temperature of the 110-foot-deep lake is generally quite cold, never rising above 50°F. A snowfield near the road along the south shore is a favorite snow-play area for

kids, but protruding rocks in late summer can be hazardous.

Just east of this snowfield is a small outcrop of highly fractured dacite. Water seeping down the vertical cracks freeze and expand, breaking the bedrock apart. A few plants, such as catchfly and Fremont's butterweed, sink their roots into the cracks, aiding in the breakdown of the rock.

11.4 Lake Helen Picnic Area: The picnic area is often snowbound until August. In 1933, just two years after completion of the main park road and the Lassen Peak Trail, the Shasta Historical Society placed a bronze plaque here to honor Helen Brodt's ascent.

Lake Helen sits in a basin scoured out of dacite bedrock, while Emerald Lake sits in a basin carved out of andesite rock that was once a part of Mt. Tehama. Andesite, which breaks down into smaller pieces, weathers differently than dacite. Andesite also releases more nutrients during the weathering process, creating soils supportive of more diverse vegetation, which is clearly evident when comparing the flora in the Lake Helen and Emerald Lake basins. The long-lasting snowfields around Lake Helen contribute to the dearth of wildflowers.

11.6 Snow Survey: A snow survey course extends from this road over to the picnic area. Snow samples are collected here in winter and spring to determine the depth and density of the snowpack. A foot of fresh snow weighs approximately one-tenth as much as a foot of water, although old, compacted snow may weigh up to half as much as an equal volume of water. By determining the volume of water in a snowpack, water managers can predict the amount of runoff expected for the upcoming season.

12.0 View of Lake Helen: This is another fine spot to view some of the remnants of ancient Mt. Tehama, including Brokeoff Mountain, Mt. Diller, Pilot Pinnacle, and Diamond Peak.

12.2 Lassen Peak Trailhead: The huge parking lot at the base of Lassen Peak is an accurate barometer of the trail's popularity. Lassen Peak, composed of dacite lava, is a plug dome, similar to Eagle Peak to the west. Geologists believe that the mountain reached its present height in several years or less, after a dramatic event that may have occurred around 27,000 years ago.

Lassen Peak is named for Peter Lassen, a Danish emigrant instrumental in bringing settlers into the region during the 1840s and 1850s. He may have been the first European to climb the peak, although the first recorded ascent is attributed to Grover K. Godfrey in 1851. The peak went through several name changes before the current appellation was applied. Upon seeing the peak in 1827, Jedediah Smith referred to the mountain and surrounding peaks as Mt. Joseph. Later, it was known locally as Snow Butte, and Peter Lassen subsequently applied the name Sister Buttes. After Lassen's death in 1859, his name became attached to the peak, first as Mt. Lassen and in 1905 as Lassen Peak.

12.5 main park road Summit: When the road was completed in 1931, this pass was recorded at an elevation of 8512 feet. Subsequent road improvements reduced the elevation to around 8500 feet. Snowstorms usually close the road for the season by late October, and the road doesn't reopen until just before the Memorial Day weekend, although sometimes the road stays closed as late as mid-July following winters of heavy snowfall. Snow banks near the summit are common until August.

12.8 Whitebark Pine Forest: In Lassen Volcanic, the whitebark pine is the most common timberline conifer, growing at higher elevations than even the mountain hemlock. On the slopes of Lassen Peak, mountain hemlocks reach an elevation of 9200 feet, while whitebark pines grow at elevations as high as 10,000 feet. While the hemlocks rely on a mantle of snow to get them through the rugged winters, whitebark pines face the harsh conditions of these wind-prone elevations without such protection. This rugged pine adapts to the harsher environments of the uppermost elevations

by taking on the form of a spreading shrub that is buried beneath winter's snowpack; its branches growing above the snow usually are killed by the cold temperatures of winter.

13.1 Lake Almanor View: Distant Lake Almanor, a reservoir of Pacific Gas and Electric Company, spreads across the flat floor of a graben, which differs from an ordinary valley as a large, fault-bordered, downthrust block, with streams playing only a minor role in carving such a landform. A number of additional grabens lie east and north of the Lake Almanor graben.

Warner Valley, 5 miles east-southeast, was formed in part due to downfaulting, although glaciers and streams performed most of the carving. At one time, glaciers extended down the canyon to within 2 miles of the western edge of the present-day town of Chester.

In 1863, William Brewer and Clarence King of the Whitney Survey proceeded across Big Meadows (presently beneath Lake Almanor) and then up Warner Valley, reaching Boiling Springs Lake and also visiting Steamboat Springs (known today as Devils Kitchen). The following day, they climbed up the canyon, perhaps passing within a few hundred yards of this viewpoint, and a day later they ascended Lassen Peak.

Mt. Harkness—which, at 8046 feet, is the highest peak on the east side of Warner Valley—is a shield volcano and was named for Harvey W. Harkness, president of the California Academy of Sciences, who explored Cinder Cone in 1874.

13.7 View of Reading Peak: Reading (pronounced "Redding") Peak is the prominent mountain about 1 mile due east, although it appears to be more of an east-west ridge than an isolated mountain. Similar to most of the park, the mountain has been glaciated more than once.

14.2 Terrace Lake Trailhead: The wide shoulder on the north side of the road acts as the parking area for the trail to Terrace, Shadow, and Cliff lakes. Snow usually remains on the ground in this subalpine realm until mid-July.

14.3 Reading Peak: At around 8030 feet, the road heads briefly south, then leaves the subalpine zone for a descent to the mixed conifer forest zone along the southwest flank of Reading Peak. Similar to Lassen Peak, Reading Peak is a volcanic dome, or plug dome volcano. Due to its composition of dacite lava, the peak is also referred to as a dacite dome. The peak itself is far from dome shaped, as glaciers have been trimming the north and south flanks of the mountain for some time. During periods of maximum glaciation, the peak was almost completely buried under ice.

Formerly known as White Mountain, the name was changed to Reading Peak to commemorate Major Pierson B. Reading's pioneering role in the settlement of the Lassen area. Reading was the first American citizen to settle in Shasta County, receiving a land grant from the Mexican government in 1844 for 26,632 acres along the Sacramento River. The current settlements of Cottonwood, Anderson, and Redding occupy the area that was included in this land grant.

15.3 Upper Kings Creek Meadow: The main park road has been descending along the top of a lateral moraine. This vantage point is about 400 feet above the floor of Upper Kings Creek Meadow, which, based on seismic measurements, lies atop a basin buried under as much as 100 feet of sediments, suggesting that a deep lake may have existed here in the past.

16.5 Road to Kings Creek Picnic Area: A short access road leads to the picnic area, which occupies the site of a former campground. The campground was closed after a 1970 USGS study reported that the area would be unsafe if Lassen Peak erupted again. In addition to the picnic grounds, a trailhead provides access to Bumpass Hell, Southwest Walk-in Campground, and Twin Meadows, as well as a very short path through the meadowlands bordering Kings Creek. Dry, gravelly slopes bordering the meadow support an abundant crop of silver-leaved lupines, which, along with other plants, support a population of Sierra pocket gophers. The gophers leave their calling cards in the form of "gopher ropes," linear tailings left by their burrowing activities when snow covers the ground. By churning the soil, the gophers improve the soil conditions much as earthworms do at lower elevations.

17.0 Kings Creek: Midway between highways 36 and 44, a glacier plowed across the terrain, heading southeast over the low divide as indicated by the direction of the glacial striations on the nearby bedrock. In contrast, Upper Kings Creek meanders east through the upper meadow and then winds through a middle meadow before reaching the lower meadow. The park's meadows are favorite haunts for deer—come early in the morning or late in the evening to catch a glimpse. Bird-watchers should look for dippers along the rapids of Kings Creek, and for spotted sandpipers along the lazy meanders.

17.6 Middle Kings Creek Meadow and Kings Creek Trailhead: The tallest lupine in the park, the large-leaved lupine, grows together with arrowhead butterweed, wandering daisy, and a host of other water-loving plants along the banks of the creek. This area sometimes overflows with cars, whose passengers are destined for the popular trail to Kings Creek Falls, just east of the bridge. Photographers should plan on a late-morning arrival at the falls for the best light, as the falls are generally shaded most of the day.

18.9 View of Kings Creek Drainage: Mt. Harkness, to the left of Lake Almanor, is the most prominent peak in the drainage and the only summit in the park that still has a staffed fire lookout on top. Saddle Mountain, below and left (northwest) of Harkness, is 5 miles to the east of the viewpoint. Other views include a north-south line of peaks near the eastern border of the park and the western border of Caribou Wilderness. Prospect Peak, at 8338 feet, is the highest peak in the park east of the viewpoint.

19.7 Red Fir Forest: Most of the park lies between 6000 and 8000 feet, which is the approximate vertical span of the red fir forest. Red firs are by far the dominant member of this conifer community, which also includes lesser amounts of western white pines, mountain hemlocks in the upper limits, lodgepole pines in wet areas, and Jeffrey pines in dry areas. The dense nature of the red fir forest limits the number of wildflowers and other plants; pinemat manzanita is the only shrub seen in significant numbers.

20.3 Lupine: Botanists can see Christine's lupine, a variety of Anderson's lupine, with pale-yellow flowers, gray-green leaves, and sometimes reddish-green stems. This lupine is common only in Lassen Volcanic and surrounding lands. The five other species of lupine found in the park all have blue flowers.

21.0 Summit Lake South Campground: Due to heavy snowfall, the two Summit Lake campgrounds usually don't open until late June. Even then, snow patches often remain on the ground until the Fourth of July or later in some years. Once open, this 48-site campground at 6695 feet, is a popular weekend destination, and the campground is usually completely full. At the south end of the campground, day-use parking is available for a trail to Corral Meadows. The lake sees perhaps too much use by swimmers, boaters, and anglers.

"Divide Lake" would be a better name than Summit Lake, as the lake sits on a flat divide and groundwater seeping from the lake flows into two river systems. Some water seeps north into East Fork Hat Creek and eventually into the Pit River, while some of it seeps south into Summit Creek and eventually into the Feather River.

21.1 Summit Lake North Campground: The north campground has 46 sites. Day-use parking is available for hikers headed for the Cluster Lakes and Echo and Twin lakes.

21.4 Summit Lake Ranger Station and Backpacker Trailhead: The ranger station may be staffed during the summer months. Wilderness permits may be obtained at the ranger station, and overnight parking is available at the end of the road, where a 0.4-mile section of trail connects to trails embarking into the wilderness from Summit Lake.

21.5 Trailhead to Cliff, Shadow, and Terrace Lakes: Easy to miss on the south side of the road is the start of the infrequently used trail climbing to these three lakes. Most hikers access these destinations via the upper trail, from the 14.2-mile mark on the main park road. Parking here is limited to a wide spot in the road.

22.7 Dersch Meadows: The Dersch family settled north of Lassen Volcanic in 1861 and grazed sheep in these meadows until the 1880s. By the turn of the century, stockmen were running tens of thousands of sheep in the park's meadows during the summer, resulting in severe overgrazing. However, after the creation of Lassen National Forest in 1905, grazing in the parklands faced increasing restrictions and was banned altogether after the designation of Lassen Volcanic National Park. Today, Dersch Meadows is a fine place to see wildflowers during the month of July. Be prepared for wet and muddy conditions and hordes of mosquitoes.

23.6 Nobles Trail: For pioneers, the Nobles Trail presented the most efficient emigrant route across northeastern California to the upper Sacramento Valley. William H. Nobles, a prospector by trade, discovered the route in 1851 on a return trip to his native Minnesota. Realizing this route was shorter and superior to Peter Lassen's 1847 route, Nobles convinced investors to back construction of a road in 1852, which carried thousands of emigrants into northern California until completion of the Transcontinental Railroad in 1869 brought about the demise of emigrant routes. Today, this section of the Nobles Trail offers hikers a serene journey along Hat Creek and over to Badger Flat.

23.8 Hat Lake Parking Area: Hat Lake was formed on May 19, 1915, when a wall of mud rumbled down the northeast slope of Lassen Peak, damming Hat Creek with logs and debris. Incoming sediments immediately began reducing the size of the lake, halving it to 10 acres by 1930 and to 1 acre by 1950. A steep, seldom-used trail climbs from the Hat Lake area to Paradise Meadow, and then continues to a junction with the trail to Terrace Lake.

23.9 Hat Mountain View: Just 2.5 miles to the east, Hat Mountain is a forested version of Lassen Volcanic's much more famous Cinder Cone. Technically, Hat Mountain, which is composed largely of lava flows, is not a cinder cone. The peak may be less than 11,000 years old, for the smooth form lends no indication that the mountain underwent any glacial erosion. Before that time, the lava plateau supporting the cone lay under an ice cap hundreds of feet thick. The plateau was substantially eroded, but the peak itself seems to have remained unscathed.

24.0 Devastated Area Interpretive Trail: Memorial Day 1914 was a day Lassen's early settlers would long remember. About 5 PM that day, Lassen Peak awoke from slumber and blasted a 25-by-40-foot crater out of the summit. By the end of March 1915, the peak had erupted about 150 times, enlarging the summit crater to a width of 1000 feet. The eruptions were phreatic explosions of old rocks and ash caused by the percolation of groundwater down to, or close to, the volcano's magma (subsurface lava), which was then converted to superheated steam. Lava never reached the surface, so the eruptions were cold and snow was not melted by falling ash.

Winds generally blow northeast in the Lassen area, and a disproportionate amount of ash accumulated in a mildly glaciated bowl on the northeast side of Lassen Peak. Somewhat protected from strong winds, this bowl also develops a snowfield that sometimes is as deep as 40 feet. Such was the case in 1915, when storm after storm brought new layers of snow, and just about every other day an eruption deposited a layer of ash on the fresh snow. By mid-May 1915, a huge accumulation of ash and snow lay in the bowl, setting the stage for catastrophe.

Around 9 PM on May 19, 1915 nearby residents noticed a glow atop Lassen Peak—lava had appeared on the mountaintop (lava may have appeared inside the crater a day or two earlier, but cloudy weather obscured the peak from view). The lava welled up to the rim of the crater, and the subsequent heat sent several small mudflows down the north and northwest slopes of the peak. Some lava spilled southwest down the western slope, creating a mudflow of moderate proportions. However, when lava spilled onto the upper-northeast slope and melted the deep snowfield in the bowl, a gigantic mudflow was created beyond anyone's imagination. The wall of mud rumbled downslope, creating so much noise that it woke up the few settlers in the valley below. Fortunately, the tremendous accumulation of ash caused the mudflow to move slowly, like wet concrete, which gave resident Elmer Sorahan enough time to alert his neighbors to the crisis, and no lives were lost.

When daylight broke on May 20, some of the settlers returned and viewed their devastated area. The flow had buried formerly luxuriant meadows under a pile of mud, rock, and snags that approached a thickness of 18 feet in some places. Almost every tree in the path of the mudflow was lost, and thousands of downed trees littered the landscape. The flow breached Emigrant Pass—the low, broad divide currently occupied by the Devastated Area Interpretive Trail and parking lot—and sent a wall of mud about 0.3-mile wide and 10 to 20 feet thick north for 4 miles down Hat Creek before it significantly diminished in volume over the next 3 miles. The flow northwest down the Lost Creek drainage was of similar proportions.

As bad as this mudflow was, the worst was yet to come. Around 4:30 PM on May

22, Lassen Peak produced its largest explosion—the 174th recorded—sending an ash cloud 30,000 feet into the atmosphere and turning the sky dark as far east as northwestern Nevada. Almost simultaneously, a blast of superheated air traveled downslope northeast, totally leveling a 1-by-3-mile swath of forest. This hot blast, creating what is now referred to as the Devastated Area, blew trees over like matchsticks, all pointing away from the origin of the blast. The air in the blast was hot enough to scorch the timber and to start at least one small fire.

Thanks to the passing of time, the Devastated Area doesn't appear so devastated anymore, as reforestation has progressed rapidly. Aspens, which propagate mainly from roots and seldom from seeds, were among the first trees to appear, as their roots and lower stems survived the mudflow. Water-loving lodgepole pines will eventually replace most of the aspens. Jeffrey pines cover the landscape in areas with less groundcover. Bear in mind that all of these trees have grown since 1915 or later.

After the May 22 eruption, volcanic activity declined, although significant eruptions occurred sporadically through the end of the year. Only four significant eruptions occurred in 1916, from late October through mid-November. Many more eruptions occurred from January through June of 1917, but then activity ceased, although the volcano smoked and steamed on and off until February of 1921. Although considered dormant today, a future eruption cannot be ruled out.

26.2 Hot Rock: This is one of the many hot rocks from Lassen Peak's summit area that was transported by the May 19, 1915, mudflow. This particular rock is about 4.5 miles from its source. When Benjamin Loomis and others visited the area on May 22, only hours before the hot blast, they noted water still boiling around some of the larger rocks. One rock was even hot enough to ignite wood nearby. When the Loomis party viewed Lassen Peak from these hot rocks, not a tree blocked their view, unlike today.

This hot rock most likely weighs a few hundred tons, assuming that half of the rock is buried, which is a fair assumption, as the rock would have settled on the floor of the buried valley after the mud ceased to flow. The valley floor at this location lies beneath around 5 to 10 feet of mud. This rock, composed of dacite lava with feldspar crystals, is part of the lava flow that spilled northeast onto the snow-and-ash field. This lava may have been as hot as 1000°F when molten—no wonder the larger hot rocks stayed hot for days.

26.6 Lost Creek Bridge: The 1915 mudflow was the last of a series of sediments to pass through the area. In roughly 900 AD, give or take a hundred years, a series of four pyroclastic flows swept down through this area. A pyroclastic flow is similar in nature to Lassen Peak's hot blast, except that a great deal of volcanic material accompanies the gas. Such horizontally directed blasts, composed of extremely hot, incandescent fine ash, coarser rock fragments, and hot gases, are referred to as *nuees ardentes* (pronounced "new-ay' ar' dawn," French for "burning clouds"). They can travel downslope at up to 200 miles per hour, and hence are far more threatening than slowly moving mudflows. These pyroclastic flows were the first products of a series of eruptions foreshadowing the extrusion of several dacite domes, known as the Chaos Crags.

Chaos Crags aren't the only dacite domes seen in this area. A 1200-foot-high, unnamed, forested peak, standing due west, is but one of a cluster of several domes that the road will take 5 miles to drive around.

26.7 West Boundary of May 1915 Mudflow: The mudflow continued several miles down this canyon. Trees in the canyon were broken from their roots, and some stumps remain buried to this day. Similarly, trees were destroyed by the four pyroclastic flows mentioned in the Lost Creek Bridge entry.

For the last 3 miles, the main park road has more or less followed the route of the Nobles Emigrant Trail. In about another 250 yards, the historic wagon road branches right and then parallels the mudflow down the canyon. That road is closed to motor vehicles but open to hikers and equestrians, although, being viewless and waterless, the route has few takers.

28.2 Burned Area: Fires have long been a part of nature's cycle. When an area such as this one is burned, the resulting open space at this elevation is usually invaded first by greenleaf manzanita, tobacco brush, and other shrubs. Jeffrey pines and sugar pines likely follow, eventually shading out some of the shrubs. As shade increases, white firs invade and prosper, virtually shading out all of the shrubs. Given enough time, the firs ultimately shade out the pines, for pine seedlings require sunny ground to get established. However, another fire, a strong wind, a volcanic eruption, or disease may open the forest once again and begin another cycle of succession.

28.7 Sugar Pine: At 5690 feet, sugar pines approach the upper end of their range. In the Lassen area, sugar pines are generally found between 3000 and 6000 feet, elevations occurring mainly outside the park. The sugar pine is easily the largest of Lassen Volcanic's three species of white pines, and identifying the large cones (10 to 16 inches long) is the easiest way to distinguish them in the forest. Historically, the Atsugewi, or "Hat Creek," Native Americans visited this part of the park from about June through October, eating the sugar pine's sweet, white resin as candy. However, in large quantities, the resin acts as a laxative.

28.9 Lost Creek Group Camp: Advanced reservations are necessary for use of this campground.

29.1 Crags Campground: This campground was developed after Manzanita Lake Campground was temporarily closed in 1974 due to safety concerns. Crags Campground is one of the least-used campgrounds in the park.

29.2 Ponderosa Pine: In addition to three species of white pines, Lassen Volcanic has two species of yellow pine: ponderosa and Jeffrey, both of which have needles in bunches of three. Only ponderosa and Jeffrey pines are common.

This linear stretch of road parallels a fault, which lies immediately southwest (left) of the road. Since erosion occurs more quickly along faulted, fractured rocks than along bedrock, a former stream cut a gully along this fault. Today, the flow of water is entirely subterranean, and the ponderosa pine, growing where a creek ought to flow, is probably tapping this underground water source.

29.7 Table Mountain Fault: Curving through the gully, the road crosses the previously mentioned fault, which slices northwest through the lower, northeast slopes of Table Mountain. Two more similarly oriented faults slice through the mountain, one on each side of the main summit.

Lassen Peak lies at the highly active crossroads of three geologic provinces, along the western edge of the Great Basin (which is composed of hundreds of northwest-oriented, fault-generated mountains and valleys), near the southern end of the Cascade Range, and close to the northern edge of the Sierra Nevada.

30.6 Sunflower Flat: A bronze plaque marks the route of the Nobles Emigrant Trail, first used by emigrants in 1852. Sunflower Flat is so named because of the one-time abundance of mountain mule ears, large-leaved sunflowers that produce a curious aroma. The shady forest of today has diminished the number of these once abundant flowers.

30.8 Nobles Pass: Ill-defined Nobles Pass lies almost a mile up the Nobles Trail, which climbs about 50 feet higher than necessary, passing through a low gap about 200 yards north of a slightly lower gap. Nevertheless, Nobles Emigrant Trail was an easy, fairly direct route from the high desert of Nevada to the upper Sacramento Valley, unlike many other California pioneer trails that crossed the mountains. William Nobles, a gold miner, was either a very keen scout or a very lucky man when he discovered this route in 1851. At the time, no map of the area existed. In 1975, the park's section of the Nobles Trail was recorded in the National Register of Historic Places.

31.3 Chaos Jumbles: These deposits are the results of a series of three or more rockfall avalanches that probably occurred in rapid succession around 1670 AD. Molten rock beneath the northwest base of Chaos Crags apparently got close enough to the surface to superheat the groundwater, producing a steam explosion that triggered the rockfall avalanches. Rocks altered by superheated water are found in the source area, indicating that the area had been steaming for some time. When the supposed blast occurred, millions of tons of rock came crashing down, compressing a layer of air that geologists theorize then acted as a suitable lubricant for the mass to rush downslope at speeds of 100 to 200 mile per hour. These rockfall avalanches moved with such great momentum that they climbed as much as 400 feet up the slopes of Table Mountain. By the end of the last rockfall avalanche, which may have been only minutes after the first, about 200 million cubic yards of debris lay strewn across the landscape. In a way, the event may have been similar to the May 18, 1980, collapse of the north side of Mt. Saint Helens, but without the accompanying eruption and ash cloud, for Chaos Jumbles rocks were cool or cold when they came to rest. No evidence of a fire exists.

31.9 Chaos Crags: The gray, lifeless mountain mass to the southeast is Chaos Crags, a series of four or more plug domes. The formation of these domes was preceded by violent volcanic activity that may have occurred sporadically over some years. These eruptions of very hot ash and rock were then followed by the extrusion of dacite lava, a thick and pasty substance that accumulated on the spot rather than flowing far from the vents. Each dome may have taken only months or, at most, several years to form, the earliest one having been formed about 900 AD. Whether all the domes formed around this time or some formed centuries later is not known.

32.9 Road to Manzanita Lake Campground: The Crags Lake Trail begins about 200 yards up this road at a bend. About 0.5 mile farther is the Manzanita Lake Picnic Area on the right, with an access point for the loop trail around the lake, and a boat launch for nonmotorized watercraft. A short distance farther is the Manzanita Lake Camper Service Store and the entrance to the 179-unit campground (the farthest loop is for tent camping only).

33.0 Loomis Museum and Lily Pond Nature Trail: In 1926, Benjamin Loomis, an early settler who probably took more photographs of Lassen Peak erupting than anyone else, purchased 40 acres of private land near Manzanita and Reflection lakes. The following year, he and his wife financed the construction of the Mae Loomis Memorial Museum, dedicated to the memory of their only child. The museum and the land were donated to the park in 1929. Recorded in the National Register of Historic Places, the magnificent rock structure was closed in the mid-1970s due to concerns of a potential rockslide avalanche from Chaos Crags. Fortunately, the Loomis Museum was restored and reopened in 1993. The Lily Pond Nature Trail begins across the road from the museum.

33.1 Reflection Lake: Reflection Lake formed in a large depression within Chaos Jumbles; two other ponds north of the lake and hidden from the road have a similar origin. Groundwater flows beneath Chaos Jumbles and surfaces at these depressions. Similarly, Manzanita Lake probably receives a larger contribution from groundwater than from Manzanita Creek. During early morning and late afternoon, if the water is still, both Reflection and Manzanita lakes offer mirrored views of Lassen Peak and Chaos Crags.

33.3 Manzanita Lake: After parking along the shoulder, visitors can walk along the shoreline trail. Similar to Reflection Lake, Manzanita Lake came into existence when the Chaos Crags rockfall avalanches swept through the area and came to a halt about three-quarters of a mile west of the 44/89 junction. The deposits dammed Manzanita Creek, giving rise to the lake. The rumpled surface along the north shore represents the southern edge of Chaos Jumbles. In May 1915, some small mudflows poured down Lassen Peak into Manzanita Creek, which contributed tons of sediments to the lake.

33.5 Manzanita Lake Entrance Station: Fees are collected at this station—if you paid at the southwest entrance, make sure you can produce your receipt or pass. The shoreline trail around Manzanita Lake passes nearby and grants a view of the low dam on the west side, which only raised the level of the lake several feet. The Northern California Power Company built the dam in 1911, hoping to significantly raise the lake level, but the volcanic sediments used to build the dam proved to be too porous, causing it to leak like a sieve. Nowadays, a healthy, dense root network of mature alders and willows growing on the dam prevents erosion and greatly reduces the seepage.

34.0 Lassen Crossroads: Past the park boundary the main park road becomes Highway 89 again and shortly leads to a right-hand turnoff into Lassen Crossroads, complete with visitor information and restrooms.

34.1 Crossroads Junction

Segment 2: Highway 44 from Crossroads Junction to Old Station

0.0 Highway 44/89 Junction: Here, the road log turns north to follow Highway 44 toward Old Station. Westbound, Highway 44 descends 45 miles to a junction

with Interstate 5 in Redding. Driving east from Redding up Highway 44, visitors will encounter the following features: Around 27.5 miles is Shingletown, the last opportunity to obtain gas, food, and supplies until Old Station. About 3 miles from town is a rest area on the left, followed by a KOA Campground in 1.2 miles. Viola, a tiny, easy-to-miss community, is another 7 miles up the road. A paved road branches right from Viola near a curve, passing homesites and then becoming a graded road that climbs to USFS Road 17, 3.6 miles from Highway 44.

From the curve in Viola, Highway 44 winds 5.4 miles to a junction with Road 17, which one can take 21.7 miles south to Highway 36, 1.1 miles west of Lassen National Volcanic Park headquarters. Road 17 provides access to South Fork Digger Creek Trail to Heart Lake. Just 1.1 miles past the Road 17 junction is the junction of Highways 89 and 44.

1.3 Eskimo Hill Summit: The highway reaches 5933 feet at Eskimo Hill Summit, where a snow play parking area is on the west side.

2.9 Road to Battle Creek Campground: A dirt road leads 5 miles to a Pacific Gas & Electric campground.

4.1 USFS Road 16: Road 16 is the main road for the southern trailheads into Thousand Lakes Wilderness. Ashpan Snowmobile Park is just off the highway to the north.

8.3 USFS Road 32N12: Branching right, this road leads to primitive campsites at Twin Bridges Campground near Hat Creek.

8.4 Vista Point: Back when this area was developed as a vista point, the trees of the Deer Hollow-Badger Mountain Plantation that currently block the view were much shorter. Fortunately, a short path leads out of the trees to a decent viewpoint. A very short nature trail with interpretive signs also loops through the area, providing tidbits about the local ecology. The area is equipped with vault toilets and picnic tables.

9.0 USFS Road 32N13: This road leads to Big Pine Campground, a half mile from the highway.

9.7 Big Spring Road: Big Spring flows year-round, pouring water into Hat Creek. During fall and winter, this large spring often contributes more water to Hat Creek than the creek itself. Big Spring, with gushing, pure water, is a fine picnic spot.

10.6 Hat Creek Resort: The rustic resort is a favorite with anglers, providing a store, cabins, post office, and gas pumps.

12.2 Hat Creek Campground and Spattercone Nature Trail: This large, 75-site campground is situated between the highway and Hat Creek and is a popular spot with anglers. Across from the campground entrance, on the east side of the highway, is the campground's dump station and the parking area for the Spattercone Nature Trail.

12.4 Hat Creek Picnic Area: This pleasant, creekside, day-use area is immediately north of Hat Creek Campground.

13.1 Rim Rock Ranch: The guest ranch offers housekeeping cabins, two motel-type units, and four bed-and-breakfast rooms, as well as a small but well-stocked store. Because fishing is the primary emphasis (license required), live bait and a large selection of tackle are available at the store.

13.5 Old Station Chevron and J.J.'s Cafe: With a credit or debit card, gas is available 24 hours a day. The small convenience store has a limited selection of groceries and supplies. Next door is a small cafe, open for breakfast and lunch only.

13.7 Old Station Visitor Center: Open limited hours between April and December, the visitor center provides information about Lassen National Forest, along with a small selection of books and gifts.

13.8/00 Highway 89 and 44 Junction: At this junction, Highway 89 heads northwest toward McArthur-Burney Falls Memorial State Park and Mt. Shasta (see Section 5 on page 50), while Highway 44 travels southeast toward Susanville.

Segment 3: Highway 44 from Old Station to Highway 36 Junction

0.0 Junction with Highway 89

2.8 Hat Creek Rim Overlook and Pacific Crest Trail Trailhead: Motorists can stop and enjoy the wide-ranging view across Hat Creek Valley from Lassen Peak to Mt. Shasta. The overlook is equipped with vault toilets and picnic tables. Not far from the highway, a dirt road travels a short distance to a PCT trailhead.

11.3 Butte Lake Road: Branching right, the graveled Butte Lake Road passes the primitive Butte Creek Campground before crossing onto Park Service land and continuing to the Butte Lake area, complete with ranger station, campground, picnic area, and trailheads.

15.6 Poison Lake: This is generally a lake only during spring and early summer, and a mucky meadow thereafter.

23.7 Bogard Rest Area and Work Station: The rest area, renovated in 2006, is on the right side of the highway, and the work station is on the left.

23.8 USFS Road 10 and Road 32N08: Road 10 heads southwest from just below the rest area, providing access to trailheads for the Caribou Wilderness and campgrounds and picnic areas near Silver Lake. Road 32N08 heads northeast to Crater Lake Campground.

25.7 USFS Road 31N26: This road, branching right, provides access to the primitive Bogard Campground.

28.6 County Road A21: Paved road A21 provides an 18-mile shortcut between highways 44 and 36, reaching Highway 36 in the small community of Westwood. This road also offers a route to the Silver Lake area via County Road 110.

35.1 McCoy Flat Reservoir

38.7 Hog Flat Reservoir

39.9 Goumaz Road: USFS Road 30N03 offers a route to Goumaz Campground.

46.9 Junction of Highway 36: Highway 44 ends at this junction, where Highway 36 travels west toward Lake Almanor and Chester.

Segment 4: Highway 44 Junction to Highway 89 Junction West of Mineral

0.0 Highway 44/36 Junction: Heading east, Highway 36 comes to a junction with County Road A1, which leads to campgrounds, picnic areas, trailheads, and a marina at Eagle Lake. A few more miles to the east is the full-service community of Susanville.

1.6 Devils Corral Trailhead: The first leg of the Bizz Johnson Trail travels from downtown Susanville to this trailhead.

3.6 USFS Road 29N03: By following this road south, campers will reach Roxie Peconom Campground in a few miles.

7.4 Fredonyer Pass: The ascent from Susanville ends at this pass before Highway 36 descends toward Lake Almanor.

15.8 Westwood and Junction of A21: The small community of Westwood offers limited services, but the full-service community of Chester is only 13 miles west. In the heart of Westwood, County Road A21 provides an 18-mile shortcut to Highway 44 and southern access to Silver Lake and the east side of Caribou Wilderness.

18.8 Junction of County Road 147: From this junction, County Road 147 provides access to the east side of Lake Almanor.

24.2 Junction of County Road A13 and USFS Road 10: A13, branching left, provides a shortcut between Highway 36 and County Road 147. Road 10, branching right, is the southern gateway to the Caribou Wilderness and Silver Lake area.

25.3 Rest Area: This rest area offers the usual accommodations, along with a fine view of Lake Almanor.

27.1 Road to Last Chance Campground: This road leads to a Pacific Gas & Electric campground near the northernmost tip of Lake Almanor.

29.0 East Side of Chester: Coming from the east, motorists encounter the historic section of Chester, a full-service community offering plenty of amenities for even the most discriminating traveler.

29.2 Junction of County Road 312: Near the fire station, a road branches right (west-northwest) and ultimately leads to the Juniper Lake and Warner Valley roads into the park, as well as Forest Service Road 29N18, providing access to several trailheads and campgrounds on Forest Service and Park Service lands.

31.1 Chester Ranger District: Toward the west end of Chester is the Chester Ranger District office.

32.0 Junction of Highway 89: From this junction, Highway 89 heads south along the west and south sides of Lake Almanor, past campgrounds, picnic areas, and trailheads, and continues toward the small community of Greenville.

37.4 Pacific Crest Trail Crossing: Here, the PCT crosses Highway 36. Upgrades in 2006 have improved parking and trail access.

39.3 St. Bernard Lodge: This lodge features seven bed-and-breakfast rooms, as well as a dining room, bar, and stables.

40.6 Deer Creek Lodge and Restaurant

42.6 Junction of Highway 32: This state highway winds through the mountains and foothills toward Chico, providing access to Elam Creek, Alder Creek, and Potato Patch campgrounds situated along pleasant stretches of Deer Creek.

44.3 Fire Mountain Store and Lodge

45.0 Gurnsey Creek Campground: This 32-unit campground is situated beneath shady conifers.

48.6 Wilson Lake Road

50.0 Spencer Meadows Trailhead

50.3 Childs Meadow Resort: This all-year resort features cabins, motel units, a general store, and a cafe.

51.4 Junction of Highway 172: Highway 172 loops back to Highway 36 near the town of Mineral. The Mill Creek Resort is an all-year facility with cabins, campground, restaurant, general store, and a post office. The highway provides access to Hole in the Ground Campground and the Mill Creek Trailhead.

54.9 Morgan Summit and Highway 89 Junction: Here, the Lassen Scenic Byway turns north toward Lassen Volcanic National Park (see Segment 1 on page 36). About 5 miles west of this junction is the town of Mineral, home of Lassen Mineral Lodge, an all-year resort with gift shop, general store, lodging, and a restaurant. The town also offers a gas station/convenience store, an RV campground, cabin rentals, laundromat,

and Lassen Volcanic National Park headquarters. West of town about a mile is Battle Creek Campground, the last Forest Service campground along Highway 36.

Segment 5: Highway 89 from Old Station through Hat Creek Valley

0.0 Junction of Highway 44

0.3 Subway Cave and Cave Campground: If you have time for only one stop in the Hat Creek area, make that stop at the self-guided tour through Subway Cave, a large lava tube located near a picnic area on the right (east) side of the highway, opposite the entrance to Cave Campground. The campground is the southern trailhead for the 4-mile Hat Creek Trail.

3.3 Rocky Campground: As trailers are not advised at this small campground, tent campers may find this an attractive option. Lying along one of the nicer stretches of Hat Creek, the eight sites go quickly, especially on weekends. A bridge across the creek provides access from the campground to the Hat Creek Trail.

4.0 Bridge Picnic Area and Campground: The picnic area is on the right side of the highway, and the campground entrance is on the left. The northern trailhead for the Hat Creek Trail is in the campground.

7.9 USFS Road 33N25: This road, branching left, leads to the Tamarack Trailhead on the east side of the Thousand Lakes Wilderness.

9.1 Honn Campground: This primitive campground has six sites along the bank of Hat Creek.

10.9 USFS Road 26: Immediately north of the Hat Creek Work Center, Road 26 heads south and west, providing access to the Cypress Trailhead just north of Thousand Lakes Wilderness.

11.1 South Junction of County Road 6R200: This road loops back to Highway 89, but first passes a private drive into the Hat Creek Hereford Ranch RV Park & Campground, and then USFS Road 22, which leads to the Hat Creek Radio Astronomy Observatory. From a store and gas station near the junction, drive a quarter mile to the Hat Creek Hereford Ranch and proceed to the campground, which has conveniences not found in the typical USFS campgrounds, such as hot showers, laundry, and a trout pond. Also, campsites are far enough away from the highway that traffic noise is not bothersome. Of course, such amenities come at higher prices than what the USFS campgrounds typically charge.

To reach the observatory, follow the loop road 1.4 miles from the southern junction of Highway 89 to USFS Road 22 (if coming from the north, this road is 0.9 mile from the northern junction of 89). Head east on 22 about 1.8 miles to the observatory entrance and continue south for three-quarters of a mile to the office. Operated by the University of California, the observatory is usually open to the public on weekdays. Berkeley's Radio Astronomy Lab selected this site because of its relative isolation from artificial radio waves. From the observatory entrance, Road 22 continues east about a half mile before turning north and switchbacking up the faulted escarpment of Murken Bench, crossing over the route of the PCT about 4 miles from the observatory entrance.

12.8 North Junction of County Road 6R200: See above entry.

21.7 Junction of Highway 299: The town of Fall River Mills is northeast, and the town of Burney is southwest of this junction.

27.5 Entrance to McArthur-Burney Falls Memorial State Park

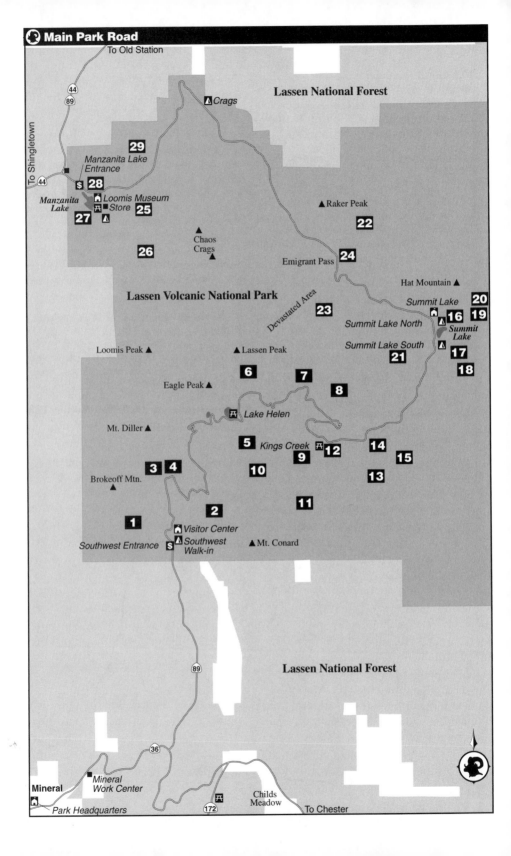

Chapter 5

Lassen Scenic Byway Trips

As detailed in the previous chapter, the Lassen Scenic Byway is a 185-mile loop that courses through and around Lassen Volcanic National Park via a combination of state highways and the main park road. This loop provides the principal access to the majority of trailheads for trips described in this guide, as well as a preponderance of tourist attractions. The trip descriptions that follow begin near the southwest entrance to Lassen Volcanic and proceed through the park to the Crossroads Junction, just outside the northwest entrance, near Manzanita Lake. From there, the descriptions follow the clockwise route of the byway as described in Chapter 4, following State Hwy. 44/89 to Old Station; then Hwy. 44 to the junction with State Hwy. 36, just west of Susanville; and finally continuing westbound on Hwy. 36 to the 36/89 junction, just south of the southwest entrance to Lassen Volcanic.

Introduction to the Main Park Road

The main park road—a 34-mile section of paved road within the park that connects to State Highway 89 outside the park boundaries—is the lifeline of Lassen Volcanic, traversing some of the park's finest scenery and delivering throngs of tourists each summer day to a wide variety of the park's major features, including Lassen Peak and Bumpass Hell. Invariably, anyone who has been to Lassen Volcanic has done so by driving at least a part of this road. Along the route, visitors are exposed to dramatic mountaintops, flower-filled meadows, crashing cascades, sulfurous fumaroles, placid lakes, and serene flats. The steep and winding road is not the route to take for motorists who wish to cover the distance in the shortest possible time; the trans-park journey takes at least an hour. Unhurried travelers will find enough diversions along the way to take up the better part of a day. In winter, the main park road is closed between the Kohm Yah-mah-nee visitor center and Manzanita Lake. Plowing of the road usually begins in early spring, with parking areas opening at the Devastated Area, Sulphur Works, and Bumpass Hell as crews make progress.

The trans-park byway provides access to several trails. Driving north from the park boundary, you first reach the Brokeoff Mountain Trailhead, a moderately difficult 3.5-mile hike to summit views that rival those from the park's namesake attraction. Just past the southwest entrance, the 1.6-mile Mill Creek Trail leaves the Southwest Walk-in Campground and heads toward the park's highest waterfall, Mill Creek Falls. A mile up the road is the trailhead for the very steep but short trail to Ridge Lakes, and the easy, self-guided nature path through Sulphur Works. Higher still is the large parking lot with access to the easy, 1.4-mile trek over to Bumpass Hell, the park's most active hydrothermal area. Immediately before the road summit is the even larger parking lot for the 2.3-mile Lassen Peak Trail.

Shortly beyond the Lassen Peak Trailhead, the road begins to descend and soon comes to a trailhead for a path to Terrace, Shadow, and Cliff lakes. A little farther below is Kings Creek Meadows, where branching trails radiate to a variety of interesting destinations from two trail-heads—one from the upper meadows and one from the lower meadows. Farther on, three trails radiate from the Summit Lake area: one south toward Drakesbad, one east to the park's lake-studded backcountry, and one west up to Cliff, Shadow, and Terrace lakes. On the approach to Hat Creek, the road crosses the Nobles Emigrant Trail, a little-used, historic route that appeals to those who tend to shun crowds. Near the Hat Creek Bridge, a trail climbs to Paradise and Kings Creek meadows. Descending into a warm, lower-elevation forest, the main park road twice crosses the Nobles Emigrant Trail on the way toward the Manzanita Lake area and its five trails: a popular path around the namesake lake, a trail up Manzanita Creek to fields of wildflowers, a route to Crag Lake at the foot of dramatic Chaos Crags, the Lily Pond Nature Trail loop, and another section of the Nobles Emigrant Trail. Beyond Manzanita Lake, the main park road terminates at the north-west entrance and continues a very short distance as Highway 89 past the Lassen Crossroads information area to the junction with Highway 44.

Access

The main park road section through Lassen Volcanic is subject to winter closure between the Kohm Yah-mah-nee visitor center and Manzanita Lake. During spring, the Park Service opens the section of road between Manzanita Lake and the Devastated Area and then works on opening the section of road from the southwest entrance to Sulphur Works and the Bumpass Hell park-ing area. Depending on snow conditions, the main park road may be opened as early as May 10 or as late as mid-July.

Amenities

The small town of Mineral, about 5 miles west of the junction of highways 36 and 89,

is home to Lassen Volcanic National Park headquarters and the Lassen Mineral Lodge (530-595-4422), an all-year resort that includes a general store, restaurant, motel, and gift shop. The town also offers cabin rentals, gas station/convenience store, a post office, and an RV campground. Services are limited within the national park to the Kohm Yah-mah-nee visitor center near the southwest entrance, set to open in October of 2008, and the Loomis Museum and the Manzanita Lake Camper Store (laundry and showers), near the northwest entrance. Inside the park, gasoline is available only at the Manzanita Lake Camper Store.

Ranger Stations and Visitor Information

Backcountry information and wilder-ness permits for overnight stays in Lassen Volcanic National Park are available at park headquarters in Mineral, the visitor center near the southwest entrance, and the Loomis Museum near Manzanita Lake. Permits can be requested online at www.nps.gov/lavo but require two weeks to process. Currently, there are no quotas or fees required for wilderness permits. Self-registration permits are available at Butte, Warner Valley, and Juniper Lake ranger stations, as well as the southwest and north-west entrance stations, depending on the time of year.

Good to Know Before You Go

All parties entering Lassen Volcanic National Park via roads without staffed entrance sta-tions, including Butte Lake, Juniper Lake, and Warner Valley, are expected to pay the $10-per-vehicle fee at the self-registration stations by cash or check. This includes the Brokeoff Mountain trailhead, which is before the southwest entrance but still inside the park. Those holding Interagency Annual, Senior, and Access passes must still register.

Campgrounds

Campground	Fee	Elevation	Season	Restrooms	Running Water	Bear Boxes
Southwest (Walk-in)	$14	6700´	Open all year	Flush	Yes	Yes
Summit Lake South (15.6 miles from sw entrance)	$16	6695´	Early July to early September	Vault	Yes	Yes
Summit Lake North (15.7 miles from sw entrance)	$18	6695´	Early July to early September	Flush	Yes	Yes
Crags (5 miles from Highway 44)	$12	5700´	Early June to early September	Vault	Yes	Yes
Manzanita Lake (1.2 miles from Highway 44)	$18	5890´	Mid-May to late September	Flush and vault	Yes	Yes

SOUTHWEST ENTRANCE TRAILHEADS

Trip **1**

Brokeoff Mountain

MS ✓ DH

DISTANCE:	7 miles out and back
ELEVATIONS:	6635/9235, +2700/-2700
SEASON:	Mid-July to October
USE:	Moderate
MAP:	*Lassen Peak*

INTRODUCTION: A stiff, 3.5-mile climb (which may feel more like 5 miles) leads to one of Lassen Volcanic's more dramatic vistas, from the summit of 9235-foot Brokeoff Mountain, so named for the ruggedly sheer north face of the peak. Not only will successful summiteers enjoy a superb view of Lassen Peak; this is also the best vantage point for examining the remnants of ancient Mt. Tehama's caldera. The scenery extends to the southern Cascades (including Mt. Shasta), northern Sierra, Sacramento Valley, and the coastal mountain ranges. Also notable is the trail itself, which travels through serene forest, passes by flower-covered meadows, visits dancing streams, and offers a short side excursion to the quiet surroundings of shallow Forest Lake.

Although far less popular than the Lassen Peak Trail, plenty of hikers set their sights on Brokeoff Mountain, whose small summit can seem a bit crowded with more than a handful of hikers. Snow lingers on the upper slopes of the mountain until midsummer—if you plan to climb earlier in the season, consider bringing an ice ax. Water is available from tributaries of Mill Creek along the first half of the route only; make sure to pack plenty of water for the second half of the ascent, which is exposed to the sun at relatively high altitudes. Valley dwellers should watch for signs of altitude sickness, and everyone should make a hasty retreat from the upper slopes when

thunderstorms are threatening. A 1.25-mile trail connecting the Brokeoff Mountain and Heart Lake trails is shown on some maps, but it has long been abandoned. These cautions aside, the trip to Brokeoff Mountain is one of the park's best adventures.

DIRECTIONS TO TRAILHEAD: Follow the main park road 0.5 mile from the south boundary (5 miles from Highway 36) to the well-marked parking area on the east shoulder. The parking area is 0.4 mile south of the southwest entrance station, so self-registration is required for entry into Lassen Volcanic National Park; fee envelopes are provided at the parking area.

DESCRIPTION: On the opposite shoulder from the parking area, wood steps lead west up the hillside and past a trailhead signboard before a single-track trail continues the climb through verdant patches of wildflowers and tall thickets of alders, well watered by spring-fed tributaries of an unnamed creek that drains Forest Lake and the southeast slopes of Brokeoff Mountain.

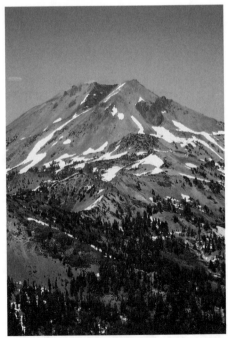

Lassen Peak from Brokeoff Mountain

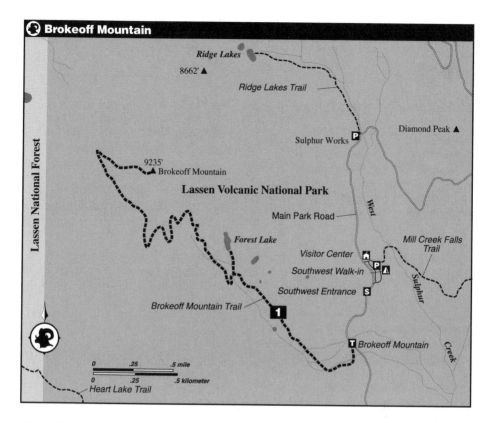

Brokeoff Mountain

Ridge Lakes
8662' ▲
Ridge Lakes Trail
Diamond Peak ▲
Sulphur Works 🅿
9235'
▲ Brokeoff Mountain
Lassen Volcanic National Park
Main Park Road
West
Forest Lake
Mill Creek Falls Trail
Visitor Center
Southwest Walk-in
Southwest Entrance 🆂
Brokeoff Mountain Trail
1
🅃 Brokeoff Mountain
Creek
Sulphur
Lassen National Forest
0   .25   .5 mile
0   .25   .5 kilometer
Heart Lake Trail

The trail crosses these rivulets a few times while proceeding up the slope through a mixed forest of western white pines, lodgepole pines, and firs. The grade momentarily eases near a pond/meadow in a shallow depression on the left. Resuming the climb, you eventually reach a small, flower-filled meadow, where Brokeoff Mountain makes the first in a series of fleeting appearances. Just before the path bends to cross the main branch of the creek, an unmarked, lesser-used trail veers right (north) to Forest Lake, 1.2 miles from the trailhead.

🆂 **SIDE TRIP TO FOREST LAKE:** Without any remarkable scenery, decent swimming, or trout, Forest Lake won't make anyone's list of must-see destinations. However, in early summer, the short stroll may attract wildflower enthusiasts who don't mind dealing with the corresponding hordes of mosquitoes. Follow the right-hand path north from the unmarked junction alongside a

tiny stream about 200 to 250 yards to the shallow, log-strewn lake. As few of the hikers bound for Brokeoff Mountain's summit take this diversion, Forest Lake's principal attraction may be a healthy dose of solitude. **END OF SIDE TRIP**

From the junction, hop across the main branch of the creek and continue the steady climb up the left side of the drainage onto the southeast slope of Brokeoff Mountain. Wind up the slope through diminishing forest, which now includes mountain hemlocks, to gain the south ridge. Although the route up the pinemat manzanita-covered south ridge would seem to be the most logical line to the summit, the trail follows the steep ridge for only a short stretch before beginning a lengthy, ascending traverse across the virtually shadeless, gravelly southwest side of the peak. Along with a few stunted whitebark pines, tufts of subalpine and alpine plants higher upslope maintain a foothold in the otherwise sterile-looking soil; in early season, a colorful display of widely scattered wildflowers lines the trail. The trail eventually switchbacks near the mountain's west ridge and then proceeds on another traverse, nearly as long as the previous one, above timberline to the ridge crest, where you'll have a prelude to the incredible vista at the top. A short climb from there leads to the summit.

Not surprisingly, the dominant feature of the 360-degree view from the summit is Lassen Peak, situated at the culmination of a sinuous ridge that winds northeast from your viewpoint. Other notable peaks to the northeast include Mt. Diller, Pilot Pinnacle, Ski Heil Peak, and Eagle Peak. Geologists theorize that this ridge is what remains of a collapsed caldera, a remnant of ancient Mt. Tehama, an 11,000-foot stratovolcano that once dominated the surrounding landscape. However, Lassen Peak is not one of Tehama's leftovers, but a plug dome volcano that formed on the ancestral mountain's northern flank. Additional points of interest visible from the top of Brokeoff Mountain include Chaos Crags and Mt. Shasta to the north, giant Lake Almanor to the south, and, on clear days, the Sacramento Valley back-dropped by the Coast Range to the west and Klamath Mountains to the northwest.

R Fires are prohibited.

> **LOOKOUTS**
>
> After the 1914 eruption destroyed a recently built lookout on top of Lassen Peak, a replacement was constructed on the summit of Brokeoff Mountain during that same year. Most of the fire lookouts in the Cascades (and Sierra) were decommissioned after the advent of satellite imagery, although the lookout on top of Mt. Harkness is one of the few still being staffed (see Trip 56). Forget about searching for any relics, as all evidence of the former Brokeoff Mountain lookout has been removed from the summit area.

Trip **2**

Mill Creek Falls

Ⓜ ∕ DH

DISTANCE: 3.2 miles out and back

ELEVATIONS: 6725/6490, +935/-935

SEASON: Mid-June to mid-October

USE: Moderate (light beyond falls)

MAP: *Lassen Peak*

INTRODUCTION: Seventy-five-foot Mill Creek Falls is the tallest waterfall within Lassen Volcanic, but it actually consists of three separate falls: East Sulphur Creek and Bumpass Creek tumble 25 to 30 feet into a swirling pool before their combined waters plunge another 50 feet to the base of Mill Creek Falls. When viewed during the height of snowmelt, usually mid-June to early-July, the falls put on a dramatic display of watery grandeur. Photographers will find the best light at midday.

Most hikers starting from the Southwest Walk-in Campground go no farther than the falls, even though the trail continues another 3.5 miles to Kings Creek Picnic Area. However, those interested in visiting Cold Boiling and Crumbaugh lakes and Conard Meadows will find the hike from the picnic area a better alternative (see Trip 9). If you do plan to hike from the campground to the picnic area—especially in early season when the creek is full of snowmelt—be wary of a potentially difficult crossing of East Sulphur Creek just beyond the falls overlook (packing along a pair of water shoes would be prudent for those times).

DIRECTIONS TO TRAILHEAD: Follow the main park road to the parking lot for the Southwest Walk-in Campground, immediately beyond the southwest entrance.

DESCRIPTION: From a hiker emblem sign near campsite 19, head northeast from the

Mill Creek Falls

Sulphur Works

Diamond Peak ▲

▲ 7879'

West

Creek

Creek

Main Park Road

Bumpass

Sulphur

Viewpoint

Conard Lake

Mill Creek Falls

Conard Meadows

Visitor Center

Mill Creek Falls Trail

Sulphur

Southwest Walk-in

Lassen National Volcanic Park

Southwest Entrance

Creek

East

2

0   .25   .5 mile

0   .25   .5 kilometer

Mt. Conard ▲

parking lot to descend a wide, paved path a short distance to a sharp, right-hand bend, where a trail sign marks the start of the dirt, single-track trail to Mill Creek Falls. Continue descending through red fir forest to a bridged crossing of alder-lined, turbulent West Sulphur Creek, made milky in appearance by mineral deposits from Sulphur Works a mile upstream.

Briefly climb away from the creek and then begin a descending traverse across open slopes carpeted in early summer with a stunning display of yellow blossoms from acres and acres of calf-high mule ears. Eventually, the path heads into a mixed forest of western white pines and firs on an undulating traverse around the nose of a ridge separating the West Sulphur Creek drainage from the East Sulphur Creek drainage; along the way you boulder hop a verdant, seasonal stream.

As the roar of East Sulphur Creek below and the waterfall ahead become more pro-

nounced, the conifers part enough to allow a view into the deep cleft of the canyon. A short distance farther, you reach the shaded overlook, perched right at the edge of the canyon wall (watch your footing), from which you can gaze across the narrow chasm at silvery Mill Creek Falls.

For an even closer falls view, continue northeast on a maintained trail to the west bank of East Sulphur Creek and follow a short use trail downstream to the brink of the falls. Here, East Sulphur and Bumpass creeks tumble down their respective channels before joining in a swirling pool and vaulting over the lip of the rock wall to form the main part of the falls. Watch your footing here, too, especially when the rock is wet and slippery. Instead of heading upstream to the main trail, follow a less obvious dirt path from the lip of the falls to a rock scramble that reaches the trail just above the overlook.

R Fires are prohibited.

Trip **3**

Ridge Lakes

S ✓ DH, BP

DISTANCE: 2 miles out and back

ELEVATIONS: 6950/7975, +1025/-1025

SEASON: July to mid-October

USE: Light

MAP: *Lassen Peak*

INTRODUCTION: Despite its location next to the popular Sulphur Works, the trail to Ridge Lakes is lightly used due to a steep climb to the lakes that averages a 20 percent grade. Even though the trail is only a mile long, the 1000-foot climb, which forgoes switchbacks in favor of a direct route up the hillside, is more than enough to deter all but determined hikers in reasonable condition. Those who tackle the ascent will appreciate the beautiful scenery around Ridge Lakes, a pair of high-altitude tarns surrounded by a scattered forest of red firs and mountain hemlocks in a rosy red cirque basin with volcanic slopes. A straightforward cross-country climb to the ridge crest above the lakes offers additional views.

DIRECTIONS TO TRAILHEAD: Take the main park road to the Sulphur Works/Ridge Lakes parking area, 1 mile north of the southwest entrance. The trailhead is equipped with a vault toilet, and trash and recycling bins.

DESCRIPTION: The trail begins just behind the restroom and climbs northwest across a flower-filled slope to the crest of a ridge that divides the main branch of West Sulphur Creek from a western tributary. Make an unrelenting, stiff climb along this ridge through red firs and western white pines, with views of Sulphur Works beyond the west side of the canyon. Higher up the trail, you may spy an old water tank to the left and, higher still, an active fumarole in the hillside on the right. At 0.3 mile, a very short side trail heads to the right, bending over to a lovely stretch of the creek, which is lined with tall grasses and alders, a good access point for acquiring water for the remainder of the climb.

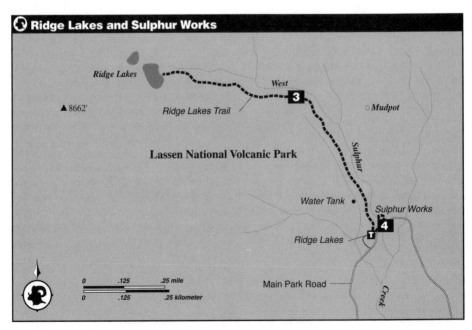

Ridge Lakes and Sulphur Works

Ridge Lakes

▲ 8662'

Ridge Lakes Trail

West

3

○ Mudpot

Lassen National Volcanic Park

Sulphur

Water Tank ●

Sulphur Works

4

Ridge Lakes

T

0   .125   .25 mile

0   .125   .25 kilometer

Main Park Road

Creek

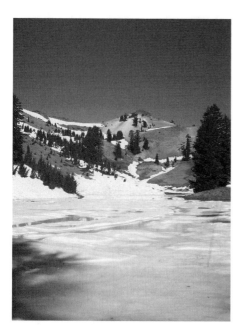

Ridge Lakes

Continue the stiff ascent, where droopy-topped mountain hemlocks join the mixed forest, and eventually top out at the cirque basin containing the two Ridge Lakes. In early season, when melting snow banks drape the cirque walls and the water level is high, the two lakes merge into one. By midsummer, the larger, lower lake is separated from the smaller, upper lake by a thin isthmus. Although the larger lake is suitable for swimming, the nearly 8000-foot elevation means chilly waters. Backpackers hardy enough to lug their gear up the steep trail will find passable campsites amid widely scattered red firs above the northeast shore.

[O] The mostly open terrain above the lakes is well-suited for an off-trail scramble up the cirque walls to the crest, from where you'll have fine views of two glaciated canyons, the nearly vertical north face of Brokeoff Mountain, and the less imposing south face of Mt. Diller, as well as numerous landmarks farther afield.

[R] Wilderness permits are required for overnight stays, and fires are prohibited.

SOUTHWEST ENTRANCE TRAILHEADS

Trip **4**

see map on p. 60

Sulphur Works

E ◯ DH

DISTANCE:	0.2 mile loop
ELEVATIONS:	6935, Negligible
SEASON:	June to mid-October
USE:	Heavy
MAP:	*Lassen Peak*

INTRODUCTION: Once restoration of the boardwalk is complete, this short, easy, self-guided nature trail will include interpretive signs situated between two branches of West Sulphur Creek. Sulphur Works, easily the most accessible active hydrothermal area in Lassen Volcanic, is one of the most frequented features in the park—an early morning or early evening visit will help to minimize the crowds. The boardwalk provides safe passage around the hydrothermal features that scientists believe are the remains of the central vent of ancient Mt. Tehama.

DIRECTIONS TO TRAILHEAD: Take the main park road to the Sulphur Works/Ridge Lakes parking area, 1 mile north of the southwest entrance. The trailhead is equipped with a vault toilet, and trash and recycling bins.

DESCRIPTION: From the large parking lot, follow a short section of sidewalk northeast along the main park road to the start of the boardwalk. With fumaroles steaming, mudpots bubbling, and hydrogen-sulfide gas permeating the air, the presence of vegetation seems something of a wonder, yet near the start of the trail you will find low pinemat manzanita and spiny-seeded chinquapin—two shrubs that are common to fir forests. Labrador teas, as usual, thrive near the stream and are easily identified by the turpentine odor from their leaves. Red firs and western white pines compose the forest.

SULPHUR WORKS

In the 1930s the geologist Howel Williams theorized that Sulphur Works is the remnant of the central vent of the ice age volcano Mt. Tehama, which may have reached a maximum height of 11,000 feet. At the time, Lassen Peak and other prominent mountains in the park today were nonexistent, and the volcano reigned as a solitary landmark similar to Mt. Hood, an equal-size volcano in present-day Oregon. After the central portion of the volcano collapsed and subsequently eroded, Brokeoff Mountain became the highest remnant of the old mountain. Today, the steaming is referred to as the last dying gasps of the ancient volcano, but this activity is perhaps better viewed as a sign of ongoing volcanism; a future eruption anywhere in the Lassen area cannot be discounted.

Here at Sulphur Works, andesitic rocks are being decomposed by hot, acidic water, which, at this elevation, boils at around 195°F (90°C). However, the acidic water is under pressure below ground, which results in superheated temperatures that are extremely corrosive. It's no wonder, then, that the andesite is readily broken down into easily erodible residues; kaolin and opal are the most common byproducts.

The amount of steam you witness at hydrothermal areas such as Sulphur Works corresponds to the amount of groundwater present. Hot pools exist when water is plentiful, but as the amount of water diminishes, the pools evolve into mudpots, which in turn evolve into dry vents, or fumaroles. The obvious rotten egg odor at Sulphur Works is from escaping hydrogen sulfide gas. Fortunately, the gasses, while nasally offensive, are not strong enough to pose any health hazards.

Upon completion of the loop, you can carefully cross the main park road for a scenic view of additional steam vents above the steep ravine of West Sulphur Creek canyon.

Trip 5

Bumpass Hell to Kings Creek Picnic Area

Ⓜ / DH

DISTANCE: 4 miles point to point

ELEVATIONS: 8200/8410/7375, +400/-1200

SEASON: July to mid-October

USE: Heavy

MAPS: *Lassen Peak, Reading Peak*

INTRODUCTION: With a wide array of steaming fumaroles, gurgling mud pots, and boiling hot springs, the 16-acre hydrothermal site known as Bumpass Hell is one of Lassen Volcanic's more interesting areas, a fact evidenced by the packed parking lot between the Fourth of July and Labor Day holidays. The largest of the park's hydrothermal areas, Bumpass Hell is the result of fissures that connect to volcanic heat as far as 3 miles beneath the earth's crust. Interpretive signs along a boardwalk explain the interesting hydrothermal activity. But that activity is not the only highlight of the trail, which includes excellent views of Lake Helen, Lassen Peak, and additional summits across the deep cleft of Little Hot Springs Valley.

Due to the high elevation and aspect of the trail from the parking area to Bumpass Hell, snowfields tend to linger here well into summer. Although the Park Service recommends decent footwear and hiking poles when snow is present, tourists wearing flip-flops routinely make the journey to Bumpass Hell and back without any severe misfortune. Several warning signs remind visitors to stay on the boardwalk and off the fragile ground around the hydrothermal features.

Very few souls continue past Bumpass Hell, missing out on some very rewarding scenery on the way to Kings Creek Picnic Area. Stunning views abound, and some of the most vivid wildflower displays in the park are found on the slopes above Crumbaugh Lake. Although it lacks the sweeping drama of Bumpass Hell, Cold Boiling Lake offers a final hydrothermal oddity before the end of the trail. If you arrange for pickup at Kings Creek Picnic Area, the majority of the hike is downhill.

DIRECTIONS TO TRAILHEAD: START: Follow the main park road to the Bumpass Hell parking area, 5.7 miles above the southwest entrance and 1.1 miles below the Lassen Peak Trail parking lot. The parking area is equipped with a vault toilet, and trash and recycling receptacles.

END: Take the main park road and turn off on the spur road to the Kings Creek Picnic Area, 4.25 miles east of the Lassen Peak Trail turnoff and 4.5 miles southwest of

Summit Lake Campground (unfortunately, the road to the trailhead may not be marked except by a stop sign). Follow the road about 0.3 mile to a turnaround at the end of the picnic area. The trailhead is equipped with a vault toilet, and the neighboring picnic area has picnic tables, barbecues, and trash and recycling bins.

DESCRIPTION: Take the short, concrete, rock-lined path that leads northeast from the busy parking area to a wide, dirt trail that winds through a sparse covering of dwarf, wind-battered hemlocks and whitebark pines, with patches of pine-mat manzanita hugging the ground. Soon reach a saddle with a picturesque view of Lake Helen back-dropped by majestic Lassen Peak. From this vista, the trail turns south to traverse a hillside with good views between the conifers of Little Hot Springs Valley and Mt. Conard, Brokeoff Mountain, and Pilot Pinnacle. At 0.75 mile

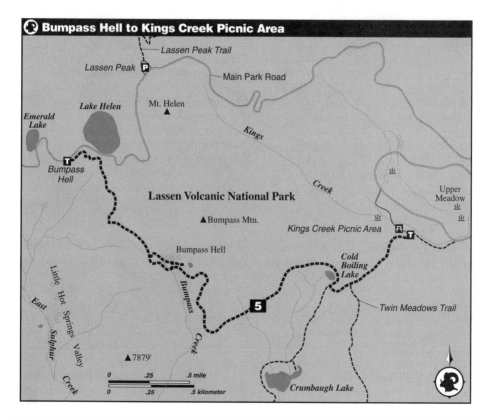

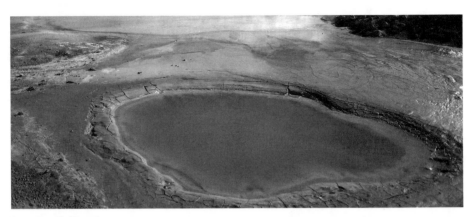

Bumpass Hell pools

from the trailhead, a short side trail leads right to a vista point complete with interpretive signs about ancient Mt. Tehama. Another quarter mile of mildly ascending trail leads to the high point of the trip at a saddle (at approximately 8400 feet) with good views (and strong smells) of Bumpass Hell steaming below.

Follow moderately descending trail for a quarter mile to a bridge over Bumpass Creek and an unmarked T-junction on the far side with an abandoned trail. Turn right and walk a short distance along the milky creek to a second junction, 1.4 miles from the trailhead, where you should proceed ahead onto the boardwalk to visit some of Bumpass Hell's unique features.

The boardwalk, complete with interpretive signs, leads to a multicolored variety of mudpots, fumaroles, and hot springs. Bumpass Hell is considered the principal release valve for the extensive underground hydrothermal system in the greater Lassen area. Photographers may want to plan an early-morning arrival at Bumpass Hell, when the cooler air temperatures mean more steam will be visible from the hydrothermal vents, and the area will be much less crowded. Restoration of the boardwalk was completed in September 2007.

To continue to Kings Creek, return to the junction, cross a small bridge over Bumpass Hell's outlet, and make a short climb to a view-packed saddle with one final look at Bumpass Hell's churning cauldron of

BUMPASS HELL

A cowboy named Kendall Vanhook Bumpass is responsible for the unusual name of this area. Bumpass came here in the 1860s and badly scalded his leg when he broke through the thin crust above a mud pot. Upon his return to civilization, he characterized the area as "hell," capturing the interest of a newspaper editor who convinced Bumpass to take him along on a return visit. Some lessons need to be learned more than once, as Bumpass repeated his performance, which unfortunately resulted in the eventual amputation of his twice-scalded leg. Signs placed in various locations throughout Bumpass Hell warn visitors from following—literally—in the namesake's footsteps.

hydrothermal activity. A short way from the overlook, more far-ranging views open up of Saddle Mountain and Mt. Harkness on the northeast rim above Warner Valley, and the sprawling surface of Lake Almanor to the southeast.

A short traverse through subalpine flora of mountain hemlocks and widely scattered patches of heather leads to the start of a 1.25-mile descent that takes you away from the Bumpass Creek drainage and into the drainage of North Arm Rice Creek. With the initial drop in elevation, heather gives way to silver lupine and pinemat manzanita, and through openings in the forest, you have fine views of Brokeoff Mountain and Mt. Conard. Farther on, Crumbaugh Lake appears ringed by verdant meadows. The remainder of the descent provides stunning scenery as well, as you travel through wild-flower-covered meadows alternating with stands of conifers. Hop across a trio of lushly lined streams on the way to the floor of Cold Boiling Lake's basin. Gently graded trail wraps around the east shore of the lake, which may appear to be more of a wet meadow than a bona fide lake.

Reach a signed junction with a trail southwest to Crumbaugh Lake (see Trip 9) and northeast to Kings Creek. To visit the unique feature for which the lake is named, follow the extremely short path north of the junction to the marshy edge of Cold Boiling Lake. From there, highlighted by a decaying sign, you can see the cold springs bubbling through the surface of the shallow water. Although the springs may be boiling hot deep down within the earth's crust, by the time they reach the surface, the water temperature has cooled considerably. While wading through gooey mud in order to fully experience the springs is permissible, you better have an effective plan for cleaning your feet afterward.

Return to the junction, and follow pleasantly graded trail northeast for 0.2 mile to a junction with a lesser-used trail to Twin Meadows on the right (see Trip 11). Continue the easy stroll past a large clearing carpeted with lupine in midsummer before entering a light forest of ponderosa pines, lodgepole pines, and mountain hemlocks. Head up a broad, low ridge, from which a very short, steep drop brings you to the trailhead at the Kings Creek Picnic Area.

R Fires are always prohibited, and camping is prohibited within a quarter mile of the trail between the trailhead and Bumpass Hell.

ROAD SUMMIT TRAILHEADS

Trip **6**

Lassen Peak

S / DH

DISTANCE:	5 miles out and back
ELEVATIONS:	8500/10,457, +1957/-1957
SEASON:	Mid-July to early October
USE:	Heavy
MAP:	*Lassen Peak*

INTRODUCTION: Reaching the 10,457-foot summit of Lassen Peak is the supreme draw for many hikers visiting the park. The 2.5-mile maintained trail follows a zigzagging course to the summit for an unparalleled view of northern California that stretches all the way into southern Oregon. Prior to the 1980 eruption of Mt. Saint Helens in Washington State, Lassen Peak was the last volcano to erupt in the continental US, in 1921. Although nature has done a great deal of healing in the subsequent decades, a trip along the Lassen Peak Trail still exposes visitors to countless volcanic wonders.

The Lassen Peak Trail rivals the nearby Bumpass Hell Trail in popularity, so don't expect solitude. Certainly, more people start up the trail than finish, but even the summit area can seem overly crowded on pleasant summer weekends. The well-maintained trail to the top is a cakewalk by mountaineering standards, although hikers must be in reasonable shape and be prepared to deal with the effects of altitude. The 2.5-mile trail, completed with the main park road in 1931, averages a steep 15-percent grade nearly the entire way and, when combined with the high elevation, this distance may feel considerably farther. However, the Lassen Peak Trail is the least difficult route to the top of any major volcano in the Cascade Range.

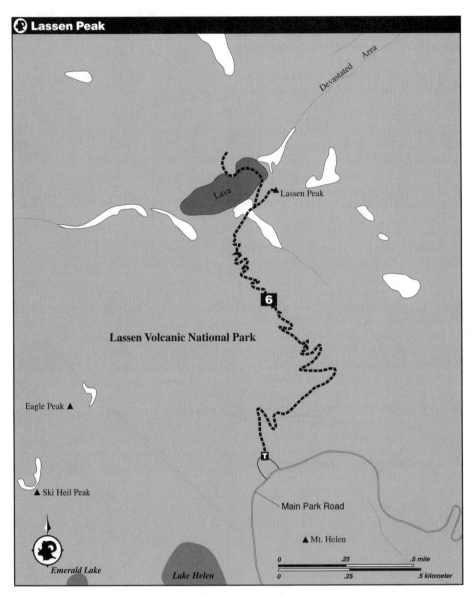

All hikers planning to summit should carry extra food and water, sunglasses, sunblock, a hat, and a Gore-Tex shell, at minimum. At the first sign of thunderstorms, beat a hasty retreat, as the mountain offers virtually no protection from lightning strikes. Snow often covers parts of the trail well into summer, creating an additional hazard for those unaccustomed to safely negotiating snow-covered slopes.

For mountaineers used to traveling over snow and ice, a spring ascent of the mountain can be quite rewarding, offering a nearly continuous glissade from the summit rim back to the Lassen Peak Trail or Devastated Area parking lots.

DIRECTIONS TO TRAILHEAD: Take the main park road to the Lassen Peak Trail parking lot, a quarter mile from the road summit and 6.75 miles from the southwest entrance. The large parking area is equipped with vault toilets as well as trash and recycling receptacles.

DESCRIPTION: Begin climbing moderately right from the start of the Lassen Peak Trail to a switchback; the short climb is daunting enough to discourage many tourists who set out from the parking lot from continuing any farther. In the past, many hikers have shortcut the trail here, creating a boot-beaten scar extending up the hillside. A well-placed interpretive sign with this scar digitally removed from a photograph makes a compelling case for remaining on the trail. Continue the unrelenting climb through low-growing plants, such as Davis' knotweeds, and widely scattered, wind-battered mountain hemlocks and whitebark pines, all the while enjoying the improving views of the surrounding terrain. Beyond the next switchback, the grade increases and remains steep all the way to the summit.

At about 9200 feet, you pass the last of the dwarf mountain hemlocks and enter the alpine zone. Silver lupine is the most widespread of wildflowers, but keep your eyes peeled for more than a dozen species of alpine flowers, including Davidson's penstemon, Freemont's butterweed, and Dwarf Mountain groundsel. As you get closer to the summit, you may notice the diminishing stature of these plants.

In all likelihood, most hikers will have only a passing interest in the flowers but may be wondering, "How much farther to the top?" A mixture of interpretive signs and old wood posts with mileages show your progress, or lack thereof. The spectacular vistas provide you with some visual refreshment while you stop to catch your breath.

The views momentarily depart where the trail climbs through a small alcove at about 10,000 feet, providing a good, nearly wind-free place to rest before the final half-mile climb to the top. Because this area is protected from the elements, relatively abundant flora thrive, including the park's highest sedges and some very stunted

> **MT. TEHAMA**
>
> Try to visualize Mt. Tehama, an 11,000-foot volcano whose summit once stood about 2 miles south-southwest. Only parts of Tehama's flanks can be seen today, with Brokeoff Mountain, about 4 miles southwest, and Mt. Diller, the long sloping ridge north of Brokeoff, two of the most prominent remnants. Between the two peaks, large glaciers from Tehama's upper slopes flowed northeast. Those glaciers gnawed into Tehama's flanks, bringing about its demise, and then smaller glaciers formed on the remaining ridges. One such glacier descended south from the Lassen Peak area, scraping out the basin now holding large, orbicular, 110-foot-deep Lake Helen. More recently, dacite lava erupted at this site, destroying the glacier and building up Lassen Peak in a comparatively short geologic time.

whitebark pines. Beyond this high-elevation oasis, a true alpine environment awaits.

A pair of signs on the next stretch of trail provides an ominous warning to hikers who may be tempted to cut the trail: The Park Service has threatened to close the mountain to all unguided parties unless the trail cutting is curtailed. So, please stay on the trail at all times, as such drastic measures would significantly alter the experience of climbing Lassen Peak, making it both restrictive and costly.

Reach the summit rim, where an expansive view welcomes you to the high-altitude aerie. Pass an area closed for plant restoration on the way to a large flat with a number of interpretive signs. Many hikers go no farther than this flat, but the true summit lies to the northeast. Proceed to the base of the summit rocks, usually over a snowfield, and then follow a route commonly marked by flags on an easy scramble to the top. For those who want to extend their wanderings,

CLIMBING HISTORY

The first recorded ascent of Lassen Peak, in 1851, is attributed to a miner, Grover Godfrey, but Peter Lassen, for whom the peak, park, county, and national forest are named, may have ascended the peak sometime earlier. William H. Brewer, a notable botanist, was on the peak's second recorded climb in September of 1863. The third party known to have ascended the peak did so in August 1864 and included the first white woman to reach the top, Helen Brodt, after whom Lake Helen was named.

Over the course of four weeks, William H. Brewer and members of his geological survey journeyed from Sacramento northward through Grass Valley, Quincy, Big Meadows (nowadays inundated by Lake Almanor), and Warner Valley to a base camp possibly near Lake Helen. On September 26, 1863, they climbed the peak in bad weather, then arose at 1:30 AM three days later under the bright light of a nearly full moon to repeat the ascent. By 2:45, the party was on its way, reaching the summit between 4:30 and 5 AM, just as the eastern horizon was beginning to glow red. On this occasion, Brewer recorded one of the best descriptions yet of Lassen's summit view:

> As we gaze in rapture, the sun comes on the scene, and as it rises, its disk flattened by atmospheric refraction, it gilds the peaks one after another, and at this moment the field of view is wider than at any time later in the day. The Marysville [Sutter] Buttes rise from the vapory plain (Sacramento Valley), islands in a distant ocean of smoke, while far beyond appear the dim outlines of Mount Diablo and Mount Hamilton, the latter 240 [217] miles distant.

> North of the Bay of San Francisco, the Coast Range is clear and distinct, from Napa north to the Salmon Mountains near the Klamath River. Mount St. Helena, Mount St. John, Yallo-balley (Yolla Bolly). Bullet Chump (Bully Choop Mountain), and all its other prominent peaks are in distinct view, rising in altitude as we look north.

> "But rising high above all is the conical shadow of the peak we are on, projected in the air, a distinct form of cobalt blue on a ground of lighter haze, its top sharp and its outlines well defined as are those of the peak itself—a gigantic, spectral mountain, projected so high in the air that it seems far higher than the original mountain itself—but, as the sun rises, the mountain sinks into the valley, and, like a ghost, fades away at the sight of the sun.

> The snows of the Salmon Mountains (specifically, the Trinity Alps) glitter in the morning sun, a hundred miles distant. But the great feature is the sublime form of Mount Shasta towering above its neighboring mountains—truly a monarch of the hills. It has received some snow in the late storms, and the snow line is as sharply defined and as level as if the surface of an ocean had cut it against the mountainside.

a trail has evolved over the years over to the crater on the north rim.

Today, successful summiteers will find the view from Lassen Peak to be as rewarding as Brewer's description (see sidebar on opposite page), although the western sky would have been significantly clearer in his day, without the haze from the pollution generated by millions of Californians. Be sure to pack a large enough map to help identify the many points of interest visible from the top.

Brewer recognized the volcanic nature of the Lassen countryside, but he may have been unaware that the area contained examples of all four types of the world's volcanoes—stratovolcano (composite), plug domes (volcanic domes), shield volcanoes,

LASSEN PEAK ERUPTIONS

A fire lookout was built on the summit in 1913, providing someone with the enviable job of surveying the scenic countryside, as well as witnessing the glorious sunrises and sunsets (nowadays, the trail and summit area are closed to camping, but with a very early start, one could catch a sunrise from the summit). The lookout was short-lived, for Lassen began a series of eruptions in May of 1914, totally destroying the lookout by October. In May of 1915, the mountain erupted again, leaving behind the lava rock that now occupies the summit area. This eruption was followed by a major explosion that destroyed several square miles of forest to the northeast, now known as the Devastated Area. Gazing across the summit area, you'll see the dark 1915 lava flow, spilling both southwest and northeast down the peak's uppermost slopes. A pre-1914 crater is buried under the western part of this flow; the flow itself emanated from a crater more centrally located. The crater visible on the flow's north edge developed after the tremendous May 22, 1915, explosion. To the northwest lies yet another crater, this one blown out in 1917, the last year of significant volcanic activity. The mountain steamed actively until 1921.

and cinder cones. Shasta is the prime example of a stratovolcano, although Sugarloaf Peak and Burney Mountain, both west of Hat Creek Valley, appear to be stratovolcanoes in the making. Lassen Peak and Chaos Crags are excellent examples of plug domes. Prospect Peak, Mt. Harkness, Sifford Mountain, and Raker Peak are the park's four shield volcanoes, while Cinder Cone and Hat Mountain are two of the more prominent cinder cones.

O A few hardy souls travel cross-country from the Lassen Peak Trailhead west to boggy-shored Soda Lake, then traverse north to a saddle at the foot of Vulcans Castle. From there, they can drop north to the meadows of upper Manzanita Creek and then follow the Manzanita Creek Trail downstream to the Manzanita Lake Campground, reversing the description in Trip 27. Excellent scenery and a wildflower display that includes more than 50 species are the chief rewards. Snow patches may hinder progress before mid-July and route-finding can be a bit tricky; it's easy to mistake Blue Lake canyon for Manzanita Creek canyon.

R Fires and camping are prohibited on Lassen Peak.

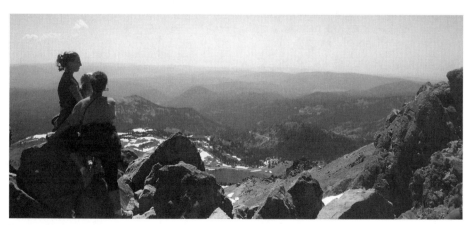

Lassen Summit view

ROAD SUMMIT TRAILHEADS

Trip **7**

Paradise Meadow

Ⓜ ⟋ DH

DISTANCE: 3.4 miles out and back

ELEVATIONS: 8050/7025, +1075/-1075

SEASON: July to early October

USE: Light

MAP: *Reading Peak*

INTRODUCTION: Paradise Meadow is one of the supreme wildflower gardens in the park. Despite this distinction, the trail is lightly used; instead, the majority of hikers who leave the Terrace Lake Trailhead are bound for the trio of lakes to the south (see Trip 8). The trail drops moderately from the trailhead almost all the way to the meadow, so reserve some energy for the climb back, although the less than 2-mile distance should be manageable by hikers in good condition. While Paradise Meadows offers an abundance of wildflowers, the number of mosquitoes in midsummer is equally as impressive—don't forget the repellent.

DIRECTIONS TO TRAILHEAD: Take the main park road to milepost 27, 2 miles east of Lassen Peak Trail parking lot and 6.8 miles southwest of Summit Lake Campground. A sign reading TERRACE LAKE marks the trailhead on the north shoulder of the road.

DESCRIPTION: From the road, the trail descends through open, subalpine forest, principally composed of mountain hemlocks, with periodic views of the massive east flank of Lassen Peak to your left.

Note the rock-walled canyon at the foot of the peak, which was cut by a glacier, or series of glaciers, prior to Lassen's eruption. Scattered patches of silver lupine grace the trail on the way to a Y-junction (at 0.2 mile) with a trail to Terrace, Shadow, and Cliff lakes (see Trip 8).

Proceed ahead (northeast) from the junction, continuing a steady descent toward the cirque basin that holds Paradise Meadow. Switchbacks lead down the slope through stands of timber, across drainage swales, and over a series of benches. Continue through an open forest of hemlocks and pines to a bench overlooking the meadow, and then drop into the meadow's cirque basin, reaching a bridged crossing of nascent Hat Creek near the 1.5-mile mark.

Just across the creek is a signed junction, where the left-hand (north) trail makes a stiff descent toward Hat Lake, but your trail turns right (south) for the very short stroll to the north edge of Paradise Meadow. Back-dropped by the rocky cliff of the cirque's headwall and topped by the slopes of Reading Peak, the symmetrically oval meadow is ablaze with color from a host of wildflowers, which typically reach the height of bloom from late July to early August. Species include gentian, paintbrush, lupine, clover, penstemon, larkspur, and Parish's yampah. Slow-moving Hat Creek sinuously courses through the boggy meadow from its birthplace at a spring. Be prepared for hordes of mosquitoes until late summer.

[O] A nice option for extending your trip is to continue on the trail downstream alongside Hat Creek 1.3 miles to Hat Lake. However, make arrangements for pickup at Hat Lake, as the return trip from there to the Terrace Lake Trailhead is quite steep.

[R] Fires are prohibited.

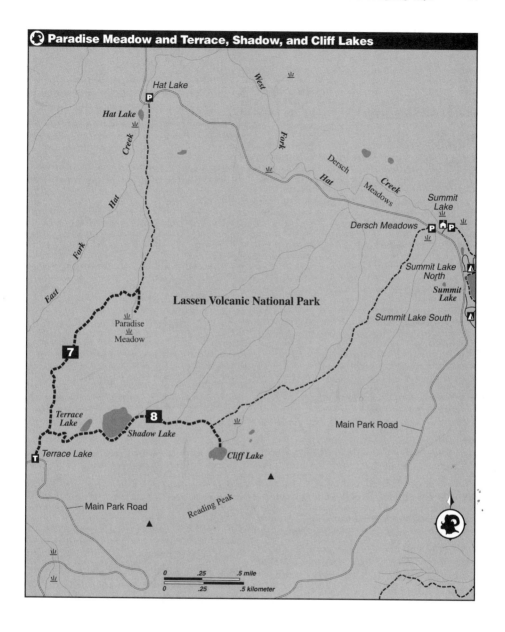

Paradise Meadow and Terrace, Shadow, and Cliff Lakes

Hat Lake

West

Hat Lake

Creek

Fork

Hat

Dersch

Creek

Meadows

Summit
Lake

Fork

Dersch Meadows

East

Summit Lake
North

Lassen Volcanic National Park

Summit
Lake

Paradise
Meadow

Summit Lake South

7

Main Park Road

Terrace
Lake

8

Shadow Lake

Terrace Lake

Cliff Lake

Main Park Road

Main Park Road

Reading Peak

0   .25   .5 mile
0   .25   .5 kilometer

ROAD SUMMIT TRAILHEADS

Trip **8**

see
map on
p.71

Terrace, Shadow, and Cliff Lakes

Ⓜ ↗ DH

DISTANCE: 3.4 miles out and back

ELEVATIONS: 8050/7345, +705/-705

SEASON: Mid-July to early October

USE: Light

MAP: *Reading Peak*

INTRODUCTION: Three picturesque lakes accessed by a trail less than 2 miles long would normally be a recipe for severe overuse. Although a camping ban has long been in place due to their proximity to the main park road, this trio of lakes sees far fewer visitors than one might expect. Lying in the shadow of Reading Peak, Terrace, Shadow, and Cliff lakes usually remain trimmed with snow until mid-July. Before then, the initial descent to Terrace Lake may be one big snow slide. With shuttle arrangements, backtracking could be avoided by continuing to Dersch Meadows, a one-way distance of 3.7 miles.

DIRECTIONS TO TRAILHEAD: Take the main park road to Post 27, 2 miles east of Lassen Peak Trail parking lot and 6.8 miles southwest of Summit Lake Campground. A sign reading TERRACE LAKE marks the trailhead on the north shoulder of the road.

DESCRIPTION: From the road, the trail descends north through open, subalpine forest, principally composed of mountain hemlocks, with periodic views of Lassen Peak's massive east flank to your left. Note the rock-walled canyon at the foot of the peak, which was cut by a glacier, or series of glaciers, prior to Lassen's eruption onto the scene. Scattered patches of silver lupine grace the trail on the way to a Y-junction (at 0.2 mile) with a trail to Paradise Meadow and Hat Lake (see Trip 7).

Turn right (southeast) at the junction, drop into a rocky cleft, stroll past a meadow, and proceed through an open forest of western white pines and mountain hemlocks to Terrace Lake. The shallow, rockbound lake, with its droopy-topped hemlocks and gray cliffs around the shoreline creating a subalpine feel, possesses a sublime beauty distinctly different from the majority of the park's forest-rimmed lakes.

The trail skirts the heather-lined shore of Terrace Lake, and then makes a very short climb to the top of a rise overlooking Shadow Lake, where you can gain a picturesque view of the lake by following a short use trail on the left to a former campsite. Follow an arcing descent to the lake, which is much larger and deeper than Shadow Lake, and stroll along the lakeshore to the east side, where Lassen Peak is reflected in the azure surface. A mixed forest of western white pines, mountain hemlocks, lodgepole pines, and red firs surrounds the lake.

Initially, gently graded trail heads away from Shadow Lake before a more moderate descent delivers you to a boggy meadow with a small pond. Cross a tiny stream lined with a verdant patch of grasses and sedges, and then stroll past a lupine-covered flat and a seasonal pond before returning to forest cover on the way to a signed T-junction.

Turn left (south) at the junction and descend through tangled woodland to the north shore of picturesque Cliff Lake, complete with a tree-studded island and massive cliffs rising toward Reading Peak. Though shallow, the lake is one of the coldest in the park, as snow patches tend to tarry long into the season around the south shore.

Ⓞ With shuttle arrangements, hikers can return to the junction above Cliff Lake and then follow a continuous, 2.2-mile descent northeast to the Dersch Meadow Trailhead, just northwest from the turnoff into the Summit Lake ranger station.

Ⓡ Fires and camping are prohibited at Terrace, Shadow, and Cliff lakes.

KINGS CREEK MEADOWS TRAILHEADS

Trip **9**

Cold Boiling Lake and Crumbaugh Lake

E / DH

DISTANCE: 2.4 miles out and back

ELEVATIONS: 7380/7225, +305/-305

SEASON: July to mid-October

USE: Moderate to light

MAPS: *Reading Peak, Lassen Peak*

INTRODUCTION: This trip travels to two very different lakes. The first is the geologically interesting Cold Boiling Lake, where superheated gases deep underground cool considerably on an upward journey before bubbling into the air at the shallow lake's surface. The second stop, Crumbaugh Lake, reposes regally in a meadow-rimmed basin that puts on one of the park's best midsummer wildflower displays. While quite a few tourists find their way to Cold Boiling Lake, far fewer continue to Crumbaugh Lake, despite the relatively short distance. Therefore, visitors to Crumbaugh Lake can expect some solitude to enjoy the beautiful surroundings.

DIRECTIONS TO TRAILHEAD: Take the main park road for and turn south on the spur road to the Kings Creek Picnic Area, 4.25 miles east of the Lassen Peak Trail turnoff and 4.5 miles southwest of Summit Lake Campground. Follow the road about 0.3 mile to a turnaround at the end of the picnic area. The trailhead is equipped with a vault toilet, and the neighboring picnic area has picnic tables, barbecues, and trash and recycling bins.

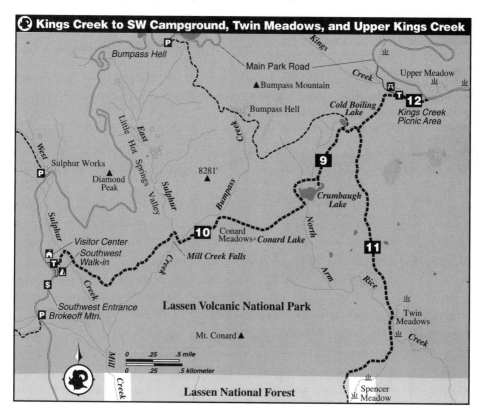

Kings Creek to SW Campground, Twin Meadows, and Upper Kings Creek

DESCRIPTION: A steep but very brief climb southwest leads away from the trailhead to the top of a low, broad ridge, before a virtually level stretch of wide trail heads through a scattered to light forest of hemlocks, western white pines, and lodgepole pines. Pass a large, lupine-covered clearing on the way to a junction with the trail to Twin Meadows on the left, 0.4 mile from the trailhead.

Proceed ahead (west) from the junction, still on pleasantly graded trail, a quarter mile to the basin of Cold Boiling Lake and another junction just south of the lake itself. Here, a very short lateral heads north to the marshy edge of Cold Boiling Lake (and then continues up to Bumpass Hell). An old sign points out the cold springs bubbling through the surface of the shallow water. Although the springs may be boiling hot deep within the earth's crust, by the time they reach the surface, the water temperature has cooled considerably. While it's permissible to wade through gooey mud in order to fully experience the springs, you better have an effective plan for cleaning the muddy goop off your feet afterward.

Head back to the junction and proceed generally south on a leisurely, 0.75-mile descent toward Crumbaugh Lake. While in the vicinity of Cold Boiling Lake, you may notice opal, whitish, decomposed rocks that readily form in areas of hot springs activity. This rock's presence indicates that at some point in the not too distant past, Cold Boiling Lake was steaming away similar to how Boiling Springs Lake (see Trip 67) does today. Soon, you reach the open meadows surrounding Crumbaugh Lake and a signed junction between the continuation of the main trail toward Conard Meadows and a usually boggy lateral to the northeast arm of the lake. By following the main trail across a pair of inlets on the north side of the lake, you can immerse yourself in one of the most extensive wildflower gardens in the park.

[O] If you wish to continue past the lake, see Trip 10.

[R] Fires and camping are prohibited at Cold Boiling and Crumbaugh lakes.

Trip **10**

see map on p.73

Kings Creek to Southwest Campground

M / DH

DISTANCE: 4.8 miles point to point

ELEVATIONS: 7380/6725, +700/-1360

SEASON: July to mid-October

USE: Light

MAPS: *Reading Peak, Lassen Peak*

INTRODUCTION: Four different features lure hikers to this trip, which begins at the Kings Creek Picnic Area and ends at the Southwest Walk-in Campground. Cold Boiling Lake is the first stop, where volcanic gasses from deep below the earth's crust bubble forth from a shallow pond. The next two destinations are something of opposites: Crumbaugh Lake is a large body of water bordered by flowery meadows, while the sprawling vegetation around Conard Meadows hides a tiny pond. Lastly, 75-foot Mill Creek Falls, the park's highest waterfall, will delight passersby with a thunderous display of watery splendor in early summer. With interesting geology, scenic lakes, wildflowers, and a waterfall, the trail packs a large amount of stunning scenery into a relatively short distance.

The area around Kings Creek Meadows often holds onto patches of snow until mid-July, so be prepared to cross snowfields earlier in the season. Also, insect repellent is necessary during the peak of wildflower bloom, which unfortunately corresponds to the height of the mosquito population. The crossings of Bumpass Creek and especially East Sulphur Creek may be hazardous during peak runoff; it's wise to pack a pair of water shoes in early season.

DIRECTIONS TO TRAILHEAD: START: Take the main park road and turn south on the spur road to the Kings Creek Picnic Area, 4.25 miles east of the Lassen Peak Trail turnoff and 4.5 miles southwest of Summit Lake Campground. Follow the road about 0.3 mile to a turnaround at the end of the picnic area. The trailhead is equipped with a vault toilet, and the neighboring picnic area has picnic tables, barbecues, and trash and recycling bins.

END: Follow the main park road to the parking lot for the Southwest Campground, immediately beyond the southwest entrance.

DESCRIPTION: A steep but very brief climb southwest leads away from the trailhead to the top of a low, broad ridge, before a virtually level stretch of wide trail heads through a scattered to light forest of hemlocks, western white pines, and lodgepole pines. Pass a large, lupine-covered clearing on the way to a junction with the trail to Twin Meadows on the left, 0.4 mile from the trailhead.

Proceed ahead (west) from the junction, still on pleasantly graded trail, a quarter mile to the basin of Cold Boiling Lake and another junction just south of the lake itself. Here, a very short lateral heads north to the marshy edge of Cold Boiling Lake (and then continues up to Bumpass Hell). An old sign

points out the cold springs bubbling through the surface of the shallow water. Although the springs may be boiling hot deep within the earth's crust, by the time they reach the surface, the water temperature has cooled considerably. While it's permissible to wade through gooey mud in order to fully experience the springs, you better have an effective plan for cleaning the muddy goop off your feet afterward.

Head back to the junction and proceed generally south on a leisurely, 0.75-mile descent toward Crumbaugh Lake. While in the vicinity of Cold Boiling Lake, you may notice opal, whitish, decomposed rocks that readily form in areas of hot springs activity. This rock's presence indicates that at some point in the not too distant past, Cold Boiling Lake was steaming away similar to how Boiling Springs Lake (see Trip 67) does today. Soon, you reach the open meadows surrounding Crumbaugh Lake and a signed junction between the continuation of the main trail toward Conard Meadows and a usually boggy lateral to the northeast arm of the lake.

Follow the main trail across a pair of inlets on the north side of the lake through one of the most extensive wildflower gardens

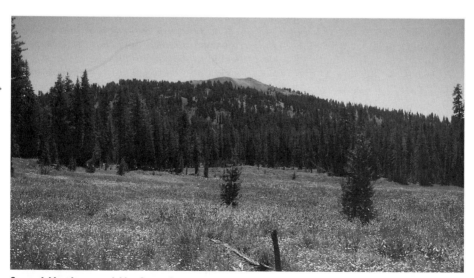

Conard Meadows and Mt. Conard

in the park. The trail swings above the west shore and then away from the lake, turning southwest through mostly shady forest before proceeding a half mile to verdant Conard Meadows, which is back-dropped by 8204-foot Mt. Conard. Tiny Conard Lake lies out of sight, hidden near the head of the meadows by an extensive covering of tall grasses and wildflowers. Toward the northwest end of the meadows, cross the flower-lined stream draining the meadows.

Beyond the stream crossing, occasional views open up of Brokeoff Mountain, Mt. Diller, and Pilot Pinnacle, along with a section of the main park road curving around the slopes of Diamond Peak. Volcanic rock cliffs on the ridge of Peak 7879 provide additional visual interest, as the trail drops steeply into the deep cleft of Bumpass Creek canyon. Tight switchbacks lead down to the crossing of the creek. From there, continue a short distance to cross East Sulphur Creek.

Across the creek, the main trail leads shortly to an overlook of thundering Mill Creek Falls. However, a use trail heads downstream along the west bank a short distance to the brink of the falls, where East Sulphur and Bumpass Hell creeks tumble down their respective channels to a swirling pool, where they vault over the lip of the rock wall to tumble form the main part of the falls. Watch your footing, especially if the rock is wet.

From the overlook, the trail makes an undulating traverse through forest cover out of the Bumpass Creek drainage into the drainage of East Sulphur Creek. In early summer, you break out of the forest onto slopes carpeted with the yellow blossoms of thousands of mule ears. After a bridged crossing of East Sulphur Creek, make a moderate climb up a hillside to the parking lot on the edge of the Southwest Walk-in Campground.

R Fires are prohibited, and camping is prohibited within a quarter mile of Crumbaugh Lake.

Trip **11**

see map on p.73

Twin Meadows

M DH, BP

DISTANCE: 4.6 miles out and back

ELEVATIONS: 7380/6725, +750/-750

SEASON: July to mid-October

USE: Light

MAP: *Reading Peak*

INTRODUCTION: Even though this relatively short trail leads to picturesque meadows, the majority of hikers heading out from the Kings Creek Picnic Area follow the trail to Cold Boiling Lake and points beyond, rather than the trail to Twin Meadows—a definite plus for solitude seekers. The serene meadows are covered with a tangle of tall grasses and wildflowers, which bloom here through midsummer (be prepared to encounter numerous mosquitoes).

DIRECTIONS TO TRAILHEAD: Take the main park road and turn south on the spur road to the Kings Creek Picnic Area, 4.25 miles east of the Lassen Peak Trail turnoff and 4.5 miles southwest of Summit Lake Campground. Follow the road about 0.3 mile to a turnaround at the end of the picnic area. The trailhead is equipped with a vault toilet, and the neighboring picnic area has picnic tables, barbecues, and trash and recycling bins.

DESCRIPTION: A steep but very brief climb southwest leads away from the trailhead to the top of a low, broad ridge, before a virtually level stretch of wide trail heads through a scattered to light forest of hemlocks, western white pines, and lodgepole pines. Pass a large, lupine-covered clearing on the way to a junction with the trail to Cold Boiling Lake on the right, 0.4 mile from the trailhead.

Following signs for Twin Meadows, veer left (south) onto a less-used path lined with silver lupine. After a short stretch of gently graded trail, you begin a moderate descent that continues all the way to Twin Meadows, passing through alternating stands of shady forest and open areas where pinemat manzanita flourishes. Along the way, some of the open areas provide views of Mt. Conard. Eventually, the grade eases as the trail skirts well to the west of the meadows. Just before the south meadows and across a small stream to the left are the remains of an old cabin. Shortly, you emerge from the trees onto the broad clearing of the south meadows amid a lush tangle of grasses and wildflowers.

The trail is easily lost in the thick vegetation, although infrequently placed, round, yellow markers may help keep you on track. The route immediately crosses North Arm Rice Creek (with a brief upstream view of Lassen Peak) and then travels near the west edge of the lower meadows, sometimes across the meadow itself and other times along the outskirts through stands of forest.

Beyond the far (south) end of the meadows, a short use trail on the left leads to shady campsites, while the main trail bends to the right and traverses through open terrain to an overlook of Spencer Meadow to the south. From the overlook, the path drops through forest cover to the verdant floor of a seasonal stream's side canyon on the way to the fenced park boundary.

O From the park boundary, you could continue south on the Spencer Meadow Trail (see Trip 77).

R Wilderness permits are required for overnight stays. Fires are prohibited and camping is prohibited in Upper and Lower Kings Creek meadows.

KINGS CREEK MEADOWS TRAILHEADS

Trip **12**

see map on p.73

Upper Kings Creek

E ✔ DH

DISTANCE:	0.6 mile out and back
ELEVATIONS:	7380/7330, Negligible
SEASON:	July to mid-October
USE:	Light
MAP:	*Reading Peak*

INTRODUCTION: This very short trail follows a stretch of Kings Creek downstream from the picnic area to the main park road.

DIRECTIONS TO TRAILHEAD: Take the main park road south on the spur road to the Kings Creek Picnic Area, 4.25 miles east of the Lassen Peak Trail turnoff and 4.5 miles southwest of Summit Lake Campground. Follow the road about 0.3 mile to a turnaround at the end of the picnic area. The trailhead is equipped with a vault toilet, and the neighboring picnic area has picnic tables, barbecues, and trash and recycling bins.

DESCRIPTION: From the Kings Creek Picnic Area turnaround, a short path parallels Kings Creek for a quarter mile southeast along the base of a low glacial moraine. Where the moraine dies out, the trail follows the creek east-northeast to the main park road. Along this brief trail, note the contrast between wet, creek-bank vegetation and dry, morainal vegetation. Monkeyflowers, elephants heads, marsh marigolds, and other water-loving plants grow only a few feet away from drought-tolerant, silver-leaved lupines and Davis' knotweeds.

KINGS CREEK MEADOWS TRAILHEADS

Trip **13**

Sifford Lakes

E ✓ DH, BP

DISTANCE: 5.4 miles out and back

ELEVATIONS: 7285/6965/7200, +750/-750

SEASON: July to mid-October

USE: Moderate

MAP: *Reading Peak*

INTRODUCTION: This easy trail provides access to a lightly forested bench that holds a handful of scenic lakes suitable for both dayhikers and backpackers. Swimmers should find the water temperatures quite satisfactory for an afternoon dip. Steep cliffs

forming the edge of the bench provide fine vistas of the surrounding terrain.

DIRECTIONS TO TRAILHEAD: Follow the main park road to the trailhead parking area on the south shoulder of the road, 5.5 miles east of the Lassen Peak Trail turnoff and 3.5 miles southwest of the Summit Lake Campground.

DESCRIPTION: Wood steps lead southeast from the edge of the road to a dirt trail paralleling meadow-lined Kings Creek through a mixed forest of western white pines, lodgepole pines, and red firs. Proceed around Lower Kings Creek Meadows, which harbors a small pond in early summer, to a junction, 0.5 mile from the trailhead.

Turn right (southeast) and head toward a pair of logs over Kings Creek. The creek tends to overflow here in early season, rendering the logs useless and requiring hikers to make a lengthy, calf-deep ford. Climb

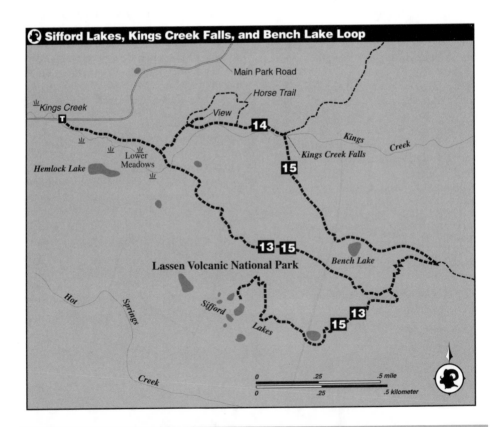

Sifford Lakes, Kings Creek Falls, and Bench Lake Loop

HEMLOCK LAKE

Away from the trail, Hemlock Lake lies hidden behind a low ridge to the south, encircled by a forest of red firs and mountain hemlocks. Labrador tea is also present, insuring plenty of mosquitoes through midsummer. The lake, best reached cross-country from the west end of the road bridge over Kings Creek, may offer a refreshing swim throughout most of August.

away from the creek and then follow a gentle course southeast across forested terrain. About a mile from the trailhead, a moderate descent ensues, leading across forested benches and open areas covered with rock and manzanita. At 1.7 miles, you reach the Sifford Lakes junction.

Turn right again and follow a slightly undulating path that curves west and then southwest through widely scattered conifers and thick patches of pinemat manzanita. After a half mile, the first lake appears suddenly over a low rise, rimmed by open forest. The small lake is fairly shallow but deep enough for swimming. Thanks to the open terrain, the lake is often snow-free by mid-June, warming up to decent swim-

ming temperature by early July. From mid-July through late August, the temperature remains in the mid- to upper 60s, ranking the lake as one of the park's warmest. Passable campsites with excellent views across Warner Valley are found near the edge of a rock cliff south of the lake.

To reach the upper lakes, follow a fairly well-defined path generally north-northwest for 0.4 mile to the top of the bench. Soon, reach the first of the upper lakes, lined with heather and low-growing shrubs beneath an open forest of mountain hemlocks, red firs, lodgepole pines, and western white pines. A pair of good campsites will lure overnighters. A rock cliff above the southeast shore offers a fine view of Lassen Peak, Reading Peak, Warner Valley, and Lake Almanor in the distance. The remaining Sifford Lakes can be accessed via short cross-country jaunts to the northwest.

[O] After retracing your steps to the Sifford Lake junction, for variety, you could follow the route of a partial loop back to the trailhead by heading to Bench Lake and then past Kings Creek Falls to the junction near Lower Kings Creek Meadows.

[R] Wilderness permits are required for overnight stays. Fires are prohibited and camping is prohibited in Upper and Lower Kings Creek Meadows.

KINGS CREEK MEADOWS TRAILHEADS

Trip 14

see map on p.78

Kings Creek Falls

M ✓ DH

DISTANCE: 2.2 miles out and back

ELEVATIONS: 7285/6810, +475/-475

SEASON: July to mid-October

USE: Heavy

MAP: *Reading Peak*

INTRODUCTION: It's exhilarating to visit Kings Creek Falls when the creek is swollen with snowmelt, as a riotous display of whitewater careens hell-bent down a narrow and steep chasm of rock, and the thunderous waterfall drops 50 feet in full force. The trail places hikers in prime locations for viewing the watery splendor, right alongside the cascades and at the brink of the falls—parents with small children will need to keep an eye on their progeny at all times. A short overlook trail offers additional views of the cascades, as well as more distant vistas. The trail descends all the way from the trailhead to the falls and, although the path is short, the section along the cascades is quite steep.

DIRECTIONS TO TRAILHEAD: Follow the main park road to the trailhead parking area on the south shoulder of the road, 5.5 miles east of the Lassen Peak Trail turnoff and 3.5 miles southwest of the Summit Lake Campground.

DESCRIPTION: Wood steps lead southeast from the edge of the road to a dirt trail paralleling meadow-lined Kings Creek through a mixed forest of western white pines, lodgepole pines, and red firs. Proceed around Lower Kings Creek Meadow, which harbors a small pond in early summer, to a junction, 0.5 mile from the trailhead.

Continue straight ahead on the left-hand trail and travel northeast over a low ridge. Drop slightly to a signed, four-way junction. Equestrians should follow the left-hand trail on a well-graded route that bypasses the steep, hiker-only trail alongside Kings Creek Cascades. The middle path offers a 170-yard climb to a fine overlook of the cascades crashing down a narrow, rocky gorge below. You'll also enjoy more far-ranging views across the forested slopes of Flatiron Ridge to Mt. Harkness, the most prominent peak on the horizon. Saddle Mountain is to the left and, farther away, a ridge topped by Red Cinder Cone marks the eastern border of the park.

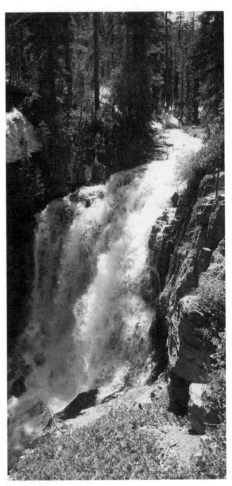

Kings Creek Falls

From the junction, take the right-hand trail east down the rocky gorge alongside Kings Creek Cascades. The steeply descending trail is cut right into the slope immediately adjacent to the turbulent creek, which puts on quite a display in early season. Watch your step, as the scenery is distracting, with the creek tumbling downstream in a series of a dozen or so minor falls before reaching a crescendo at a larger, final cascade. Below the cascades, the trail veers away from the creek slightly and descends more mildly through a mixed forest of western white and lodgepole pines. After it reunites with the horse trail, the grade eases on the way to a junction with the trail from Bench Lake, which crosses Kings Creek on a dual, log-plank bridge. Proceed a short distance beyond the junction to the Kings Creek Falls viewpoint.

Situated on the very brink of the falls and guarded by a cable, the overlook provides a fine perch from which to gaze at the 50-foot cascade. Some visitors scramble down the steep slope to the base of the falls, but this is a very steep, unmaintained route that plunges down the wall of the canyon—exercise extreme caution if you choose to descend the potentially loose and slippery rocks. Because of the fall's aspect, photographers should plan on a visit between late morning and shortly after noon, as these are the only times when the falls are bathed in sunlight.

R Fires are prohibited, and camping is prohibited in Upper and Lower Kings Creek meadows and within a quarter mile of Kings Creek Falls.

KINGS CREEK MEADOWS TRAILHEADS

Trip **15**

see map on p.78

Kings Creek Falls and Bench Lake Loop

M **DH**

DISTANCE: 8.4 miles semiloop

ELEVATIONS: 7285/6750/7285, +770/-770

SEASON: July to mid-October

USE: Heavy to Falls, light for semiloop

MAP: *Reading Peak*

INTRODUCTION: On this trip, hikers can enjoy the beauty of Kings Creek Cascades and Falls, as well as the seclusion and serenity found on the other 3-plus miles of trail. This semiloop passes quiet Bench Lake and a junction with the trail to Sifford Lakes, which provides an additional diversion for hikers with extra time and energy.

DIRECTIONS TO TRAILHEAD: Follow the main park road to the trailhead parking area on the south shoulder of the road, 5.5 miles east of the Lassen Peak Trail turnoff and 3.5 miles southwest of the Summit Lake Campground.

DESCRIPTION: Wood steps lead southeast from the edge of the road to a dirt trail paralleling meadow-lined Kings Creek through a mixed forest of western white pines, lodgepole pines, and red firs. Proceed around Lower Kings Creek Meadow, which harbors a small pond in early summer, to a junction, 0.5 mile from the trailhead.

Continue straight ahead on the left-hand trail and travel northeast over a low ridge. Drop slightly to a signed, four-way junction. Equestrians should follow the left-hand trail on a well-graded route that bypasses the steep, hiker-only trail alongside Kings Creek Cascades. The middle path offers a 170-yard climb to a fine overlook of the cascades crashing down a narrow, rocky gorge below. You'll also enjoy more far-ranging views across the forested slopes of Flatiron Ridge to Mt. Harkness, the most prominent peak on the horizon. Saddle Mountain is to the left and, farther away, a ridge topped by Red Cinder Cone marks the eastern border of the park.

From the junction, take the right-hand trail east down the rocky gorge alongside Kings Creek Cascades. The steeply descending trail is cut right into the slope immediately adjacent to the turbulent creek, which puts on quite a display in early season. Watch your step, as the scenery is distracting, with the creek tumbling downstream in a series of a dozen or so minor falls before reaching a crescendo at a larger, final cascade. Below the cascades, the trail veers away from the creek slightly and descends more mildly through a mixed forest of western white and lodgepole pines. After it reunites with the horse trail, the grade eases on the way to a junction with the trail from Bench Lake, which crosses Kings Creek on a dual, log-plank bridge. Proceed a short distance beyond the junction to the Kings Creek Falls viewpoint.

Situated on the very brink of the falls and guarded by a cable, the overlook provides a fine perch from which to gaze at the 50-foot cascade. Some visitors scramble down the steep slope to the base of the falls, but this is a very steep, unmaintained route that plunges down the wall of the canyon—exercise extreme caution if you choose to descend the potentially loose and slippery rocks. Because of the fall's aspect, photographers should plan on a visit between late morning and shortly after noon, as these are the only times when the falls are bathed in sunlight.

Few hikers continue past the falls, so you can expect solitude and serenity from here to the junction with the Pacific Crest Trail near Corral Meadows. Retrace your steps 100 yards or so to the junction and head south across the bridge over Kings Creek. Climb briefly to the base of a long cliff with an extensive talus slope. At about 0.6 mile from the junction, the trail tops a low spot in the lateral moraine that dams chest-deep, forest-rimmed Bench Lake.

From the lake, descend a gully between two moraines, reaching a junction after 0.4 mile. Turn right and make a curving, 0.3-mile climb to a small flat carpeted with silver lupine. Reach a junction with the trail to Sifford Lakes (see Trip 13 if you choose to visit the lakes).

Continue northwest for a moderate, 0.75-mile ascent through open forest and patches of manzanita and wildflowers. After the climb, gently graded trail leads across a bench before a short drop brings you to a crossing of Kings Creek near the edge of Lower Kings Creek Meadows. A pair of logs provides an easy way across, except in early season when snowmelt swells the stream outside its banks. Across the creek, a short stroll leads to a junction and the close of the loop. From there, retrace your steps a half mile to the trailhead.

R Fires are prohibited, and camping is prohibited in Upper and Lower Kings Creek Meadows and within a quarter mile of Kings Creek Falls.

Trip **16**

Summit Lake

E ♀ **DH**

DISTANCE:	1.5 miles semiloop
ELEVATIONS:	6685/6685, negligible
SEASON:	July to mid-October
USE:	Heavy
MAP:	*Reading Peak*

INTRODUCTION: This easy stroll around the mostly forested shoreline of Summit Lake is suitable for hikers of all ages. The popular trail is a favorite for campers staying at the two lakeside campgrounds, as well as picnickers, boaters, and anglers. It's possible to access this 0.75-mile loop from either the Summit Lake North or Summit Lake South campgrounds, but the 1.5-mile description that follows begins from the parking area near the Summit Lake ranger station.

DIRECTIONS TO TRAILHEAD: Take the main park road 0.3 mile north of the entrance to Summit Lake North Campground to the road to the Summit Lake ranger station and turn northeast. Proceed past the ranger station to the overnight parking area.

DESCRIPTION: From the overnight parking area, follow a boardwalk east across a spongy clearing, a finger of Dersch Meadows, into a mixed forest of red firs and western white and lodgepole pines. Cross a lush swale, briefly ascend a low hill, and reach the northeast shore of Summit Lake near a junction with a lateral from the Summit Lake North Campground. Proceed ahead on the shoreline trail, enjoying a fine view of Lassen Peak towering above the lake, and soon pass a second junction with a trail on the left to Twin Lakes and then an unmarked junction on the left with a short spur to the Summit Lake Amphitheater. At the south end of the lake, cross a boardwalk and head toward the Summit Lake South Campground. Follow the shoreline past the campground to a section of the trail tightly sandwiched between the main park road and the west shore. Reach the North Campground and proceed to the close of the loop, where you can retrace your steps to the parking lot.

R Fires and camping around Summit Lake are prohibited, except in developed campgrounds.

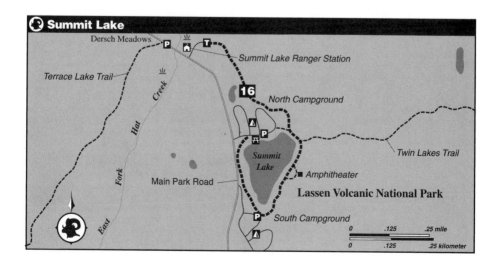

Trip **17**

Corral Meadow

M / DH, BP

DISTANCE: 5.0 miles out and back

ELEVATIONS: 6685/6035, +650/-650

SEASON: July to mid-October

USE: Light

MAP: *Reading Peak*

INTRODUCTION: Corral Meadow may not be one of Lassen Volcanic's famous flower-filled, open meadows, but this meadow—actually more of a forested flat today—offers pleasant walking and camping along a serene stretch of Kings Creek. Corral Meadow, or at least the immediate vicinity,

is known today by Pacific Crest Trail backpackers as a place to find a decent campsite. The trail from Summit Lake to the meadow, which drops 650 feet in the 2.5 miles, is all uphill on the return leg.

DIRECTIONS TO TRAILHEAD: Take the main park road to the Summit Lake South Campground entrance, and park in the day-use lot along the access road.

DESCRIPTION: Work your way to the southernmost part of the campground to the "E" loop and find the beginning of singletrack trail heading south near Campsite 10. Follow the gently descending trail alongside alternating groves of conifers and pockets of meadow fed by tiny Summit Creek. Soon the descent becomes slightly steeper, and the trail crosses lushly lined, spring-fed tributaries on the way to the log crossing of a more vigorous side stream, which the trail follows for about a quarter mile to a T-junction

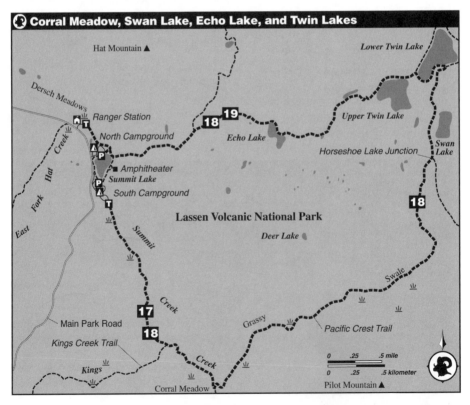

Corral Meadow, Swan Lake, Echo Lake, and Twin Lakes

with the Kings Creek Trail, 1.8 miles from the parking area.

Turn left, following signed directions to Corral Meadow, and soon reach the crossing of a thin rivulet just prior to a pair of old logs spanning the vigorous side stream you previously followed. From there, proceed through the trees a short way to a significant crossing of the main branch of Kings Creek, near its confluence with Summit Creek. A set of small logs placed between two large boulders may provide safe transport across the tumbling stream. Otherwise, plan on a wet ford. Mildly descending trail parallels the creek, usually at a distance, on the way toward Corral Meadow. Just before a junction with the Pacific Crest Trail, this trail makes a short, steep climb across the hillside above the creek. To the east, you have a brief, filtered view through the trees of a picturesque cascade on Grassy Swale Creek, just above its confluence with Kings Creek.

From here, the trail makes another short, steep drop to a narrow flat directly above Kings Creek, where Corral Meadow campsites will tempt backpackers with the prospect of falling asleep to the melodious sound of the creek. Although this area is generally referred to as Corral Meadow, what remains of the meadow proper lies away from the trail to the southwest. Although thick grasses still cover the flat, the encroaching forest appears to be well on the way to completely overtaking the meadow. Directly south of the camp area is the well-signed PCT junction, 2.5 miles from the parking lot.

R Wilderness permits are required for overnight stays, and fires are prohibited.

SUMMIT LAKE TRAILHEADS

Trip **18**

see map on p.84

Corral Meadow–Swan Lake Loop

Ⓜ ↻ DH, BP

DISTANCE:	11.9 miles loop
ELEVATIONS:	6670/5980/7155/6670, +1520/-1520
SEASON:	July to mid-October
USE:	Light to moderate
MAP:	*Reading Peak*

INTRODUCTION: Dropping approximately 700 feet in the first 3.3 miles, this trip offers the easiest approach to the spacious campsites along the west margin of Corral Meadow. From there, hikers and backpackers will enjoy the serenity of lushly vegetated Grassy Swale on a section of the Pacific Crest Trail, followed by a more popular circuit through some of the area's most noteworthy bodies of water: Swan, Lower Twin, Upper Twin, and Echo lakes.

DIRECTIONS TO TRAILHEAD: Take the main park road 0.3 mile north of the entrance to Summit Lake North Campground, turn northeast on the road to the Summit Lake ranger station, and continue to the overnight parking area at the end of the road.

DESCRIPTION: From the overnight parking area, follow a boardwalk east across a spongy clearing, a finger of Dersch Meadows, into a mixed forest of red firs and western white and lodgepole pines. Cross a lush swale, briefly ascend a low hill, and reach the northeast shore of Summit Lake, near a junction with a lateral from the Summit Lake North Campground. Proceed ahead on the shoreline trail, enjoying a fine view of Lassen Peak towering above the lake, and soon pass a second junction with a trail on the left to Twin Lakes (your return route), and then an unmarked junction with a short spur to the Summit Lake Amphitheater. At the southern end of the lake, cross a boardwalk and head into the Summit Lake South Campground.

Work your way to the southernmost part of the campground to the "E" loop and find the beginning of single-track trail heading south near Campsite 10 (dayhikers can park in the South Campground day-use parking lot). Follow the gently descending trail alongside alternating groves of conifers and pockets of meadow fed by tiny Summit Creek. Soon the descent becomes slightly steeper, and the trail crosses lushly lined, spring-fed tributaries on the way to the log crossing of a more vigorous side stream, which the trail follows for about a quarter mile to a T-junction with the Kings Creek Trail, 1.8 miles from the parking area.

Turn left, following signed directions to Corral Meadow, and soon reach the crossing of a thin rivulet just prior to a pair of old logs spanning the vigorous side stream you previously followed. From there, proceed through the trees a short way to a significant crossing of the main branch of Kings Creek, near its confluence with Summit Creek. A set of small logs placed between two large boulders may provide safe transport across the tumbling stream. Otherwise, plan on a wet ford. Mildly descending trail parallels the creek, usually at a distance, on the way toward Corral Meadow. Just before a junction with the Pacific Crest Trail, this trail makes a short, steep climb across the hillside above the creek. To the east, you have a brief, filtered view through the trees of a picturesque cascade on Grassy Swale Creek, just above its confluence with Kings Creek.

From here, the trail makes another short, steep drop to a narrow flat directly above Kings Creek, where Corral Meadow campsites will tempt backpackers with the prospect of falling asleep to the melodious sound of the creek. Although this area is generally referred to as Corral Meadow, what remains of the meadow proper lies away from the trail to the southwest. Although thick grasses still cover the flat,

the encroaching forest appears to be well on the way to completely overtaking the meadow. Directly south of the camp area is the well-signed PCT junction, 3.3 miles from the parking lot.

Turn left and follow the northbound PCT to a ford of Kings Creek—look downstream for snags and logs for a dry crossing. A short, moderate climb leads over a hillside into the Grassy Swale drainage, where the forested trail initially stays a good distance away from the creek. The forest is broken by a trio of meadows filled with boggy vegetation, but well-placed boardwalks span the gooey ground to help keep hikers out of the muck and off the fragile plant life. About 1.5 miles from the junction, the trail crosses to the north bank of Grassy Swale Creek and heads up the drainage with much better views of the lushly lined stream. Mildly rising trail leads to a junction, at 5.7 miles, where the trail ahead leaves the PCT and travels up Grassy Swale to a connection with the trail northwest from Horseshoe Lake.

Remaining on the PCT, veer left and follow the north bank of the creek for 0.3 mile until the trail bends and makes a stiff ascent up a low side canyon. Climb out of the canyon through charred forest, and then follow nearly level trail to a three-way junction with the previously mentioned trail from Horseshoe Lake. Continue ahead (north) on the PCT and drop into thicker forest on the way toward Swan Lake. Backpackers should look for passable campsites above the south shore or on an east-shore bench. The trail almost reaches the northwest shore of the lake, then immediately crosses the barely discernible outlet before dropping 0.5 mile to a junction near the southeast shore of lodgepole-fringed Lower Twin Lake. Turn left and pass along the south shore of Lower Twin Lake for 0.4 mile to a junction with the west shore trail, 8.3 miles from the parking lot.

Bear left at the junction, following signed directions to Upper Twin and Summit lakes. Follow the usually dry outlet uphill a short distance to Upper Twin Lake. The trail skirts the north shore along the base of a steep slope that limits potential campsites to the west, south, and east shores.

A moderately steep climb incorporating a few short switchbacks leads out of Twin Lakes basin and past a fair-size pond, where the grade momentarily eases. A long, gentle ascent, followed by a short, stiff climb brings you to another pond, this one back-dropped by a talus slope. More climbing precedes a short drop to Echo Lake, which displays a fine forest-lake ecotone, a transition zone between forest plants and lakeshore plants. Pinemat manzanita, characteristic of well-drained forest slopes, gives way to red mountain heather only a few feet from the shore. In turn, the heather gives way to a thin band of shoreline species, notably western blueberry, primrose monkeyflower, and moss. Sedges flourish along the shoreline and advance into the shallow water near the edge of the lake. Due to its close proximity to the trailhead, camping is not allowed at Echo Lake.

A mild climb across the floor of Echo Lake's basin is followed by a steeper climb of a shrub-covered slope, where tobacco brush, chinquapin, and manzanita flourish. Where the grade eases, you stroll across the top of a lightly forested bench to a junction, 11 miles from the parking area.

The gentle stroll continues across the bench through open forest and pinemat manzanita before the trail begins a plunge toward Summit Lake, with views of Lassen Peak to the west and Crescent Crater on the north flank. A moderate descent along a ridge and a gully leads into thicker forest on the way to the junction near the northeast shore of Summit Lake. From there, turn northwest to retrace your steps 0.5 mile to the trailhead at the overnight parking lot near the Summit Lake ranger station.

R Wilderness permits are required for overnight stays. Fires are prohibited, and camping is prohibited from Echo Lake to Summit Lake.

SUMMIT LAKE TRAILHEADS

Trip **19**

see map on p.84

Echo and Twin Lakes

Ⓜ ⟋ DH, BP

DISTANCE: 7.4 miles out and back

ELEVATIONS: 6685/7160/6550, +1225/-1225

SEASON: July to mid-October

USE: Moderate

MAP: *Reading Peak*

INTRODUCTION: Summit Lake is both a popular campground and a departure point for hikers and backpackers bound for the central part of Lassen Volcanic National Park. This popular trip visits dreamy Echo Lake, with its droopy-tipped mountain hemlocks and dark rocks ringing the shoreline, and the larger Twin Lakes, whose deep-blue surfaces act as mirrors for the thick forests surrounding their shorelines. At Echo Lake, which has more of a subalpine ambiance than the park's average backcountry lake, overnight camping is not allowed, due to its proximity to the trailhead. However, camping is permitted at the Twin Lakes.

DIRECTIONS TO TRAILHEAD: Take the main park road to the entrance of Summit Lake North Campground and park in the day-use lot on the south side of the access road. If you're doing this trip as a backpack, take the main park road 0.3 mile north of the entrance to Summit Lake North Campground, turn northeast on the road to the Summit Lake ranger station, and continue to the overnight parking area at the end of the road.

DESCRIPTION: From the day-use parking lot, walk toward the east end of the campground and find the start of the trail near a sign marked AMPHITHEATER. Follow dirt trail southeast past some trail signs and across a boardwalk over a marshy stretch of

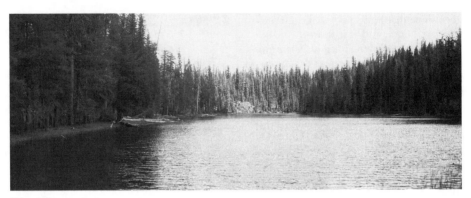

Echo Lake

ground to a junction with the trail from the ranger station trailhead. (Backpackers can reach this spot from the overnight parking area by following a boardwalk east across a spongy finger of Dersch Meadows, crossing a lush swale, and briefly ascending a low hill to the junction at the northeast shore of Summit Lake.) A short distance ahead, near the northeast finger of the lake, is a well-signed Y-junction with a trail to Corral Meadow on the right and your trail to Echo Lake on the left.

A moderate climb travels up a gully and then up a ridge to a switchback, with the first good view of Lassen Peak due west and Crescent Crater on the peak's north flank. Continue climbing through open forest across a slope covered with pinemat manzanita and lesser amounts of greenleaf manzanita to a plateau and a junction with a trail to the Bear and Cluster lakes on the left, 1 mile from the trailhead.

Proceed ahead and follow gently graded trail across the plateau for a quarter mile before a moderate descent leads down shrub-covered slopes of manzanita, chinquapin, and tobacco brush toward the floor of Echo Lake's basin, where an easy, half-mile stroll takes you to the north shore of the lake.

Echo Lake, similar in some ways to Twin Lakes, displays a fine forest-lake ecotone, a transition zone between forest plants and lakeshore plants. Pinemat manzanita, characteristic of well-drained forest slopes, gives way to red mountain heather only a few feet from the shore. In turn, the heathers give way to a thin band of shoreline species, notably western blueberry, primrose monkeyflower, and moss. Sedges flourish along the shoreline and advance into the shallow water near the edge of the lake.

Echo Lake is certainly a worthy goal in itself, but most hikers descend to Twin Lakes before heading back to Summit Lake. Climb out of the depression holding Echo Lake and then drop to the east, passing a meadow and a stagnant pond before heading north through a small, flat-floored valley. The exposed lava flows that comprise the sides of the valley yield to a shallow, linear pond, from which the trail drops rather steeply down more lava flows to the west corner of Upper Twin Lake.

The trail skirts across steep slopes above the north shore of the forest-rimmed lake and then follows the rollicking outlet on a 40-foot drop to a trail junction near the southwest corner of Lower Twin Lake. The right-hand trail traverses 0.4 mile to a junction with the Pacific Crest Trail, while the left-hand trail hugs the west shore below steep slopes and semi-stable talus. You can follow either trail around the east or west shores of Lower Twin Lake from here, or simply retrace your steps to the trailhead.

R Wilderness permits are required for overnight stays. Fires are prohibited, and camping is prohibited from Summit Lake to and including Echo Lake.

SUMMIT LAKE TRAILHEADS

Trip **20**

Cluster and Twin Lakes Loop

Ⓜ ↻ DH, BP

DISTANCE: 10.8 miles loop

ELEVATIONS: 6685/7320/6480/7160/668, +1385/-1385

SEASON: July to mid-October

USE: Moderate

MAPS: *Reading Peak, West Prospect Peak, Prospect Peak*

INTRODUCTION: This nearly 11-mile loop trip samples a number of what are considered to be some of the park's best lakes—Little Bear, Big Bear, Silver, Feather,

Lower Twin, Upper Twin, and Echo. Strong hikers can complete the loop as a dayhike, but backpackers will have the opportunity to spend more time exploring the lakes and visiting far-flung destinations by way of several connecting trails. Echo is the only lake with a camping ban, but backpackers have plenty of other sites to choose from in the mostly forested backcountry. The circuit also offers occasional views of Lassen, Reading, and Prospect peaks.

DIRECTIONS TO TRAILHEAD: Take the main park road 0.3 mile north of the entrance to Summit Lake North Campground, turn northeast on the road to the Summit Lake ranger station, and continue to the overnight parking area at the end of the road.

Dayhikers may park in the day-use lot on the south side of the access road into Summit Lake North Campground.

DESCRIPTION: From the overnight parking area, follow a boardwalk east across

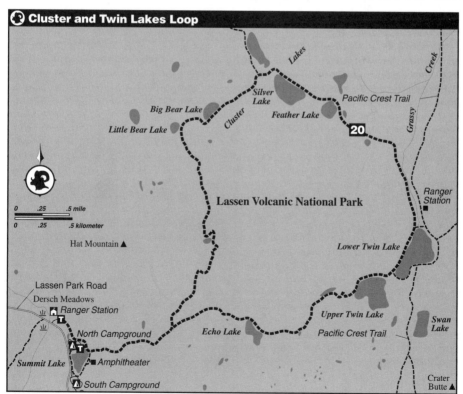

Cluster and Twin Lakes Loop

a spongy clearing, a finger of Dersch Meadows, into a mixed forest of red firs and western white and lodgepole pines. Cross a lush swale, briefly ascend a low hill, and reach the northeast shore of Summit Lake, near a junction with a lateral from the Summit Lake North Campground (day-hikers can access this junction from the day-use parking lot by walking toward the east end of the campground and finding the start of the trail near a sign marked AMPHI-THEATER). A short distance farther, near the northeast finger of the lake, is a well-signed Y-junction with a trail to Corral Meadow on the right and your trail to Echo Lake on the left.

A moderate climb travels up a gully and then up a ridge to a switchback, with the first good view of Lassen Peak due west and Crescent Crater on the peak's north flank. Continue climbing through open forest across a slope covered with pinemat manzanita and lesser amounts of greenleaf manzanita to a plateau and a junction with a trail to Echo and Twin lakes on the right, 1 mile from the trailhead.

Turn left at the junction to head toward Little Bear Lake, and make a gradual climb that soon becomes moderate. After a half mile, reach the high point of the loop atop a rumpled plateau of old lava flows. A

cross-country route heads northwest from here a nearly level half mile to the base of Hat Mountain and then more steeply to the summit. Hat Mountain's cone, with its composition of andesite lava flows, differs from the park's more famous Cinder Cone, which is composed of basalt cinders.

From the high point, descend northward to a shallow, unnamed lake that offers pleasant swimming. A half mile of gently graded trail leads across the plateau and past a tiny pond before a moderate-to-steep descent heads down a ridge separating a pair of small, glaciated canyons. The grade eases and the forest thickens on the approach to lodgepole-lined, shallow Little Bear Lake, which offers good swimming, hordes of mosquitoes through midsummer, and no campsites due to a lack of level ground.

A short but steep descent east brings you to Big Bear Lake, also ringed by trees but not quite as shallow as its smaller counterpart. Passable campsites near the northeast and south shore will tempt backpackers for an overnight stay.

Northeast of Big Bear Lake, a half mile of gently descending trail leads to a junction. The northernmost Cluster Lake is just 200 yards north, where backpackers will find good campsites near the north end. The lake loses some of its attractiveness by mid-July

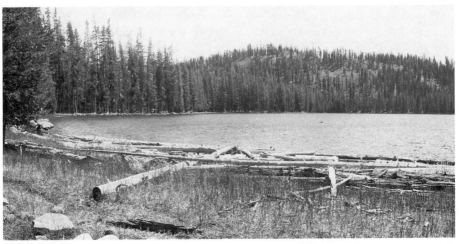

Lower Twin Lake

(when the trail to Bear Lakes is still mottled with snow), as the lake level drops about a foot and the very shallow western arm disappears entirely, reducing the lake's surface area by one-third. Before mid-July, all of the Cluster Lakes suffer from a healthy population of mosquitoes.

Reach the north shore of Silver Lake after a short stroll east of the junction. The trail hugs the northeast side of the lake and passes through a forest of western white pines, lodgepole pines, and firs. Shallow Silver Lake, the largest of the Cluster Lakes, has several campsites, but please select a site that is at least 100 feet from the lake and trail. In the early morning, sunlit Lassen Peak reflects brightly in the surface of the lake's dark, placid water.

A low drainage separates Silver Lake from Feather Lake, which is, perhaps, the best of all the Cluster Lakes. The unnamed triangular lake 200 yards to the north of Feather Lake is also quite pleasant, for despite the shallowness, the lake seems to attract fewer mosquitoes—an important consideration prior to late July. Generally, by early August, all of the Cluster Lakes, as well as Twin Lakes, drop a foot or so, creating habitat around the lakes for a narrow ring of yellow blossoms from tiny primrose monkeyflowers.

Leaving the Cluster Lakes, the trail proceeds southeast through mixed forest and past a chest-deep pond to the low point of the circuit at the usually dry, rocky swale that serves as the seasonal outlet for Twin Lakes. A short climb from there brings you to a junction with the wide path of an old road that now serves as a section of the famed Pacific Crest Trail.

On a not-too-scenic section of this often-scenic trail, you follow the roadbed past a small seasonal pond to the right, and the backcountry cabin that serves as the Twin Lake ranger station on your left. Proceed a short distance to the north shore of Lower Twin Lake. At the junction here, turn right (west), leaving the PCT, and cross a narrow, lodgepole pine-dotted isthmus separating the main body of the lake from the seasonal overflow pond to the north. The trail closely follows the west shore, as the hillside above is quite steep. Backpackers will find campsites on the east side. At the south end of the lake, come to a junction with a tail section that follows the east shore back to a connection with the PCT.

Proceed ahead (southwest) at the junction, following signed directions to Upper Twin and Summit lakes. Follow the usually dry outlet uphill a short distance to Upper Twin Lake. The trail skirts the north shore along the base of a steep slope that limits potential campsites to the west, south, and east shores.

A moderately steep climb incorporating a few short switchbacks leads out of Twin Lakes basin and past a fair-size pond, where the grade momentarily eases. A long, gentle ascent, followed by a short, stiff climb leads to another pond, this one back-dropped by a talus slope. More climbing precedes a short drop to Echo Lake, which displays a fine forest-lake ecotone, a transition zone between forest plants and lakeshore plants. Pinemat manzanita, characteristic of well-drained forest slopes, gives way to red mountain heather only a few feet from the shore. In turn, the heather gives way to a thin band of shoreline species, notably western blueberry, primrose monkeyflower, and moss. Sedges flourish along the shoreline and advance into the shallow water near the edge of the lake. Due to its proximity to the trailhead, camping is not allowed at Echo Lake.

A mild climb across the floor of Echo Lake's basin is followed by a steeper climb of a shrub-covered slope, where tobacco brush, chinquapin, and manzanita flourish. Where the grade eases, stroll across the top of a lightly forested bench to the trail junction at the close of the loop. Head generally west to retrace your steps to the trailhead.

R Wilderness permits are required for overnight stays. Fires are prohibited, and camping is prohibited at Echo Lake and from Echo Lake to Summit Lake.

Trip **21**

Dersch Meadows to Cliff Lake

M ⟋ **DH**

DISTANCE: 4.7 miles out and back

ELEVATIONS: 6665/7340, +825/-825

SEASON: July to mid-October

USE: Moderate

MAP: *Reading Peak*

INTRODUCTION: The shortest and least difficult route to Cliff Lake and the two neighboring lakes, Shadow and Terrace, is via the high route from the Terrace Lake Trailhead (see Trip 8). Except for very short, gently graded stretches near a pair of meadows, this lower route from Dersch Meadows climbs stiffly for the first 3.5 miles. When snow blankets the upper trail from the Terrace Lake Trailhead down to Shadow Lake, usually until mid- or late July, the low route is more desirable. Hikers in good condition who don't mind a bit of climbing will find the scenery and the solitude rewarding during any season.

DIRECTIONS TO TRAILHEAD: Follow the main park road 0.1 mile northwest of the turnoff to the Summit Lake ranger station.

Limited parking is available in wide parts of the shoulder near the trailhead, which is on the south side of the road.

DESCRIPTION: The trail climbs mildly to moderately southwest through thick forest. Farther up the slope, where the grade increases, a more open forest with flourishing pinemat manzanita provides filtered views of Lassen Peak. Near a tributary of East Fork Hat Creek, the forest thickens again on the way to a boulder-and-log crossing of the grass- and flower-lined stream. Stroll past a small patch of meadows near the stream and continue the ascent through the trees. After 0.2 mile, the trail reaches the creek draining Cliff Lake and heads upstream to a large meadow with sweeping views of Reading Peak. Gently graded trail passes around the north side of the meadow until a short climb brings you to the junction with the trail to Cliff Lake, 2.2 miles from the trailhead.

Turn left (south) and follow descending trail through tangled woodland to the north shore of picturesque Cliff Lake, complete with a tree-studded island and massive cliffs rising toward Reading Peak. Though shallow, the lake is one of the coldest in the park, as snow patches tend to tarry around the south shore well into the summer.

O Strong hikers bursting with additional energy can continue the climb from the Cliff Lake junction, 2.2 miles from Dersch

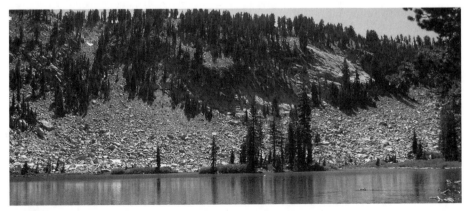

Cliff Lake

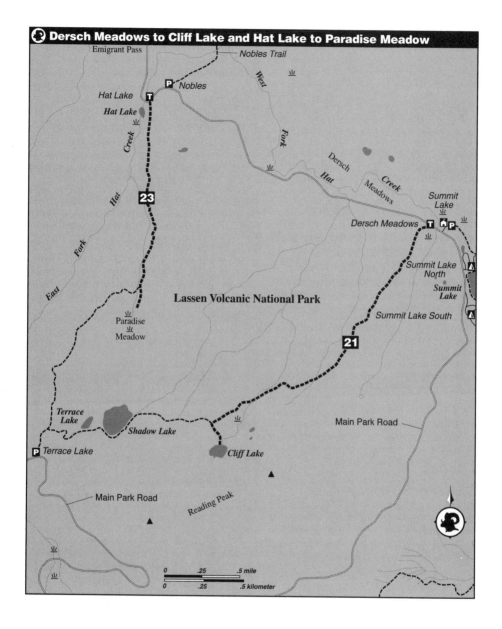

Dersch Meadows to Cliff Lake and Hat Lake to Paradise Meadow

Meadows Trailhead, to Shadow and Terrace lakes. From the spur trail to Cliff Lake, the main trail climbs briefly to a bench, passes a pond, and crosses a small stream. A short, moderate-to-steep ascent follows, leading up a moraine that hides Shadow Lake. Exceptionally deep for its size, the lake is also one of the park's coldest, as is beauti-

ful Terrace Lake, to the west, whose basin harbors long-lasting snow patches. A half-mile climb from Terrace Lake leads to the trailhead at milepost 27 on the main park road (see Trip 8).

R Fires and camping are prohibited at Cliff, Terrace, and Shadow lakes.

Trip **22**

Nobles Trail to Badger Flat

Ⓜ / DH, BP

DISTANCE: 12.2 miles out and back

ELEVATIONS: 6480/6140/6250, +665/-665

SEASON: June to mid-October

USE: Light

MAP: *West Prospect Peak*

INTRODUCTION: Walk a bit of history along a segment of the Nobles Emigrant Trail. For nearly the first 4 miles, the old wagon road heads downstream within earshot of Hat Creek, crossing the stream a couple of times. Then the trail turns east and proceeds through serene forest for two more miles on the way to secluded Badger Flat.

DIRECTIONS TO TRAILHEAD: Follow the main park road to the gated Nobles Emigrant Trail, 0.2 mile northeast of the bridge over West Fork Hat Creek near Hat Lake. Park along the shoulder as space allows. There are no facilities at the trailhead.

DESCRIPTION: Head northeast down the closed road on a half-mile, moderate descent to a bridge over West Fork Hat Creek, the last easily obtainable water until a ford of Hat Creek, 2.6 miles away. From the bridge, nearly level trail passes around the eastern base of Raker Peak. Up to that base, the predominant shrub is Bloomer's goldenbush, a low, uninteresting bush that most hikers overlook until late August, when blossoms of golden sunflowers paint the landscape with splashes of yellow. Along Raker Peak's east base, a few aspens and Jeffrey pines add diversity to the lodgepole pine forest, as do

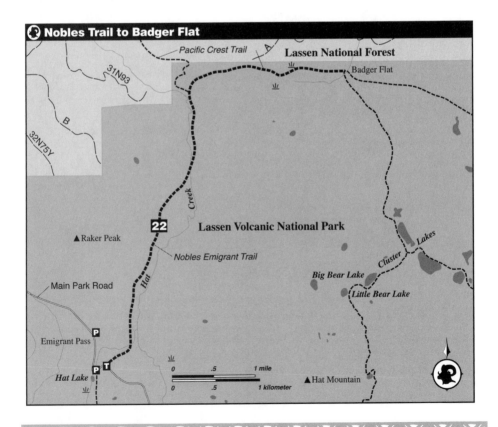

Nobles Trail to Badger Flat

Pacific Crest Trail · Lassen National Forest
31N93
Badger Flat
32N75Y
B
Creek
Lassen Volcanic National Park
22
▲ Raker Peak
Nobles Emigrant Trail
Lakes
Cluster
Hat
Big Bear Lake
Little Bear Lake
Main Park Road
P
Emigrant Pass
P T
Hat Lake
0   .5   1 mile
0   .5   1 kilometer
▲ Hat Mountain

NOBLES EMIGRANT TRAIL

In 1851, Prospector William H. Nobles discovered this natural route—which proved to be both superior to and shorter than Peter Lassen's pioneer route of 1847—on a return trip to his native Minnesota. After procuring financial backing, Nobles supervised the construction of a wagon route that opened to emigrants in late summer of 1852. Thousands took this trail until 1869, when the completion of the Transcontinental Railroad made pioneer wagon roads obsolete.

Christine's lupine, slender penstemon, coyote mint, pumice paintbrush, and catchfly.

Near the north end of the east base of Raker Peak, the road begins to drop and continues to do so for a mile down to Hat Creek. Pass a spur road on the right that leads to some park cabins, and continue a quarter mile to the ford. Keeping your feet dry at the crossing will be a real trick until late August, unless you happen upon a fallen log. Both sides of the creek offer viewless campsites.

Once on the east bank, the trail heads downstream, within earshot of the creek on a nearly level grade. About 0.9 mile from the creek crossing, an old road heads 300 yards west to a fairly large campsite near Hat Creek. This campsite used to be set aside for equestrian use, but the Park Service has decided to eliminate horse camping altogether within the park's backcountry. In 1915, a mudflow swept across this campsite, then continued more than 2.5 miles down Hat Creek, coming to a stop near Emigrant Ford, about 9.5 miles from the source of the flow.

From the road junction, a moderate, 0.3-mile climb leads up to some tall Jeffrey pines on a small flat, and a junction with the Pacific Crest Trail, 4.4 miles from the trailhead.

Turn right (northeast) and follow the shared route of the Pacific Crest and Nobles Emigrant trails on a short climb that leads to the southern base of fault-and-logging-scarred Badger Mountain, a shield volcano (a large volcano with shallow, sloping sides built from multiple flows of basalt lava) that lies just outside the park. Fortunately, the thick forest inside Lassen Volcanic obscures the extensive clear-cut on Badger Mountain from view. Another mile or so of level, featureless walking takes you past a shallow pond just north of the trail.

Soon reach a saddle, where an old spur trail veers right, dropping 275 yards south to a good campsite near the spring-fed, boggy west end of Badger Flat. The wet meadow is home to a wide variety of wildflowers, including pink-flowered Oregon checker, the off-white-flowered Newberry's gentian, and the dark-blue and violet-flowered gentian—three fairly uncommon species.

Beyond the spur trail junction, the main trail continues eastward, dropping gently to the east end of Badger Flat. Here, by the east bank of a creek that flows through mid-July, you reach a junction with a trail heading south to the Cluster Lakes, about 2.5 miles away.

[O] There are many possibilities for extending this trip. Remaining on the Nobles Emigrant Trail leads past Cinder Cone for 7 miles to a trailhead at Butte Lake. Or you can follow the PCT to a number of connecting trails to create a variety of loop trips.

[R] Wilderness permits are required for overnight stays, and fires are prohibited.

EMIGRANT PASS TRAILHEADS

Trip **23**

see map on p.93

Hat Lake to Paradise Meadow

M ✦ DH

DISTANCE: 2.8 miles out and back

ELEVATIONS: 6440/7065, +625/-625

SEASON: July to mid-October

USE: Light

MAPS: *West Prospect Peak, Reading Peak*

INTRODUCTION: The steep climb may deter the faint of heart, but hikers up to the task will enjoy the scenic cataracts of a West Fork Hat Creek tributary, as well as the verdant, grass- and flower-filled Paradise Meadow, which is cradled in a lovely cirque basin.

DIRECTIONS TO TRAILHEAD: Follow the main park road to a parking area just east of a bridge over West Fork Hat Creek, near Hat Lake. Park in the paved lot on the road's north side and look for the trail on the opposite shoulder. The parking lot is equipped with a vault toilet and an interpretive sign.

DESCRIPTION: Head south from the road on a wide, sandy, and nearly level path just east of Hat Lake, which is blocked from view by dense lodgepole pine forest. A short use trail wanders over to the lakeshore for a view of Lassen Peak and Crescent Crater.

All too soon, the trail begins the unrelenting climb toward the meadow. Fortunately, the steep ascent is shaded from a forest of firs and western white pines. Lassen Peak makes peekaboo appearances over the tops of these trees, providing psychological boosts as you labor up the trail. Footbridges span a trio of seasonal streams before the trail settles alongside the alder-lined branch of West Fork Hat Creek, which drains Paradise Meadows. Where the trail gets

> **HAT LAKE**
>
> This lake burst onto the scene on May 19, 1915, when a wall of mud rumbled down Lassen Peak's northeast slope, damming Hat Creek with logs and debris. Incoming sediments soon began reducing the size of the lake; by 1930, the lake was half its original size of 20 acres, and by 1950 it was down to a mere acre.

steeper in order to keep pace with the plummeting creek, a very short path leads to a fine view of a picturesque cascade tumbling down the narrow canyon. Tight switchbacks drag you farther up the trail, past another scenic cascade. As the forest starts to open up, lush foliage forms a carpet along the banks of the stream.

At a junction, the main trail turns right, crosses the creek, and continues climbing toward the Terrace Lake Trailhead. However, you proceed ahead (south) on nearly level trail and stroll a short distance to the north end of lovely Paradise Meadow.

Back-dropped by the rocky cliff of the cirque's headwall and topped by the slopes of Reading Peak, the symmetrically oval meadow is ablaze with color from a host of wildflowers, which typically reach the height of bloom from late July to early August. Species include gentian, paintbrush, lupine, clover, penstemon, larkspur, and Parish's yampah. Slow-moving Hat Creek sinuously courses through the boggy meadow from its origin at a spring. Be prepared for hordes of mosquitoes until late summer.

[O] With shuttle arrangements, tough hikers can continue the steep, 1.5-mile climb southwest to the Terrace Lake Trailhead, at milepost 27 on the main park road, or take the same trail 1.3 miles a junction, turn east to Terrace, Shadow, and Cliff lakes, and then continue down to the Dersch Meadows Trailhead.

[R] Fires are prohibited.

EMIGRANT PASS TRAILHEADS

Trip **24**

Devastated Area Interpretive Trail

E ↻ DH

DISTANCE: 0.4 mile loop

ELEVATIONS: 6465, Negligible

SEASON: June to mid-October

USE: Moderate

MAP: *West Prospect Peak*

INTRODUCTION: On May 19, 1915, hot lava spilled over the crater rim of Lassen Peak onto a thick snowfield layered with volcanic ash from previous minor eruptions, creating a slow-moving mudflow (*lahar*) down the northeast slope of the mountain. Three days later, a massive eruption sent a blast of superheated air (*nuee ardente*) down the same path, leveling a swath of forest 1 mile wide and 3 miles long. Thousands of downed evergreens were blown over like matchsticks, all pointing away from the source of the blast. The Devastated Area has been able to heal for nearly a century, which

has dramatically softened the appearance of a slope that was once a vivid portrait of nature's power of destruction. Over the years, a vigorous forest of aspen, ponderosa pine, and Jeffrey pine has replaced the flattened trees. Nowadays, visitors can learn about Lassen's violent past from interpretive signs along this paved loop trail. The short, gentle path is well-suited for just about anyone, especially families with young children.

DIRECTIONS TO TRAILHEAD: Follow the main park road to Emigrant Pass and the Devastated Area parking lot, 2.8 miles northwest of the Summit Lake ranger station and 9.3 miles from the Manzanita Lake entrance station. The parking area is equipped with vault toilets, picnic tables, trash and recycling receptacles, and interpretive signs.

DESCRIPTION: A level, paved trail leads away from the parking area and passes a side path to restrooms on the way to a three-way junction at the start of the loop. Turn left for a clockwise loop through scattered forest and volcanic rock, with massive, solemn Lassen Peak always looming to the southwest. Proceed past a number of interpretive signs that provide details of the area's interesting volcanic history.

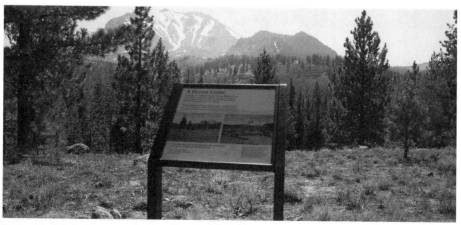

Devastated Area

Trip **25**

Crags Lake

M / DH

DISTANCE: 4 miles out and back

ELEVATIONS: 5920/6650, +990/-990

SEASON: Mid-June to mid-October

USE: Moderate

MAPS: *Manzanita Lake, West Prospect Peak*

INTRODUCTION: Although short, the trail to Crags Lake does require a moderate climb. The trip offers plenty of enticements, including a walk through a noble forest alongside delightful Manzanita Creek on the lower part, and a scenery-rich ascent through open forest on the upper part. Crags Lake, Chaos Crater, and Chaos Crags provide plenty of volcanic wonders at the trail's end.

DIRECTIONS TO TRAILHEAD: From the Manzanita Lake entrance station, drive 0.6 mile east to a junction with the road to Manzanita Lake Campground. Turn right

(south) and proceed 200 yards to the signed trailhead at a sharp bend in the road.

DESCRIPTION: Within earshot of Manzanita Creek, follow a rock-lined stretch of trail on a moderate climb through a light forest of white firs and Jeffrey pines. Watch for an easy-to-miss use trail heading to an overlook of a scenic cataract on the creek. As the trail moves away from the creek, pockets of greenleaf manzanita and tobacco brush appear before the crossing of a low glacial moraine. A shady traverse north over low, rolling moraines brings you to a small rivulet and a spring, the only water between here and Chaos Lake (the lake's water may be of dubious quality, depending on the time of year and the amount of the previous winter's snowpack).

Past the spring, the trail bends east and climbs along the forested south edge of Chaos Jumbles. Eventually, the grade increases and the trail switchbacks across more open slopes with a pleasant balance of conifers and evergreen shrubs, where red fir and western white pine intermix with chinquapin and pinemat and greenleaf manzanita.

Pass through a stand of lodgepole pines, just before reaching an exposed ridge above Chaos Crater, the pit that holds diminutive Crags Lake. This ridge provides the best view of the steep, intimidating talus

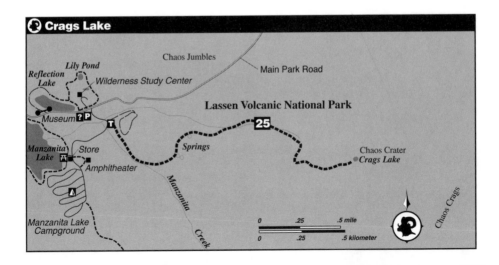

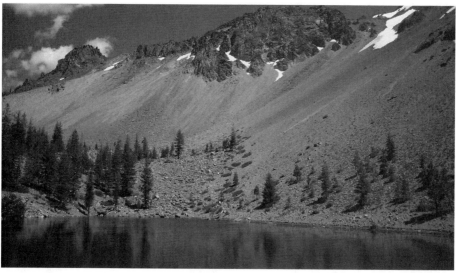

Chaos Lake

slopes of Chaos Crags and the relatively flat-topped Table Mountain, about 2 miles northwest. Standing 12 miles away, above and to the right of Table Mountain's east summit, are the clustered peaks of Thousand Lakes Wilderness, notably Magee, Crater, and Fredonyer peaks. Similar to Brokeoff Mountain and Mt. Diller, these peaks are remnants of an old, 9000-foot volcano that has been largely dissected by glaciers. Before descending to the lake, you may want to search for a couple of relatively uncommon wildflowers sometimes found among the rocks of the ridge—ballhead ipomopsis, a small, prostrate plant with a globe of miniature white flowers, and shaggy hawkweed, an equally small, upright plant, with hairy leaves and yellow sunflowers.

On poor tread, drop steeply off the ridge amid boulders and blocky volcanic rock. The unstable slopes are home to the usual assortment of talus-slope wildflowers, such as coyote mint, Davis' knotweed, silver-leaved lupine, pumice paintbrush, granite gilia, and one or more species of buckwheat. Fortunately, the descent is short-lived, and soon you stand on the rocky shore above the tiny lake.

Over the years, the size of Crags Lake has been cut in half, which is no won-

der considering that minor rockfalls occur almost daily on the very steep slopes above. In fact, chances are good you'll hear loose dacite tumbling down the slope during your stay. If you visit in early summer following winters of significant snowfall, you may see a lake in Chaos Crater. However, the lake often disappears by late summer, particularly after a dry winter.

R Fires are prohibited, and camping is not allowed at Crags Lake.

CHAOS JUMBLES

Chaos Jumbles is a series of rockfall avalanches that broke loose from Chaos Crags, each slide crashing swiftly downslope to rest against the lower flanks of Table Mountain. Lily Pond and Reflection Lake filled large hollows in this debris, while Manzanita Lake was dammed behind the southern edge of the Jumbles. The Jumbles extend approximately 0.75 mile west of the Highway 44/89 junction and nearly 3.5 miles from the source near Chaos Crater.

MANZANITA LAKE TRAILHEADS

Trip **26**

Manzanita Creek

M ✗ DH

DISTANCE: 6.6 miles out and back

ELEVATIONS: 5900/7150, +1250/-1250

SEASON: July to late October

USE: Light

MAPS: *Manzanita Lake, Lassen Peak*

INTRODUCTION: Few seem to tread this trail up the canyon of Manzanita Creek to the base of Crescent Cliff, which is a shame, as the wildflower display in the upper meadows is one of Lassen Volcanic's finest. What the trail lacks in picturesque lakes

and sweeping views is more than made up for by the serenity of the lowland forest and the outstanding floral delights of the upper canyon.

DIRECTIONS TO TRAILHEAD: From the Manzanita Lake entrance station, drive 0.6 mile east to a junction with the road to Manzanita Lake Campground. Turn right (south) and proceed past the Manzanita Lake Camper Service Store to the upper loop of the campground (tents only). The trail begins across from Campsite #31, near the close of the loop. Parking is very limited—if spots are not available, you may have to park near the store and walk to the trailhead.

DESCRIPTION: A wide, sandy path leads south from the trailhead and soon intersects the course of the old Manzanita Creek Road on a moderate climb through patches of greenleaf manzanita and stands of Jeffrey pine and white fir. Eventually,

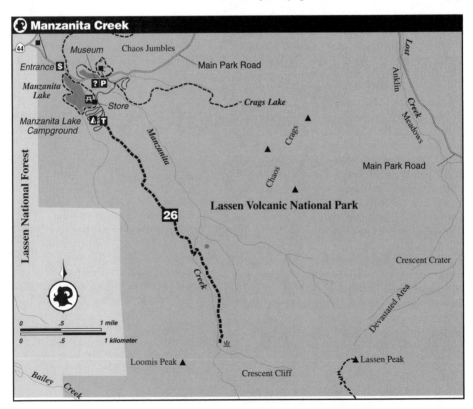

MANZANITA CREEK ROAD

In 1925, Benjamin Loomis, an early settler whose photographic record of Lassen Peak's eruptions is on display at the Loomis Museum, and a crew built a narrow road, which the trail initially follows, to the base of Crescent Cliff. From there, a 2-mile, 3000-foot trail climbed to the summit of Lassen Peak. That trail, which averaged a 30 percent grade and was twice as long as the current Lassen Peak Trail, fell into disuse after the completion of the modern-day route to the top in the 1930s.

monk's hood, arrowhead butterweed, stickseed, and cow parsnip. The wildflower extravaganza continues as the trail meanders farther upstream and disappears in a tangle of lush vegetation and very boggy soils. Here, below the base of Crescent Cliff, look for Lewis' monkeyflower, a pink-flowered plant somewhat common to the Sierra and very common in the Cascades of Oregon and Washington, but a rare find in the Lassen backcountry. Progress farther up the canyon involves cross-country travel through thick brush.

R Wilderness permits are required for overnight stays, and fires are prohibited.

the trail crosses to the west of a steep-sided gully, switchbacks out of the gully, and then climbs moderately before the grade eases on a pleasant, half-mile ascent to a notch in a morainal ridge. Although views are rare along this stretch of trail, parts of Lassen Peak and Chaos Crags can be seen through the trees. Gently ascending trail leads away from the notch across dry, gravelly, open slopes carpeted with silver-leaved lupine, coyote mint, slender penstemon, pumice paintbrush, scarlet gilia, and King's sandwort. Shadier spots sport white hawkweed, pinedrops, and white-veined wintergreen. Nearly 2 miles from its namesake feature, the Manzanita Creek Trail draws near to the stream, where a short side trail leads over to a picturesque pool. Shortly, the trail crosses the piped creek.

Continue upstream on a moderate climb through red fir forest and keep your eyes open for drab western dwarf mistletoes growing on swellings on some of the red fir branches. Nearly 3 miles from the trailhead, at about 6900 feet, the grade eases at the first in a series of meadows that grace the upper canyon. Stroll past the first meadow, an alder-filled clearing, to a copse of trees, and then proceed to a stunning, wildflower-carpeted meadow bisected by a refreshing rivulet, where flower lovers may see such varieties as corn lily, large-leaved lupine,

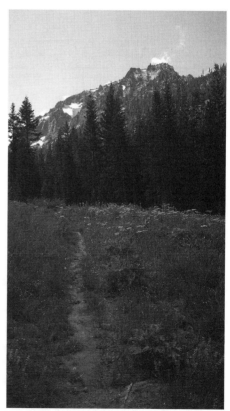

Manzanita Creek Trail

Trip **27**

Manzanita Lake

E ↻ **DH**

DISTANCE: 1.5 miles loop

ELEVATIONS: 5870, Negligible

SEASON: May to late October

USE: Heavy

MAP: *Manzanita Lake*

INTRODUCTION: Manzanita Lake is one of Lassen Volcanic's busiest hubs, and for good reason. The easy shoreline access and the relatively short loop trail around the lake are attractive for sightseers, naturalists, anglers, picnickers, hikers, and joggers.

Motorized boating is not allowed on any park lake, which contributes to a peaceful ambiance, at least away from the traffic noise generated from the main park road nearby. On most summer days, a thriving cross-section of wildlife, mainly birds, will reward visitors with keen eyes.

DIRECTIONS TO TRAILHEAD: From the Manzanita Lake entrance station, drive 0.6 mile east to a junction with the road to Manzanita Lake Campground. Turn right (south) and proceed a short distance to the picnic area parking lot, just before the campground entrance. The picnic area has restrooms and shoreline picnic tables.

DESCRIPTION: Begin at the north end of the parking lot and head north along the course of an old road. In about 90 yards is a grove of Pacific willows, some of the park's largest specimens. Turn right and travel another approximately 90 yards to a bridge span-

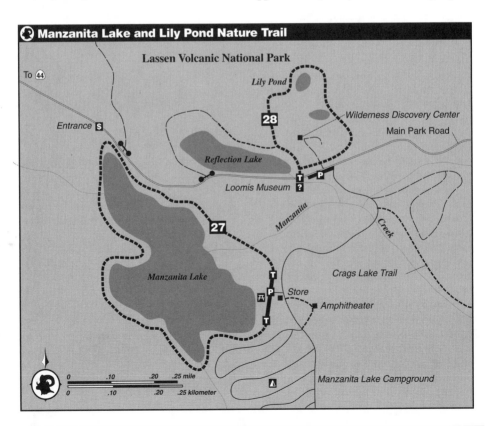

◎ Manzanita Lake and Lily Pond Nature Trail

Lassen Volcanic National Park

To ④④

Lily Pond

28

Entrance **S**

Wilderness Discovery Center

Main Park Road

Reflection Lake

Loomis Museum **?**

T **P**

Manzanita

27

Creek

Manzanita Lake

T

P

A Store

T

Crags Lake Trail

Amphitheater

0   .10   .20   .25 mile
0   .10   .20   .25 kilometer

▲

Manzanita Lake Campground

MANZANITA LAKE

Manzanita Lake came into existence around 1670, when Chaos Jumbles broke loose from Chaos Crags and dammed Manzanita Creek, forming a new environment with still water, where several aquatic plants became established. Water smartweed, the most prominent species, sprouts thumb-size clusters of tiny pink flowers, particularly in the shallow water on the lake's east side. Spiked water-milfoil is another common, though reclusive, lake "wildflower," with inconspicuous flowers but distinctly hairlike leaves that grow in whorls on rising, underwater stems.

The volume of the lake was substantially increased after the addition of a low dam in 1912. However, mudslides generated by Lassen Peak's 1915 eruptions produced tons of sediments that greatly reduced the lake's volume. Trout were introduced and stocked until the 1980s, and today catch-and-release fishing for rainbow and brown trout in Manzanita Lake lures many avid anglers. The lake's appearance may tempt swimmers, but the lake is relatively cold (considering the shallowness and low elevation), the result of cold groundwater that seeps into Manzanita Lake.

ning Manzanita Creek, then turn left and proceed 130 yards to where the shoreline trail branches left. Follow a clockwise circuit around the lake.

In addition to Pacific willows—the giants in the willow family—you'll also see large specimens of Scouler's willow, recognized by their smooth bark. Lemmon's willow is the common, shrubby willow found here and in most wet areas of the park. Another member of the willow family is the black cottonwood, with deeply furrowed bark similar to the Pacific willow but with broader leaves. Mountain alders complete the complement of deciduous, water-loving shrubs and trees around the lake. Juxtaposed against such vegetation is an open, west-shore Jeffrey pine forest with a few white firs and sugar pines; the understory is composed of greenleaf manzanita and tobacco brush. This combination of vegetation groups, along with shade, sun, marsh, and lake environments, makes the Manzanita Lake area extremely rich in habitats.

This is perhaps the best spot in the park for birdwatchers. On any given summer day, hikers can expect to see about three dozen common species in, above, or near the lake.

[R] Fires are prohibited. Mechanized boats are not allowed. Fishing is catch-and-release with single, barbless hooks and artificial lures only. Fishing is not allowed from the boat launch northwest to 150 feet west of the present inlet and 150 feet at the apex of a radius from the center of the inlet.

Trip **28**

see map on p.102

Lily Pond Nature Trail

E ↻ DH

DISTANCE: 0.75 mile loop

ELEVATIONS: 5920, Negligible

SEASON: May to late October

USE: Moderate

MAP: *Manzanita Lake*

INTRODUCTION: Less than a mile long, without much elevation change, and with varied scenery, a trip along the Lily Pond Nature Trail is a fine experience for just about anyone, from families with small children to seasoned hikers well-schooled in the natural sciences. Armed with a leaflet corresponding to the 30-plus numbered posts along the way, visitors can learn about the botany and geology of the area while enjoying the constantly changing scenery of the lakeshore, forest, pond, and meadow environments.

DIRECTIONS TO TRAILHEAD: From the Manzanita Lake entrance station, drive 0.5 mile south to the parking lot near the Loomis Museum. Water fountains and restrooms are nearby.

DESCRIPTION: Find the trail across the main park road from the Loomis Museum. Follow a very brief path downhill from the road to a box containing leaflets ($0.50) that correspond to the numbered posts along the trail. The loop starts immediately beyond the box, where you veer left (north) in a clockwise direction through mixed forest along the northeast shore of picturesque Reflection Lake.

Reach a junction after 0.1 mile, and turn right (north), away from the lake up a low rise and down to a lovely meadow drained by a tiny brook spanned by a twin-logged bridge. Leaving the meadow behind, you enter a thicker forest of lodgepole pines, white firs, incense cedars, and a few sugar pines on the way to aptly named Lily Pond, which is covered with green lily pads that sport brilliant yellow flowers in early summer. The path arcs around the scenic pond, allowing views that capture the different moods of the area. Beyond the pond, the trail passes a smaller pond/meadow and then enters drier, more open woodland of Jeffrey pines. Soon, the route crosses the paved road to the Wilderness Discovery Center and then proceeds shortly to the close of the loop.

R Camping and fires are prohibited.

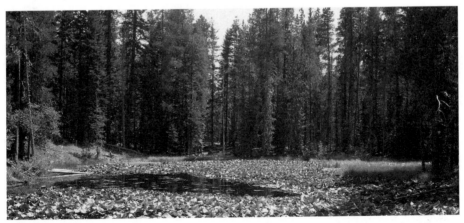

Lily Pond Lake

MANZANITA LAKE TRAILHEADS

Trip **29**

Nobles Trail to Lost Creek

Ⓜ ╱ DH

DISTANCE: 12.6 miles point to point

ELEVATIONS: 5875/6275/5645/6040, +850/-700

SEASON: June to mid-October

USE: Light

MAPS: *Manzanita Lake, West Prospect Peak*

INTRODUCTION: Probably no other maintained trail in the park receives so little use. The reasons are obvious: lack of views and lack of water. Besides devout solitude

seekers, history buffs and nature lovers are perhaps the only ones willing to explore this route. While following in the steps of pioneers, you can enjoy a quiet stroll on the mildly graded trail through serene forest.

DIRECTIONS TO TRAILHEAD: START: Find the trailhead just past the northwest entrance station near Manzanita Lake, on the north side of the main park road.

END: Take the main park road to the obscure end of the trail, about a quarter mile north of a bridge over Lost Creek and 2 miles southeast of Lost Creek Group Campground. Park along the shoulder as conditions allow.

DESCRIPTION: Beginning at a closed gate, follow a service road north for 0.6 mile to its end at the historic site of Summertown. From there, the narrower Nobles Trail strikes east up a gully separating Table Mountain from Chaos Jumbles, a huge

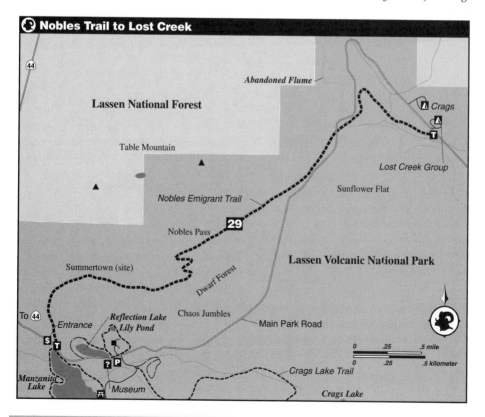

rockfall avalanche that broke loose from Chaos Crags. After about a half mile, sharp-eyed naturalists may spy a couple of prominent Douglas firs. Rare in the park, the Douglas firs here live among strange bedfellows—Jeffrey, lodgepole, and a few sugar pines. A few white firs soon appear as you progress eastward. The gully dead-ends about a mile above Summertown, forcing the trail to switchback up the slope before climbing easily over to ill-defined Nobles Pass, 2.25 miles from the trailhead.

The open Jeffrey pine forest gives way to a shadier forest of increasing white firs, as the trail follows a moderate descent that eventually leads to the main park road. Reach a crossing of the road at 3.5 miles and find the continuation of the Nobles Trail about 45 yards northeast down the road.

The next stretch of trail, just 1.2 miles long, begins among white firs but soon reaches brushy slopes dominated by green-leaf manzanita and tobacco brush; both shrubs are starting to overgrow the trail. Reenter the forest just before a shady flat and, near an ephemeral stream, you may be fortunate to see tiny, ankle-high western prince's pines, evergreen members of the wintergreen family. A nearly level stroll through a mature forest of white firs and Jeffrey, ponderosa, and sugar pines leads to the second crossing of the main park road at 4.7 miles.

When you reach the road, about 0.1 mile southeast of Lost Creek Group Campground, walk about 200 yards southeast along the pavement to the resumption of the Nobles Trail. This last stretch, approximately 1.8 miles long, follows a closed gravelly and/or sandy service road, making it perhaps the least inviting of the three segments. The road climbs just over a mile to a spur road down to Lost Creek, then continues for another 0.75 mile to where the tread is obliterated by the main park road, a point about a quarter mile north of the bridge across Lost Creek.

R Fires are prohibited.

Introduction to the Hat Creek Recreation Area and Thousand Lakes Wilderness

The Hat Creek area is a recreation bonanza with seven campgrounds, four picnic areas, and a bevy of attractions, including Subway Cave, Hat Creek Rim Overlook, Hang Glider Launch, Panorama Vista Point, West Prospect Fire Lookout, and Old Station Visitor Information Center, all managed by the Forest Service. Additional points of interest include the University of California Hat Creek Radio Observatory and Crystal Lake State Fish Hatchery. For hikers, the area boasts a couple of nature trails, a 4-mile trail along refreshing Hat Creek, and a stretch of the famed Pacific Crest Trail.

The self-guided Spattercone Nature Trail is conveniently located across from the Hat Creek Campground entrance. The 1.6-mile loop, a big hit with children who like to scamper around spattercones—volcanoes that form when expanding gases tear molten lava ejected from a vent into irregular globs that fall back to earth. The circuit takes about an hour to complete, although much more time can be spent inspecting the numerous geological wonders en route. Subway Cave, another family-friendly spot, requires a lantern and a warm jacket for the dark and chilly trip through a lava tube.

The Hat Creek Trail, which closely follows a stretch of creek and provides access points for anglers, is the valley's most popular hike, although the trail rarely feels crowded. The Pacific Crest Trail, generally noted as a high-elevation route, is anything but high north of Lassen Volcanic. From Old Station, the PCT climbs to the Hat Creek Rim and then closely follows the edge of the escarpment for the next 20 miles before dropping into the north end of Hat Creek Valley. Barely over 5000 feet in elevation and without water or shade, this section of the famed trail can be unbearable during the

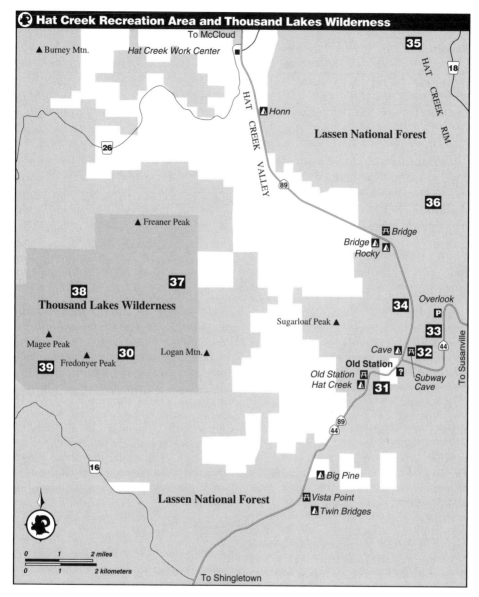

Hat Creek Recreation Area and Thousand Lakes Wilderness

To McCloud

▲ Burney Mtn.   Hat Creek Work Center   ■

35

18

HAT CREEK RIM

▲ Honn

Lassen National Forest

HAT CREEK VALLEY

26

89

36

▲ Freaner Peak

Bridge

Bridge ▲ ▲
Rocky

38   37

Thousand Lakes Wilderness

Overlook

34   P

Sugarloaf Peak ▲

33

44

To Susanville

▲
Magee Peak   30   Logan Mtn. ▲

39   ▲ Fredonyer Peak

Cave ▲   32

Old Station

Old Station   ?   Subway
Hat Creek ▲   31   Cave

89
44

16

Lassen National Forest

▲ Big Pine

Vista Point
▲ Twin Bridges

0   1   2 miles
0   1   2 kilometers

To Shingletown

hot summer—no doubt a miserable stretch for thru-hikers attempting to complete the 2650-mile route in one season. However, the open nature of the topography on the rim affords stunning views in spring, when Lassen Peak, Mt. Shasta, and the high peaks of Thousand Lakes Wilderness are cloaked in winter's mantle. From April through early June, brilliant patches of wildflowers enhance the extraordinary scenery.

Although it is about 900 lakes short of the promise in its name, the 25.5-square-mile Thousand Lakes Wilderness is a fine spot for a dayhike or two- to three-day backpack. The wilderness area has only nine named lakes, three of which are first-rate. Lake Eiler, easily the largest and most popular of these three is usually snow-free by mid-June. However, the other two, Magee and Everett, typically have snow

Campgrounds						
Campground	Fee	Elevation	Season	Restrooms	Running Water	Bear Boxes
Big Pine (4.7 miles SW of 44/89 Jct.)	$12	4600′	Late April to October	Vault	Yes	No
Hat Creek (1.5 miles SW of 44/89 Jct.)	$17	4300′	Late April to October	Flush and vault	Yes	No
Cave (0.3 N of 44/89 Jct.)	$17	4300′	Open all year	Vault	Yes	No
Rocky (3.4 miles N of 44/89 Jct.)	$11	4000′	Late April to October	Vault	No	No
Bridge (4.1 miles N of 44/89 Jct.)	$11	4000′	Late April to October	Vault	Yes	No
Honn (9.2 miles N of 44/89 Jct.)	$11	3400′	Late April to October	Vault	No	No

until early to mid-July. Of the remaining named lakes, Barrett and Durbin are waist-deep, or shallower, and become semi-stagnant by late season. The same is true of hidden Box Lake, encircled by, but unseen from, the circuit of trails beyond its shore. Upper Twin Lake barely wets the knees, although Lower Twin Lake, an easy off-trail jaunt southeast, is a great swimming hole. Hufford Lake and the small lake above it would be fine destinations if only a trail to them existed; the cross-country route is both brushy and steep.

The two dozen ponds scattered across Thousand Lakes Valley produce hordes of mosquitoes through the better part of July—perhaps the magnitude of these hordes was what led early visitors to assume there must be at least a thousand lakes nearby. By August, the mosquitoes diminish in number and the lakes enter their prime. However, with few first-rate lakes, the area can feel a bit crowded even with only two dozen groups. Fortunately, the wilderness is not near any population center, which helps keep the numbers of visitors to a manageable level.

Unlike the slightly larger Caribou Wilderness to the southeast, Thousand Lakes Wilderness is mountainous, with more diverse and photogenic scenery. Ringed by a horseshoe of peaks that includes Red Cliff, Fredonyer Peak, Gray Cliff, Magee Peak,

and Crater Peak, the scenery around Magee and Everett lakes is spectacular. A climb to the top of 8549-foot Magee Peak offers one of the best vistas in the greater Lassen area and is reason enough for a visit to the wilderness.

The wilderness is accessible via four trailheads: Cypress, near the north boundary; Tamarack, near the east boundary; Bunchgrass, near the south boundary; and Magee, near the southwest boundary. Currently, well-groomed dirt roads lead to all four trailheads, but the Forest Service has decided not to maintain the Magee Trail, which may eventually put the condition of the road to the Magee Trailhead in jeopardy.

Access

State Highway 44/89 heads east from the Lassen Volcanic vicinity to a junction near the tiny community of Old Station. From this junction, Highway 89 heads north through Hat Creek Valley, and Highway 44 continues east toward Susanville. Forest Service roads connect these two highways to trailheads.

Amenities

Eastbound from the 44/89 junction, near the northwest entrance to Lassen Volcanic, you may find an open store or cafe on the way to Old Station. Old Station itself features a gas station/convenience store, laundry and showers, small cafe, Old Station Visitor Center, Hat Creek Resort, and Rim Rock Ranch Resort. The Rancheria RV Park, with a small store and cafe, is on Highway 89, 10 miles north of the Highway 44 junction.

Ranger Stations and Visitor Information

The Old Station Visitor Center offers information, books, maps, and gifts.

Good to Know Before You Go

After the opening of fishing season, sometime during April, the campgrounds in Hat Creek Valley start to get busy on weekends. Prior to that, during warm periods of early spring, all-year Subway Campground may provide a secluded basecamp from which to enjoy some early-season hiking opportunities.

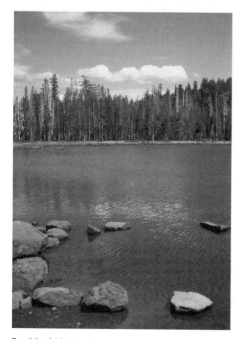

Durbin Lake

BUNCHGRASS TRAILHEAD

Trip **30**

Durbin and Barrett Lakes

M ✓ DH, BP

DISTANCE:	9.5 miles out and back
ELEVATIONS:	5860/6675/6435, +1075/-1075
SEASON:	Mid-June to late October
USE:	Light
MAP:	*Thousand Lakes Valley*

INTRODUCTION: The lightly used Bunchgrass Trail heads into the heart of Thousand Lakes Wilderness, offering hikers plenty of solitude and serenity on the way to a pair of shallow, forest-rimmed lakes. Mosquitoes are usually a nuisance until the porous volcanic soils have sucked up most of the wilderness area's surface water, usually by midsummer. From then on, the seasonal creeks run dry, with water available only at the lakes.

DIRECTIONS TO TRAILHEAD: From Highway 44/89, take National Forest Road 16, 4 miles northeast of the Crossroads Junction near Manzanita Lake and 9.4 miles southwest of the junction near Old Station. Watch for signs for the Ashpan Snowmobile Park, which has a large parking lot and restrooms near the start of the road. After 6.4 miles, turn right (northeast) onto National Forest Road 32N45, and proceed 2.1 miles to the Bunchgrass Trailhead.

DESCRIPTION: Walk northeast from the trailhead. For the first couple of miles, the moderately climbing trail stays within forest cover, following a gully separating the ancient, extinct Thousand Lakes volcano on the left from the far more recent lava flows on the right. These heavily vegetated flows hide from view Devils Rock Garden, a sparsely covered, andesite flow originating just south of Tumble Buttes. Leave the forest and proceed another mile through

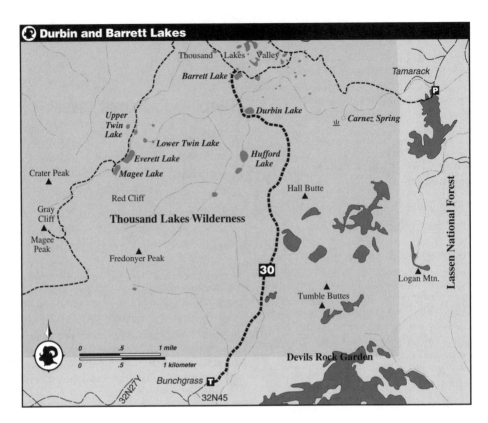

shrub-covered terrain on a climb toward Hall Butte, a cinder cone that may have erupted as recently as 500 years ago.

Forest shade returns for good as the trail veers away from Hall Butte. Soon cross an ill-defined saddle and enter a lush forest of lodgepole pines, red firs, and western white pines—the trademark forest of Thousand Lakes Wilderness. Beyond the saddle, the trail drops slightly into a flat, hanging valley, where a pleasant, half-mile traverse gives way to a brief climb to a low saddle near the entrance to Thousand Lakes Valley. A moderate, half-mile descent leads to the south shore of shallow Durbin Lake. Limited campsites are scattered around the northwest lakeshore and down a short use trail that heads west from the lake.

If Durbin Lake appears too shallow, you'll probably be disappointed with Barrett Lake, 0.5 mile north, which is also about waist deep. From early to midsummer, marauding bands of mosquitoes wait in ambush along the lodgepole pine flat between the two lakes. If you can tolerate the bloodsuckers, this is one of the better places for viewing wildflowers in the wilderness. Fair campsites can be found near the trail junction above the north shore of Barrett Lake.

With a number of connecting trails, there are many options for further wanderings in the wilderness to additional lakes and perhaps a climb of Magee Peak.

HAT CREEK TRAILHEADS

Trip **31**

Spattercone Nature Trail

E ↻ **DH**

DISTANCE: 1.6 miles loop

ELEVATIONS: 4470/4685, +215/-215

SEASON: April to mid-November

USE: Light

MAP: *Old Station*

INTRODUCTION: With just enough explosive gas to prevent a flow, but not enough to bust it into small pieces, erupting lava is ripped apart by expanding gases into hot, fluid clots called splatter. When the splatter falls back to earth, the clots merge, cool, and solidify into steep-sided humps, or spattercones. Geologists speculate that 20,000 to 30,000 years ago, volcanic lava flowed from fissures in the earth's crust and spilled across Hat Creek Valley for a distance of 16 miles.

Today, visitors can explore firsthand some of the spattercones near the locations of these fissures on the 1.6-mile Spattercone Nature Trail. The Forest Service's natural history brochure (available either by download from the Lassen National Forest website, or in person from a box at the trailhead or at the Old Station Visitor Information Station) has information linked to numbered posts on the trail. Additional geologic features along the loop include lava tubes, lava mounds, and views of cinder cones and the plug dome volcano of Lassen Peak.

The trail takes about an hour to complete, although much more time can be spent exploring all the geologic wonders. Most of the route is open and exposed, so be prepared for hot summertime temperatures and carry water, as none is available along the route. Tennis shoes are fine for those who plan to stick to the trail, but sturdy boots are recommended for those who wish to clamber over the rough volcanic rock. Children in particular love to explore the spattercones, but the loose rock means accidents are possible—parental supervision is a must. Please refrain from collecting samples or defacing the rock in any way.

DIRECTIONS TO TRAILHEAD: Take Highway 44/89 to the Hat Creek Campground, 1.5 miles southwest of the junction near Old Station. The nature trail parking area is on the opposite (east) side of the road.

DESCRIPTION: Head south on the short, easy trail through ponderosa pines that leads to

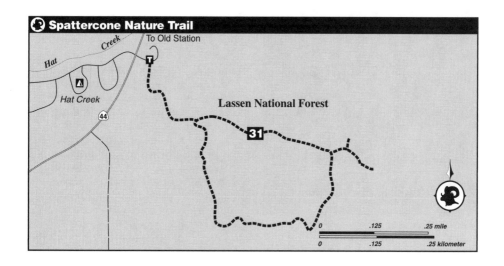

Spattercone Nature Trail

an equally short climb to open slopes carpeted with sagebrush, bitterbrush, squaw carpet, and greenleaf manzanita. Cross the unmarked Pacific Crest Trail and continue a short distance to the loop junction. Turn left to follow the brochure's recommended clockwise loop and climb past collapsed lava tubes to the first of the spattercones near post 12; nearby, short laterals split away from the loop to additional spattercones. Good views from the upper part of the loop include such notable features as Lassen Peak, Chaos Crags, Badger Mountain, and West Prospect Peak. Eventually, the trail heads downhill for the return portion of this clockwise journey back to the loop junction. From there, head west to retrace your steps 0.2 mile to the trailhead.

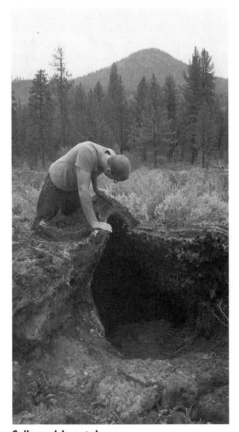

Collapsed lava tube

HAT CREEK TRAILHEADS

Trip **32**

Subway Cave

E ↺ DH

DISTANCE:	0.6 mile loop
ELEVATIONS:	4350, Negligible
SEASON:	Late May through October
USE:	Moderate
MAP:	*Old Station*

INTRODUCTION: The most popular trail in Hat Creek Valley may be the cool, self-guided walk through Subway Cave. The actual cave extends for about 2300 feet, but only 1300 feet are open to the public; the northern half is closed for safety concerns. In the open section, the ceiling ranges from about 6 to 16 feet in height, but it's lower near the sides—watch your head! The thickness of the cave's roof varies from 8 to 24 feet, obviously thinner at the entrance and exit where the roof collapsed. Bring a sweater or jacket, as the temperature inside the cave is generally around 46°F. A lantern is also essential, although a headlamp or flashlight (with extra batteries) will do in a pinch.

SUBWAY CAVE

A series of basalt lava flows emerged from fissures in the earth near the present site of Old Station and crept northward, covering the floor of Hat Creek Valley. Geologists theorize that the lava near the surface cooled and hardened while rivers of molten lava continued to flow beneath the surface. Eventually, these lava rivers drained away, leaving behind the lava tubes visible today. Subway Cave is the largest of these lava tubes. Partial collapses of the cave's roof created the present-day entrance and exit to the cave.

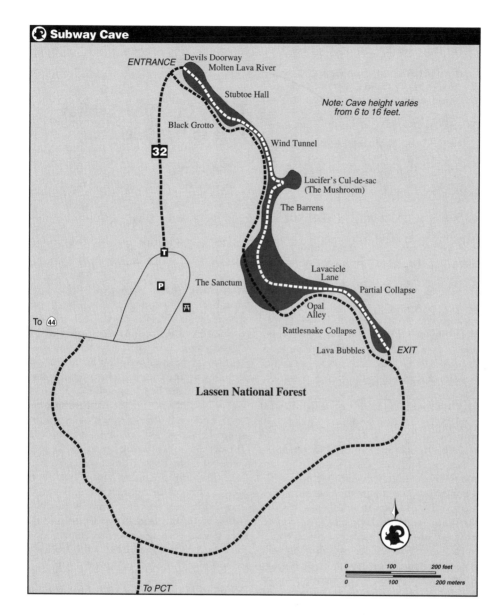

Subway Cave

ENTRANCE
Devils Doorway
Molten Lava River
Stubtoe Hall

Note: Cave height varies from 6 to 16 feet.

Black Grotto

32

Wind Tunnel

Lucifer's Cul-de-sac
(The Mushroom)

The Barrens

The Sanctum

Lavacicle
Lane
Partial Collapse

Opal
Alley

Rattlesnake Collapse

To (44)

Lava Bubbles

EXIT

Lassen National Forest

To PCT

| 0 | 100 | 200 feet |
| 0 | 100 | 200 meters |

DIRECTIONS TO TRAILHEAD: Take Highway 89 to the Subway Cave parking lot, 0.3 mile north of the Highway 44 junction near Old Station. The parking area is opposite the entrance to Cave Campground.

DECRIPTION: The cave entrance is just beyond a set of stairs in the north part of the parking loop. Descend another set of stairs to the floor of the cave, allowing time for your eyes to adjust to the dim light. About half of the traverse through Subway Cave will be in total darkness, so make sure your light source is fully operational. The first part of the cave is appropriately called Stubtoe Hall, perhaps due to visitors not expecting such a rough, uneven floor. Interpretive signs guide you past additional features, such as Black Grotto, Wind Tunnel, Lucifer's Cul-de-sac, the Barrens,

FALLOUT SHELTER

In early 1962, during the Cold War, Shasta County's Civil Defense Office considered using Subway Cave, and several smaller caves, as emergency fallout shelters. During the Cuban Missile Crisis (October 22–28, 1962), with nuclear war an imminent possibility, the shelters were almost put to use.

Trip **33**

Pacific Crest Trail: Subway Cave to Hat Creek Rim

Ⓜ / DH

DISTANCE: 3 miles point to point

ELEVATIONS: 4350/4875, +570/-40

SEASON: Late March to December

USE: Light

MAP: *Old Station*

the Sanctum, Opal Alley, Lavacicle Lane, and Rodent Rocks. Near the far end of the cave, head toward the increasing light and climb up the stairs through Rattlesnake Collapse.

Emerging from Subway Cave, you can take either a short trail winding northwest back to the entrance, or follow a longer, more obvious path on a clockwise route back to the south end of the parking loop. Along the latter trail are views to the east of Hat Creek Rim and to the west of Sugarloaf Peak. In a small flat, where this path turns from southwest to northwest, a lightly used connector trail heads south to a junction with the Pacific Crest Trail.

Vegetation in the Subway Cave environs is largely composed of a sagebrush plant community, although, given enough time, a ponderosa pine forest may spread across the breadth of Hat Creek Valley—provided there are no more lava flows, of course. Along with the ponderosa pines, other forest associates include western junipers, gray pine, and curleaf mountain mahogany. Along with varieties of sagebrush, common trailside shrubs include bitterbrush, squaw carpet, greenleaf manzanita, rabbitbrush, squaw currant, and Wood's rose. Lavender-flowered sagebrush mariposa tulips may delight passersby in May and early June, while yellow-flowered blazing stars may have a similar effect on trail users in August and September, although neither plant is all that common.

INTRODUCTION: Except for dedicated thru-hikers attempting to walk every step of the 2650-mile Pacific Crest Trail, very few hikers walk this 3-mile section of the famed route. Low elevations and intermittent shade mean this trip can be uncomfortably hot in the summer. However, a spring trip—when the high country is still buried under winter's mantle, the temperatures are mild, and wildflowers are in bloom—can be quite delightful. The scenery is superb, from the depths of Hat Creek Valley to the lofty aerie of Hat Creek Rim Overlook, with several volcanic summits visible from both near and far. Although the overlook can be reached by car, the view is more satisfying when you climb from the valley to the rim. Those who wish to avoid that climb should reverse the description and hike from the Mud Lake Trailhead to Subway Cave.

DIRECTIONS TO TRAILHEAD: START: Head north for 0.3 mile on Highway 89 from the junction with Highway 44 to the turnoff for Subway Cave, and proceed a short distance to the parking area.

END: Follow Highway 44 to the turnoff for the Hat Creek Rim Overlook, 3 miles east of the junction with Highway 89. Instead of following the road to the overlook, make an immediate right turn onto Plum Valley Road, following a sign marked PCT

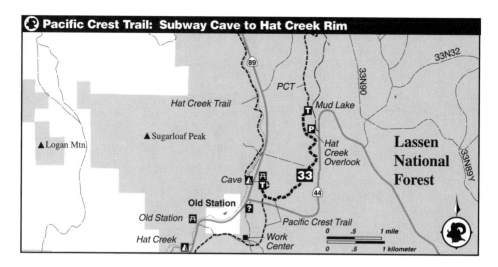

Pacific Crest Trail: Subway Cave to Hat Creek Rim

TRAILHEAD 1/2. Proceed north for 0.4 mile and turn left onto a lesser road that soon leads to the Mud Lake Trailhead, complete with pit toilet, equestrian facilities, and campsites with picnic tables and fire pits.

DESCRIPTION: The hardest part of this trip may be locating the beginning of the trail, as the path is unmarked and starts out very faint before more discernible tread is reached. Just before the parking loop, leave the access road to Subway Cave and head south across the pine-needle-covered floor of an open ponderosa-Jeffrey pine forest. With luck, you'll soon see a more defined path that cuts through the shrubs, primarily sagebrush and manzanita. The track widens about 0.1 mile from the road at an unmarked junction, where the loop around Subway Cave continues ahead, but the spur trail to the Pacific Crest Trail veers to the right (south). After a short, gentle walk, you reach the PCT, marked simply by crude writing on a post that reads: WATER, SUBWAY CAVE.

Turn left and follow the PCT along the gentle course of an old road through scattered pines, junipers, and mountain mahoganies across Devils Half Acre, a part of Hat Creek Valley covered by lava flows and towered over by Hat Creek Rim on the east and several volcanoes to the west—most prominently Sugarloaf Peak.

The PCT merges with the old highway, 1.5 mile from the Subway Cave road, which heads directly northwest to the new highway across from the long-abandoned Sugarloaf Picnic Area. Soon, the trail starts to climb up the face of Hat Creek Rim, following the course of the old highway into a thicker forest of Jeffrey and ponderosa pines, incense cedars, sugar pines, and junipers. The forest becomes more open again and the trail a bit rockier just above the junction of an old road on the right. The moderate to moderately steep climb continues across the face of the rim, within sound of the intermittent traffic on Highway 44 above. Just after the 2-mile mark, you reach an unmarked Y-junction and proceed on the left-hand road, climbing another 0.1 mile to a point where a path on the right traverses over to the shoulder of the highway at the shortest point between the PCT and Highway 44. From this path, the route of the PCT veers away from the highway and climbs to the edge of Hat Creek Rim.

Beyond a gate in a wire fence, the grade of the PCT eases to a mild climb along the edge of Hat Creek Rim through mixed forest with filtered views across Hat Creek Valley, preludes to the incredible vista at the Hat Creek Overlook. Soon, gently graded trail merges with the edge of the concrete path to the overlook, where a short stroll leads to the semicircular vista point. The 👁

magnificent view extends across the expanse of Hat Creek Valley, from the snow-capped Lassen Peak and the Chaos Crags in the south to the dominant profile of Mt. Shasta in the north. On very clear days, Oregon's Mt. McLoughlin and the Crater Lake rim may be visible to the distant right of Shasta. In between, a host of lower summits are visible, including Badger Mountain and West Prospect Peak in the south; Sugarloaf Peak, Magee Peak, and Freaner Peak in the west; and Burney Mountain in the northwest. Although the overlook is nicely equipped with modern vault toilets, picnic benches, and trash receptacles, water is not available, unless you can coax a bottle from a visiting motorist.

Find the resumption of the PCT on the far side of the parking area and follow mildly descending trail a quarter mile north and then west to the Mud Lake Trailhead, a much more rustic spot than the overlook, with wood picnic tables, barbecues, an antiquated outhouse, and a horse tie-bar.

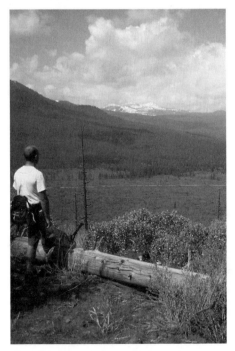

View from the Pacific Crest Trail, Hat Creek Rim

Trip **34**

Hat Creek Trail

E / DH

DISTANCE:	4 miles point to point
ELEVATIONS:	3875/4325, +450
SEASON:	March to mid-November
USE:	Light
MAP:	*Old Station*

INTRODUCTION: From its frosty origin in Lassen National Park, sparkling Hat Creek tumbles through broad Hat Creek Valley before merging with the Pit River just above Lake Britton. The stream is well-known for its good fishing and chilly temperatures; anglers use the Hat Creek Trail throughout the season to access their favorite fishing holes, while swimmers tend to venture into their preferred spots only during the oppressing summer heat. The 4-mile path described here is the only stretch of trail outside Lassen Volcanic that follows the sprightly stream, connecting three Forest Service campgrounds (Bridge, Rocky, and Cave). The trail remains within a stone's throw of Hat Creek for the duration of the hike, but access to the stream is not always guaranteed, thanks to brushy spots and steep-walled mini-gorges. Mixed forest shades the trail in spots, but a good portion of the trail is subject to open sun—midsummer visitors should plan on hiking during the early morning or early evening hours to beat the heat. The low elevation makes hiking the Hat Creek Trail a marvelous spring or fall experience.

DIRECTIONS TO TRAILHEAD: START: Follow Highway 89 to Bridge Campground, 4 miles north of the Highway 44 junction near Old Station and 17.7 miles south of the Highway 299 junction northeast of Burney. Park in the small day-use area on the east side of the road.

END: Take Highway 89 to Cave Campground, 0.3 mile north of the Highway 44 junction. The trailhead is located on the west side of the campground.

DESCRIPTION: Find the marked beginning of the Hat Creek Trail on the east edge of the campground and head south along the brink of the rushing creek's deep gorge through shady, verdant forest. Among the water-loving trees and shrubs, keen eyes may spy two large species of lily blooming during the month of June: The leopard lily, adorned with brilliant orange blossoms, may grow to head height, while the Washington lily has enormous (at least by wildflower standards) 3- to 4-inch white flowers. After 0.6 mile, reach a bridge providing access to Rocky Campground, perched on a narrow shelf above the far bank.

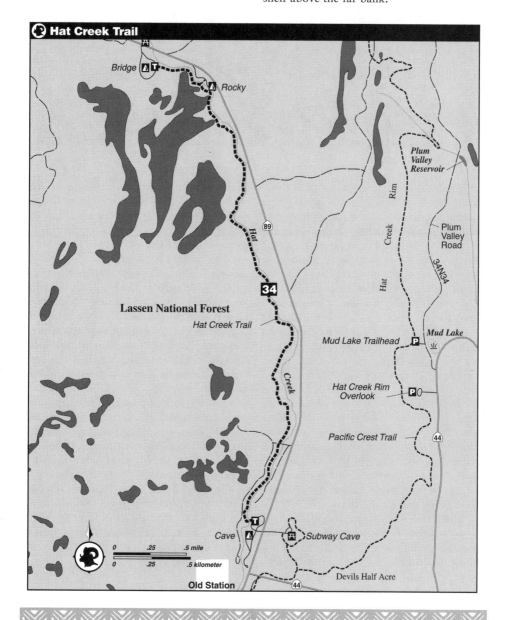

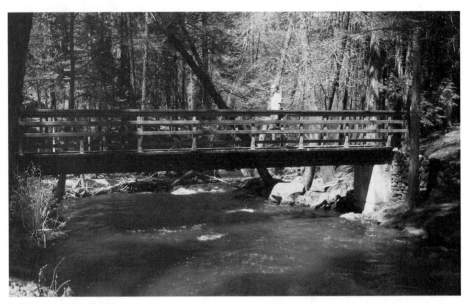

Bridge over Hat Creek

Continue south through a forested section of the Hat Creek gorge, which is prime habitat for the dipper, a small, chunky gray bird that feeds on insect larvae along the bottom of swift streams. Soon leave the shady forest behind and walk through an open section of the manzanita-covered Hat Creek Valley basalt flow, where shade is at a premium. The flow apparently originated from fissures near a series of spattercones close to the present-day site of the Hat Creek Campground. Although blisteringly hot in summer, the mostly open terrain provides fair views of Hat Creek Rim to the east and peaks within Thousand Lakes Wilderness to the west. Near the 1.5-mile mark, where the creek slows and widens for a spell, scattered conifers provide some welcome shade for a crude campsite that occupies a small neck of land near water's edge. Moist varieties of plants in this grotto include miner's lettuce, false Solomon's seal, snow plant, and thimbleberry.

Leave the forested oasis and make an open traverse through more manzanita-covered terrain for nearly a mile to the site of a destroyed footbridge that used to span

Hat Creek, formerly providing anglers easy access to the Hat Creek Trail via a 0.1-mile path from Highway 89. All that remains of the bridge today are two concrete abutments on either side of the creek.

From the site of the old footbridge, continue hiking through shadeless manzanita, broken only by the occasional juniper tree. After nearly a mile, reach a Y-junction with a path on the right that heads toward the site of the abandoned Sugarloaf Picnic Grounds. Veer left at the junction, soon passing a wild cataract, where the waters of Hat Creek are forced through a narrow gorge of volcanic rock.

Shortly past the watery grandeur, the trail crosses the access road for the old picnic grounds near a road bridge over the creek and continues upstream along the west bank. Ponderosa pines, white firs, and incense cedars bathe the path in welcome shade beyond the road crossing, as you pass primitive campsites on the right and a stream gauge on the left. Near the campground, cross a dirt road and then follow a footbridge over Hat Creek to the trailhead in Cave Campground.

FOREST ROAD 22 TRAILHEAD

Trip **35**

Pacific Crest Trail to Hat Creek Rim Lookout

M ✓ DH

DISTANCE: 5.8 miles out and back

ELEVATIONS: 4665/5125, +460/-460

SEASON: April to late November

USE: Light

MAP: *Murken Bench*

INTRODUCTION: Although a few staffed fire lookouts still operate in the southern Cascades, most notably the one atop Mt. Harkness (see Trip 56), most lookouts have gone out of service. A 1987 forest fire destroyed the lookout on the edge of Hat Creek Rim, but the view from the rim itself is still spectacular, accessible via a 3-mile section of the Pacific Crest Trail. Water is nonexistent and shade is almost as scarce, so carry water and hike during cooler hours. The hike is best done in the spring, when wildflowers are in bloom and the temperatures are well below their midsummer zenith.

DIRECTIONS TO TRAILHEAD: From Highway 89 across from the Hat Creek Work Center, 11.1 miles north of the Highway 44 junction, turn east on Doty Road Loop (County Road 6R200) and proceed 1.4 miles to a junction with Bidwell Road (County Road 6R201). Head east on Bidwell Road, past the University of California's Hat Creek Radio Observatory, to a T-intersection at 3.7 miles, where Forest Road 22 goes left. From the junction, follow graded, dirt-and-gravel Road 22 on a switchbacking climb up the faulted escarpment of Murken Bench. Remain on Road 22 at all junc-

tions until reaching the Pacific Crest Trail crossing at 7.5 miles from Highway 89. Park along the shoulder as space allows. Although it's marked by posts on either side of the road, the trail is easily missed from a passing car—if you reach a junction with Forest Road 34N18, go back 0.1 mile.

DESCRIPTION: A brief climb from the road on the southbound PCT takes you to a junction with a short use trail on the right that leads over to a crude shelter with a shady bench built among a grove of trees. In past years, plastic jugs of water have been cached here for PCT thru-hikers. The ascent continues for a short while until the trail meets the lip of Hat Creek Rim and the grade eases. Pass below a set of power lines and continue along the edge of the rim, where shrubby and rocky slopes provide sweeping views across Hat Creek Valley, from Lassen Peak in the south to Mt. Shasta in the north.

A mile or so from the road, the trail moves away from the rim and starts to climb moderately up a conifer-covered slope. Beyond a gate in a barbwire fence, the ascent continues amid a diminishing forest until all but a few widely scattered Jeffrey pines and junipers remain. Eventually, the trail returns to the edge of the rim, and a milder, half-mile ascent leads to the old lookout site. After a fire destroyed the lookout in 1987, a microwave repeater station replaced the wood structure in 1992. Although it's no longer possible to ascend the lookout steps, the view from the base is still stunning. Mt. Shasta is the preeminent peak to the north, flanked on the left by mountains of the Trinity Alps and on the right by Oregon's Mt. McLoughlin and the Crater Lake rim, while Lassen Peak and the Chaos Crags draw most of the attention in the south. In between are several volcanic summits, including Burney Mountain, Freaner Peak, Magee Peak, Logan Mountain, Sugarloaf Peak, Raker Peak, Badger Mountain, and West Prospect Peak.

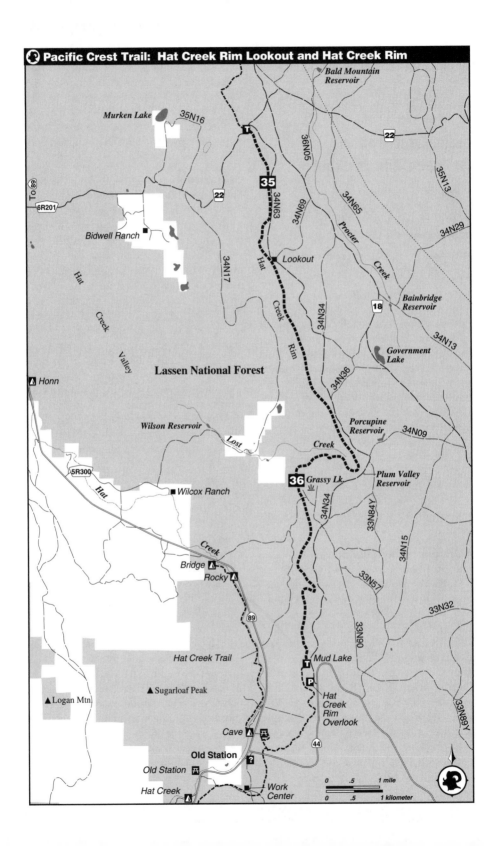

Bald Mountain
Reservoir

Murken Lake

35N16

22

36N05

35N13

To 89

6R201

22

35

34N63

34N69

34N65

Procter

34N29

Bidwell Ranch

34N17

Hat

Lookout

Creek

Bainbridge
Reservoir

18

34N34

34N13

Creek

Government
Lake

Hat

Lassen National Forest

Rim

34N36

Creek

Valley

Honn

Wilson Reservoir

Lost

Creek

Porcupine
Reservoir

34N09

Plum Valley
Reservoir

5R300

36

Grassy Lk

Hat

Wilcox Ranch

34N34

33N84Y

34N15

Creek

Bridge

Rocky

33N57

33N32

89

33N90

Hat Creek Trail

Mud Lake

Logan Mtn

Sugarloaf Peak

Hat
Creek
Rim
Overlook

33N89Y

Cave

44

Old Station

Old Station

Hat Creek

Work
Center

0   .5   1 mile

0   .5   1 kilometer

MUD LAKE TRAILHEAD

Trip **36**

Pacific Crest Trail: Hat Creek Rim

Ⓜ ╱ DH

DISTANCE: 13.5 miles point to point

ELEVATIONS: 4875/5130/4655, 675/-900

SEASON: April to mid-November

USE: Light

MAPS: *Old Station, Murken Bench*

INTRODUCTION: Pacific Crest Trail thru-hikers, who usually arrive in northern California during the height of summertime heat, have probably uttered more than one curse at sections of the famed 2650-mile trail that travel through lowland areas around Hat Creek Rim. There is very little shade here, and with relatively low elevations (4600 to 5100 feet) and little access to water, their hike through here in July and August can be brutal. However, dayhikers not tied to such a strict schedule will find this route a fine trip during other seasons, particularly in spring, when water courses through seasonal swales, an assortment of wildflowers line the path, and snow-capped peaks glisten in the abundant sunshine. No matter what the season, the mostly open terrain provides rewarding, wide-ranging views that span Hat Creek Valley, from Lassen Peak in the south to Mt. Shasta in the north.

DIRECTIONS TO TRAILHEAD: START: Follow Highway 44 to the turnoff for the Hat Creek Rim Overlook, 3 miles east of the Highway 89 junction. Instead of following the road to the overlook, make an immediate right onto Plum Valley Road, following a sign marked PCT TRAILHEAD 1/2. Proceed north for 0.4 mile and turn left onto a lesser road that soon leads to the

Mud Lake Trailhead, complete with pit toilet, equestrian facilities, and campsites with picnic tables and fire pits.

END: From Highway 89, across from the Hat Creek Work Center and 11.1 miles north of the Highway 44 junction, turn east onto Doty Road Loop (County Road 6R200) and proceed 1.4 miles to a junction with Bidwell Road (County Road 6R201). Head east on Bidwell Road past the University of California's Hat Creek Radio Observatory to a T-intersection at 3.7 miles, where Forest Road 22 goes left. From the junction, follow graded dirt-and-gravel Road 22 on a switchbacking climb up the faulted escarpment of Murken Bench. Remain on Road 22 at all junctions until the crossing of the Pacific Crest Trail at 7.5 miles from Highway 89. Park along the shoulder as space allows. Although marked by two posts, the trail is easily missed from a passing car—if you reach a junction with Forest Road 34N18, go back 0.1 mile.

DESCRIPTION: Head north from the trailhead on lightly used tread through a mixed forest of Jeffrey pines and incense cedars, with a dry understory that includes squaw carpet, bitterbrush, manzanita, and sagebrush. The month of May is the time to see a surprisingly vibrant collection of blooming wildflowers lining the path, including shooting stars and lupines. After a quarter mile, the trail merges with an old dirt road and briefly follows it to the resumption of single-track trail—pay close attention here, as the trail is not particularly well marked. A pleasantly graded, forested stroll leads to the edge of Hat Creek Rim, where views open up across Hat Creek Valley of Lassen Peak to the south, Sugarloaf Peak to the southwest, the peaks of Thousand Lakes Wilderness to the west, Burney Mountain to the northwest, and Mt. Shasta in the distant north-northwest. As you continue across the mostly open terrain with sweeping views, a few junipers join the widely scattered pines and cedars. Pass through an opening in a dilapidated barbed-wire fence and then follow the trail across an area burned in 1987 into a side drainage. Hop across a seasonal creek that drains Plum Valley Reservoir, 1.8 miles from the trailhead.

Climb out of the drainage and proceed across the extensive burn, where young conifers have yet to exceed head height. About 0.5 mile from the creek, the trail regains the edge of the escarpment for a short spell before veering into a gully and crossing another seasonal stream. Beyond the gully, the trail continues a northbound course across open terrain carpeted with dry vegetation. After crossing a fire road, the trail climbs moderately, still through burned snags, to the top of the higher rim, the result of uplift along a north-south fault. A half-mile winding traverse on the upper rim passes near a shallow depression to the east that is lined with the first mature conifers to be seen in the last couple of miles. Following wet winters, the depression is filled by shallow Grassy Lake. In previous years, the lake has been used as a watering hole for range cattle; beware of drinking this water. A stock trail used to connect Grassy Lake to Hat Creek Valley below, but scarcely a trace exists nowadays.

Beyond the vicinity of Grassy Lake, the trail continues along the rim for another half mile to the edge of the deep cleft of Lost Creek canyon, which has an audible, vigorous, spring-fed stream flowing down the lower part of the gorge. During spring, this flow may be augmented by upstream water from Porcupine Reservoir, Cone Reservoir, and Twin Ponds. The impressive view from the lip of the canyon is marred slightly by the scorching damage of the 1987 fire, but, fortunately, some of the more mature conifers were spared. The trail turns sharply east and follows the lip of Lost Creek canyon for nearly 1.5 miles to the crossing of its seasonal creek at a point where the canyon floor has steeply risen to be nothing more than a low depression at the lip of Hat Creek Rim. Just before this crossing, a stand of mature forest heralds the limit of the fire's devastation. Almost simultaneously, you pass through a gate in a barbed-wire fence, followed by a short climb up to the

boulder hop of Lost Creek, 6.25 miles from the trailhead.

Head northwest, away from Lost Creek, on rising tread, and soon reach a cyclone fence gate. An old, twin-track road follows the fence line northeast for 0.2 mile to intersect Forest Road 34N34 (which desperately thirsty hikers could take east-southeast to a junction of Forest Road 34N09 and then northeast to Porcupine Reservoir). Steadily ascending tread leads along the lip of another fault-formed rim, providing sweeping views across Hat Creek Valley of mountains near and far. The route roughly parallels ◉ Road 34N34, nearly reaching the gravel road at one point. At 7.5 miles, the trail crosses Road 34N94 (a spur road heading northwest 0.4 mile to Road 34N34A that doubles back to usually dry Little Lake). The steady ascent continues almost uninterrupted for the next couple of miles until trail tops out at around 5130 feet.

From there, drop into a saddle and then make a short climb to the site of the Hat Creek Rim Fire Lookout, 10.5 miles from the trailhead. In 1992, a microwave repeater station replaced the wood lookout that was destroyed in the 1987 fire. Although sweeping views have been available for most of the journey along the Hat Creek Rim, one can only wonder what the view might have been like from the higher vantage of the lookout. Mt. Shasta is the preeminent peak to the north, flanked ◉ on the left by mountains of the Trinity Alps and on the distant right by Oregon's Mt. McLoughlin and the Crater Lake rim, while Lassen Peak and the Chaos Crags draw most of the attention in the south. In between are several volcanic summits, including Burney Mountain, Freaner Peak, Magee Peak, Logan Mountain, Sugarloaf Peak, Raker Peak, Badger Mountain, and West Prospect Peak.

For nearly the next 3 miles, the trail plunges downhill, losing almost 500 feet of elevation in the process. Fortunately, the path stays close to the rim, offering almost continuous views. As has been the case for most of your journey, water and shade are both lacking along this arid stretch. The

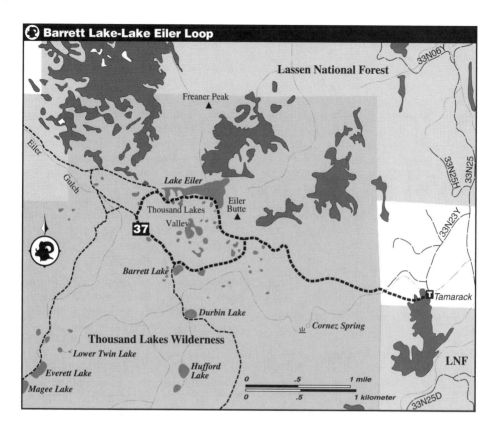

Barrett Lake-Lake Eiler Loop

Lassen National Forest

Freaner Peak ▲

Eiler Gulch

Lake Eiler

Thousand Lakes Valley

Eiler Butte ▲

37

Barrett Lake

Durbin Lake

Cornez Spring

Thousand Lakes Wilderness

Lower Twin Lake

Everett Lake

Hufford Lake

Magee Lake

Tamarack

LNF

33N06Y

33N25H

33N25

33N23Y

33N25D

0   .5   1 mile
0   .5   1 kilometer

descent bottoms out about a mile before reaching Forest Road 22.

[O] Rather than complete the route as described, an out-and-back option is possible by turning around at any convenient point along the way. Be sure to pack along extra water and plenty of sunscreen.

TAMARACK TRAILHEAD

Trip **37**

Barrett Lake-Lake Eiler Loop

E 𝒫 DH, BP

DISTANCE: 7 miles semiloop

ELEVATIONS: 5880/6540/5880, +750/-750

SEASON: Mid-June to November

USE: Moderate

MAP: *Thousand Lakes Valley*

INTRODUCTION: This relatively easy semi-loop visits the most popular water destination in Thousand Lakes Wilderness, Lake Eiler, along with small and shallow Barrett Lake, and a host of even smaller and shallower ponds. Reaching the loop portion necessitates a nearly 2-mile approach that gains almost all of the little elevation that the whole route demands. Other than the open crossing of a lava flow early into the approach, the entire trip passes through a light forest of Jeffrey, lodgepole, and western white pines, and red and white firs. Visitors will find picturesque Lake Eiler, back-dropped by volcanic Freaner Peak, to offer the best campsites and scenery, but also the greatest chance of encountering company. Lake Eiler is deep enough and large enough to offer decent swimming and fishing. Barrett Lake, although not nearly as large or scenic, would be a better choice for quieter camping. For even more solitude opportunities, Box Lake in the interior of the loop may easily be reached cross-country from any point along the trail, along with several of the other smaller "thousand lakes."

DIRECTIONS TO TRAILHEAD: Leave Highway 89 about 0.1 mile north of Wilcox Road (7.9 miles north of the Highway 44 junction and 13.8 miles south of the Highway 299 junction) and head west on Forest Road 33N25, signed THOUSAND

9. The well-signed road climbs steeply and bends sharply a couple of times on the way to an X-intersection, 2.8 miles from Highway 89. Head diagonally northwest across the intersection and continue climbing on the upper road ahead. The grade eases for a while near the 5-mile mark, but drivers should stay alert at some washouts around 6.3 miles. The climb eventually resumes and leads to a pair of signed intersections, at 7.6 and 8.2 miles, where the route continues ahead. Bend right at another intersection at 8.4 miles and then wind through an extensive lava flow to the large trailhead parking area (at 9.2 miles), which is equipped with a modern vault toilet and trailhead signboard.

DESCRIPTION: Follow nearly level trail west from the parking area through a scattered to light forest of Jeffrey pines, white firs, and a few lodgepole pines to the edge of a substantial lava flow. After crossing the lava flow, resume a forested stroll for a brief spell before a mild to moderate ascent. Eventually, the grade eases near a small patch of willows and other lush vegetation before a very brief descent leads to a junction, 1.9 miles from the trailhead.

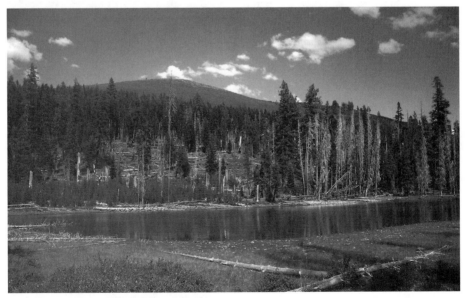

Lake Eiler back-dropped by Freaner Peak
LAKES WILDERNESS, TAMARACK TRAILHEAD

Turn right (west) at the junction on a clockwise, rising traverse across the southwest base of mostly hidden, conical Eiler Butte. Pass a handful of shallow ponds to Lake Eiler, where a use trail heads to campsites along the east shore. Such easy access to the largest and one of the most scenic lakes in the wilderness increases the odds that you'll be sharing the area with others. Successful anglers may be rewarded with foot-long rainbows. Proceed along the south shore of the large lake, with views across the surface of treeless Freaner Peak. Pass shady campsites to the west shore and reach a three-way junction with Trail 3E21, 3.2 miles from the trailhead.

Veer left (west) at the junction and follow gently rising tread past shallow ponds for 0.4 mile to a junction with Trail 3E03, which provides a connection to the Cypress Trailhead.

Turn left to head southeast, and follow gently graded tread on a lightly forested romp through lodgepole pines, western white pines, and white firs. Pass a good-size pond to the right on the way to Barrett Lake. Immediately before the lake, reach a junction with the continuation of Trail 3E03 ahead to the Bunchgrass Trailhead, at 4.25 miles (waist-deep Durbin Lake is 0.6 mile south). Although it is a good-size lake, tree-rimmed Barrett is fairly shallow. The lakeshore offers only a couple of passable campsites and, unless more solitude is the goal, overnighters will be better served by camping at Lake Eiler.

From the junction, head east above the north shore of Barrett Lake, passing to the left of a fair-size pond after 0.3 mile. Continue east-northeast on gently graded trail through light forest until the trail bends north-northeast and makes a mild climb to the junction near Eiler Butte, at the close of the loop section. From there, turn right (east) to retrace your steps 1.9 miles back to the Tamarack Trailhead.

Trip **38**

Upper Twin, Everett, and Magee Lakes, and Magee Peak

(MS) ✎ **DH, BP**

DISTANCE: 16 miles out and back

ELEVATIONS: 5515/7200, +1715/-1715

SEASON: Mid-June to November

USE: Light

MAP: *Thousand Lakes Valley*

INTRODUCTION: Lake Eiler may be the most popular lake destination in Thousand Lakes Wilderness, but Everett and Magee lakes arguably have the best lake scenery. The price to be paid for accessing such extraordinary scenery is a stiff, mostly shadeless, mile-plus climb alongside Eiler Gulch from the trailhead to the lip of Thousand Lakes Valley. After surmounting that obstacle, the remainder of the hike is mostly a mild-to-moderate ascent through mixed forest to Twin Lakes, followed by a short climb to the Everett-Magee lakes basin. A semicircle of features tower over these two subalpine lakes, including Red Cliff, Grey Cliff, Magee Peak, and Crater Peak, providing rugged mountain scenery generally lacking in the remainder of the wilderness. Everett and Magee lakes are both fairly deep, offering decent swimming and fishing, along with plenty of pleasantly shaded campsites for overnighters. A visit to the area would be incomplete without an ascent of nearby Magee Peak for the far-ranging views from a summit that once held a fire lookout. Be aware that patches of snow may still cover the upper part of the trail before mid-July.

DIRECTIONS TO TRAILHEAD: Immediately north of the Hat Creek Work Center, 10.9 miles north of the Highway 44 junction

Upper Twin, Everett and Magee Lakes, and Magee Peak

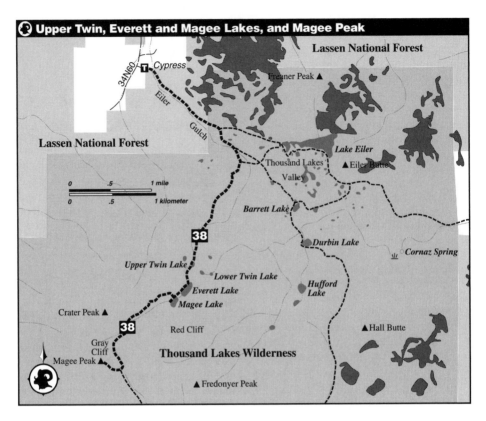

and 10.8 miles south of the Highway 299 junction, leave Highway 89 and follow well-graded Forest Road 26 3.5 miles to a four-way junction. Veer right, following a sign marked CYPRESS TRAILHEAD 7, and proceed to another four-way junction at 5 miles. Turn left, still on Road 26, and continue on the main road, ignoring logging roads that branch away. At 7.9 miles, turn left onto Road 34N60 and proceed for 2.3 miles to a somewhat confusing, unmarked Y-junction, where the correct route to the trailhead veers ahead to the left. At 10.8 miles, reach the large trailhead parking area, furnished with a modern vault toilet and trailhead signboard.

DESCRIPTION: Head southeast down a trail shaded by Jeffrey pines and white firs, and soon come to the crossing of Eiler Gulch, a broad, boulder-filled gully that carries seasonal snowmelt from Thousand Lakes Valley above—except for early in the sea-

son, the crossing should be dry. Following the north bank of Eiler Gulch along the course of an old road, the trail begins an unrelenting, stiff climb toward the lip of the valley through alternating stands of open forest and exposed, shrub-covered terrain, where manzanita, tobacco brush, and chinquapin flourish. An early-morning start is recommended during the hottest parts of the summer, as the steep ascent can be tedious when temperatures are high. Step into Thousand Lakes Wilderness at the 1-mile mark; shortly afterward, the grade mercifully eases as you approach a signed, three-way junction.

Veer right (south-southeast) at the junction, following signed directions for Magee Lake, and head into a deeper forest of white firs, Jeffrey pines, and lodgepole pines. For the most part, the grade is quite pleasant on the way to a junction with Trail 3E03, heading east at 1.75 miles.

Continue ahead (right) on mildly graded trail that soon leads to a crossing of rocky Eiler Gulch. Continue across slopes carpeted with pinemat manzanita to a junction on the left with Trail 3E21, a short connector to Lake Eiler and Trail 3E03 to Barrett Lake. A moderate to moderately steep switchbacking climb heads away from the junction through a forest of red and white firs, and lodgepole and western white pines. Where the trail gains a ridge, the climb abates and the forest becomes scattered, allowing a healthy understory of chinquapin, and pinemat and greenleaf manzanita to flourish. Tree-filtered views of Red Cliff provide hints of the stunning scenery awaiting you. Soon, the trees close in again and the climbing resumes, with mountain hemlocks now in the mixed forest. Step over the channel of a seasonal stream that drains the lakes ahead and continue the ascent into the Twin Lakes basin, 3.5 miles from the trailhead.

Along with the two lakes, Twin Lakes basin also holds a couple of shallow, lake-size ponds. According to the USGS and Forest Service maps, both Upper Twin Lake and Lower Twin Lake lie away from the trail; the body of water just to the left of the trail is simply one of the unnamed ponds. Although either of the twins is only a short, cross-country jaunt away, Everett and Magee lakes, just a short distance farther up the trail, are much more desirable destinations, with deeper waters, more extraordinary scenery, and superior campsites.

A brief climb leads out of the Twin lakes basin and into the basin holding Everett and Magee lakes. The dramatic rock face of Red Cliff offers a stunning backdrop to the green-hued waters of Everett Lake, as the trail passes above the northwest shore. Plenty of decent campsites ring the shoreline. Reach a junction just past the far end of Everett Lake, where the right-hand trail heads toward the summit of Magee Peak. A short walk on the path ahead leads to Magee Lake, near the base of Red Cliff. As with Everett Lake, a mixed forest rims the shoreline and shades several good campsites. Both lakes are fairly deep, offering refreshing swimming and good fishing.

To reach Magee Peak, return to the junction above the northwest shore of Magee Lake and climb moderately to moderately steeply up the hillside through open forest carpeted with pinemat manzanita, with occasional views of the surrounding peaks. Higher up the slope, as you continue the stiff ascent, mountain hemlocks and occasional western white pines diminish in both stature and quantity, improving the views. Tightly winding switchbacks lead across gray, gravelly slopes to the crater rim, where usually snow-capped Lassen Peak appears to the southeast. Soon reach a junction with the unmaintained trail from the Magee Trailhead (see Trip 39) and then continue along the narrow rim toward the summit, as Mt. Shasta pops into view in the northwest.

On a clear day, the expansive vista from the old lookout site stretches for hundreds of miles in virtually every direction—make sure to pack along a big enough map to help identify some of the surrounding landmarks. Closer at hand, the Thousand Lakes Wilderness spreads out around you, including Crater Peak, which, being 127 feet higher, obscures Burney Mountain, a young volcano 8 miles to the north. An unrestricted view is available by ambling 0.75 mile along the windy crest to the summit of Crater Peak. Even better views can be had from Peak 8446 to the east, from where you have an unencumbered vista of Thousand Lakes Valley, the semicircular Magee Peak crest, and the lands from Lassen Volcanic north past the Hat Creek Rim escarpment to Burney Mountain. Also visible is the line of cinder cones extending south from Freaner Peak, starting with Eiler Butte and ending, past desolate Devils Rock Garden, with Bear Wallow Butte. By descending 0.5 mile northeast to Point 8224 at the brink of Red Cliff, you can look straight down at Twin, Everett, and Magee lakes.

Trip **39**

Magee Peak

S ✗ DH

DISTANCE: 6 miles out and back

ELEVATIONS: 6140/8549, +2399/-2399

SEASON: Mid-June to November

USE: Light

MAP: *Thousand Lakes Valley*

INTRODUCTION: The stiffly graded Magee Trail was originally designed not for hikers but for pack mules that resupplied the fire lookout on top of the peak. Since the lookout is now gone, and so are the mules,

the Forest Service has elected not to maintain the trail for hikers, which is a shame. Although steep, rocky, and waterless, the trail offers hikers in good shape the opportunity to reach one of the area's best views, including Lassen Peak and the Mt. Tehama rim. Hikers may have to clamber over and around numerous deadfalls on the lower section of trail and plow through some overgrown brush on the upper section, but the incredible view from the summit is well worth it. Without regular maintenance from the Forest Service, the Magee Trail would be more than worthy of adoption by a local trails organization.

DIRECTIONS TO TRAILHEAD: From Highway 44, near the Ashpan Snowmobile parking area, head northwest on Forest Road 16 for 10 miles and turn right onto Forest Road 32N48. Proceed 1.3 miles to the trailhead at the end of the road (no facilities).

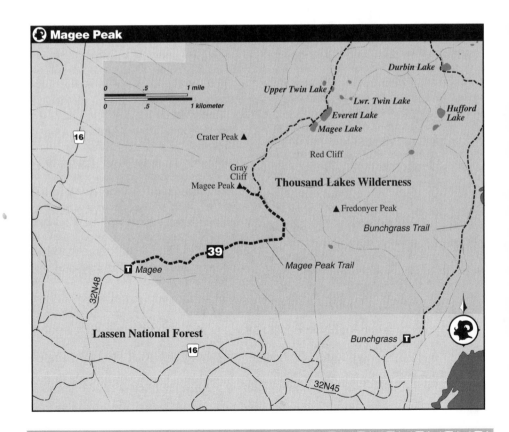

DESCRIPTION: The unmaintained trail begins to the right of a pair of 4-by-4 posts that once held the trailhead signboard and very quickly crosses the still-marked Thousand Lakes Wilderness boundary. Gently rising tread heads into a mixed forest of Jeffrey pines, white firs, and sugar pines, before a moderate to moderately steep climb that continues almost all the way to the summit. The first couple of miles constitutes a steady climb east-northeast through alternating sections of shady forest with little groundcover and more open forest carpeted mainly by pinemat manzanita with lesser amounts of chinquapin and tobacco brush. Beyond the first mile, western white pines and red firs, with a smattering of Jeffrey and lodgepole pines, replace the sugar pines and white firs of below. Before gaining the southeast ridge of the peak, a short traverse with filtered views of Lassen Peak to the south-southeast offers a momentary break in the otherwise continuous climb.

Once on the ridge, angle northwest toward the summit through a diminishing forest composed primarily of mountain hemlocks and whitebark pines above 7800 feet. Eventually, you break out of the trees to the first spellbinding views of the surrounding terrain. Continue climbing through widely scattered, weather-beaten whitebark pines and thick brush that threatens to overgrow the trail in places. At the crater rim, reach a junction with the trail from Magee Lake, turn left, and then follow the crest to the summit.

On a clear day, the expansive vista from the old lookout site stretches for hundreds of miles in virtually every direction—make sure to pack along a big enough map to help identify some of the surrounding landmarks. Closer at hand, the Thousand Lakes Wilderness spreads out around you, including Crater Peak, which, being 127 feet higher, obscures Burney Mountain, a young volcano 8 miles to the north. An unrestricted view is available just 0.75 mile along the windy crest to the summit of Crater Peak. From Peak 8446 to the east are even better views, which include Thousand Lakes Valley the semicircular Magee Peak crest, and the lands from Lassen Volcanic north past the Hat Creek Rim escarpment to Burney Mountain. Also visible is the line of cinder cones extending south from Freaner Peak, starting with Eiler Butte and ending, past desolate Devils Rock Garden, with Bear Wallow Butte. By descending 0.5 mile northeast to Point 8224 at the brink of Red Cliff, you can look straight down at Twin, Everett, and Magee lakes.

Introduction to Butte Lake and Caribou Wilderness

The Butte Lake area, located at 6100 feet, in the remote northeast corner of Lassen Volcanic National Park, features a ranger station, 101-site campground, and picnic area. The lake was created when waters backed up after lava flows dammed Grassy Creek. Several destinations can be reached from the two trailheads on the north shore of the lake, including remote areas in the eastern edge of the park. The first trail described in this section is an easy, short loop to Bathtub Lake and an adjacent, unnamed twin; both lakes provide the warmest and safest swimming in the area. Next is a 3.5-mile moderately strenuous hike to the top of Prospect Peak, the site of a former fire lookout. Dark Cinder Cone is one of the park's most distinctive features, and a self-guided nature trail, with a section of very steep but short climbing, leads to an expansive view at the summit. The next two trips are extended loops that visit some of the least-traveled parts of Lassen Volcanic. The last trail from Butte Lake visits lonely Widow Lake.

Lacking any caribou but possessing dozens of lakes and ponds, the 20,625-acre Caribou Wilderness borders the east-ern boundary of Lassen Volcanic National Park. The mostly forested area is blessed with gentle terrain with some of California's easiest trails. Of the wilderness's 25.5 miles of trail, only a half mile could be considered steep; the remainder is nearly level, slightly rising, or slightly descending. With lakes an easy hour or two from a trailhead, the lightly used wilderness is well suited for novice backpackers or families with young children. Nevertheless, be forewarned that the same gentle terrain that makes the hiking so easy also makes off-trail route-finding difficult because it lacks any significant landmarks.

Three trailheads—one each near the northern, eastern, and southern borders—provide straightforward access to a corresponding number of lake groups, which help to make the Caribou Wilderness a fine area for weekend backpack trips. Trails usually shed their snow by mid-June, with the height of mosquito season shortly behind. Just outside the eastern edge of the wilderness, Silver Lake has a couple of campgrounds and picnic areas, and a summer home community. The Trail Lake Trail connects the Silver Lake area to Echo Lake, with a section of the trail following the eastern border of the wilderness.

Access

Butte Lake is accessible from Highway 44 via the well-graded, gravel Butte Lake Road,

Campgrounds						
Campground	Fee	Elevation	Season	Restrooms	Running Water	Bear Boxes
Butte Lake	$16	6100′	Early June to mid-September	Flush and vault	Yes	Yes
Bogard	$13	5600′	Late April to October	Vault	No	No
Crater Lake	$13	6800′	June to October	Vault	Yes	No
Silver Bowl (Silver Lake)	$13	6400′	May to October	Vault	Yes	No
Rocky Knoll (Silver Lake)	$13	6400′	May to October	Vault	Yes	No

which is generally open from early June to the end of September. Good Forest Service roads provide access to Caribou Wilderness from Highway 44 to the northeast, County Road A21 to the east, and Highway 36 to the south.

Amenities

Services are completely lacking along Highway 44 between Old Station and Susanville. Chester, directly south of Caribou Wilderness, is a full-service community. Westwood, near the junction of Country Road A21 and Highway 36, has limited services.

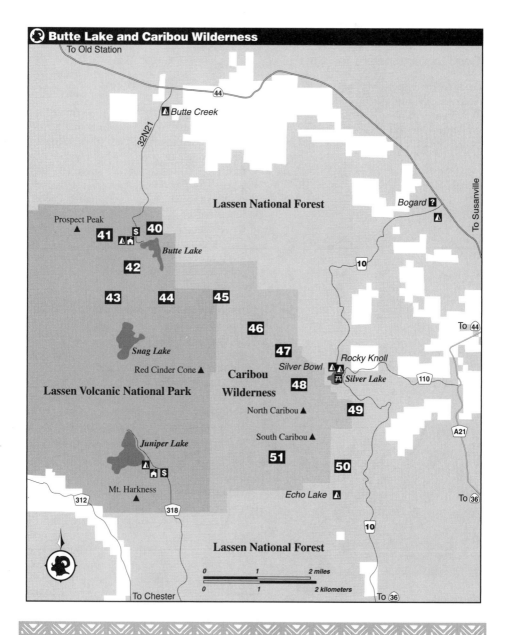

Ranger Stations and Visitor Information

The Park Service has a seasonal ranger station at Butte Lake near the campground, where wilderness permits and emergency services may be obtained. The closest Forest Service stations are the Old Station Visitor Information Center, Lassen National Forest headquarters in Susanville, and the Almanor Ranger District office in Chester.

Good to Know Before You Go

Backpackers planning to enter Lassen Volcanic National Park from Caribou Wilderness trailheads must still obtain a wilderness permit to legally camp in the park.

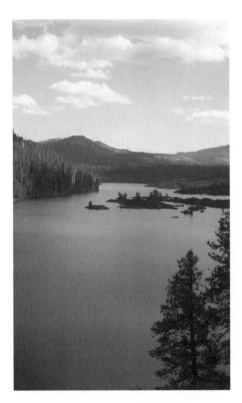

Butte Lake

BUTTE LAKE TRAILHEADS

Trip **40**

Bathtub Lake Loop

E **↻** DH

DISTANCE: 2.3 miles loop

ELEVATIONS: 6085/6215/6085, +300/-300

SEASON: Early June to October

USE: Moderate

MAP: *Prospect Peak*

INTRODUCTION: This short loop trail passes a pair of shallow lakes quite suitable for a midsummer swim, and then follows a short stretch of lovely Butte Creek before returning along the north shore of Butte Lake. The Butte Lake Picnic Area near the trailhead provides a nice setting for a picnic lunch before or after the hike. Most of the day users and campers from the nearby campground go to Bathtub Lake and no farther, which means you'll likely have some solitude and serenity on the remainder of the loop.

DIRECTIONS TO TRAILHEAD: Leave Highway 44 11 miles east of the Highway 89 junction and 16.8 miles westbound of the junction of County Road A21, and head south on well-graded gravel Forest Road 32N21, signed for Butte Lake. Pass a turnoff for the primitive Butte Creek Campground and proceed to the Butte Lake area. After stopping at the self-pay registration station, continue to the left-hand turn into the day-use parking area, equipped with restrooms and a nearby picnic area.

DESCRIPTION: Leave the north edge of the parking area and follow the volcanic soil tread of a single-track trail northeast through scattered ponderosa pines well above the north shore of Butte Lake. Cresting a low rise, the unnamed lake southeast of Bathtub Lake pops into view. Briefly descend to an area above its west

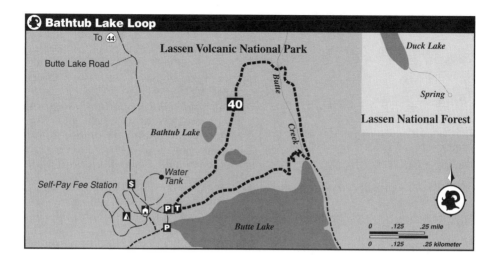

Bathtub Lake Loop

side. In order to reach Bathtub Lake, you must leave the trail and easily stroll over to the east shore. Charred timber from a controlled burn scattered around the twin lakes diminishes their scenic appeal a bit, but relatively warm swimming is a possibility from mid-July to mid-August, when the water temperature usually is in the high 60s and occasionally the low 70s. Bathtub Lake is barely deep enough for good swimming, but its more popular (albeit more shallow), unnamed twin offers significantly better swimming. However, be alert for submerged logs and rocks on the bottom of the lake. Camping is not allowed at either lake.

Make a rising climb out of the lake basin, followed by a descending traverse to the crossing of delightful Butte Creek on a pair of log bridges. Briefly walk through the lush vegetation bordering the creek, and then head upstream on a moderate climb through shady red fir forest. The grade eases

a bit on the approach to Butte Lake; at a junction with the east shore trail, a picnic bench nearby beckons you to sit and admire the fine scenery.

From the junction, head west across a tangle of logs choking the outlet and walk downstream to pick up the trail on the far side (avoid the tendency to look for the resumption of trail in the rocks near the shoreline). A steep, winding climb leads high above the rocky cliff, from where you're afforded a good view across the lake to the edge of the Fantastic Lava Beds. A gentler descent follows well above the north shore of Butte Lake until the trail swings down to lake level on the way to the trailhead. Pass the picnic area and soon reach the parking lot.

R Camping is not allowed, and fires are prohibited.

BUTTE LAKE TRAILHEADS

Trip 4I

Prospect Peak

(MS) DH

DISTANCE: 7 miles out and back

ELEVATIONS: 6075/8338, +2263/-2263

SEASON: Early July to October

USE: Light

MAP: *Prospect Peak*

INTRODUCTION: In the past, a fire spotter lived at the lookout atop Prospect Peak, scanning the wide-ranging vista from above the 8338-foot summit. All that remains of the lookout today are some pieces of broken glass and decaying bits of lumber, but the view is still remarkable, despite a maturing and thriving forest along the rim of the young cinder cone. After the first half mile, the ascent becomes increasingly stiff, but the trail passes through interesting and changing patterns of vegetation, with a pine forest, followed by a red fir belt, and then an open, subalpine forest. The climb to Prospect Peak is one of the more physically taxing trails in the Butte Lake area, providing a reasonable amount of solitude and serenity for those up to the task.

DIRECTIONS TO TRAILHEAD: Leave Highway 44 about 11 miles east of the Highway 89 junction and 16.8 miles west of the County Road A21 junction, and head south on well-graded gravel Forest Road 32N21, signed for Butte Lake. Pass a turnoff for the primitive Butte Creek Campground and proceed to the Butte Lake area. After stopping at the self-pay registration station, continue past the campground to the right-hand turn to the Cinder Cone Trailhead at the end of the road.

DESCRIPTION: Head southwest on the Cinder Cone Trail, which also doubles as a portion of the Nobles Emigrant Trail. This gently graded stroll follows the north edge of the Fantastic Lava Beds for a half mile to a signed junction with the Prospect Peak Trail.

Veer right and begin a mild climb through open forest, primarily of Jeffrey pines but with a smattering of ponderosa pines mixed in at the lower elevations. The grade soon increases to moderate near 6400 feet, where white firs start to intermix with the Jeffrey pines, and chinquapin, pinemat manzanita, and squaw currant form the understory. By 7300 feet, Jeffrey pines and white firs essentially disappear and are replaced by red firs and a lesser amount of western white pines. The white firs disappear for good as you climb onward, but Jeffrey pines continue to make sporadic appearances before temporarily yielding to a prime red fir belt.

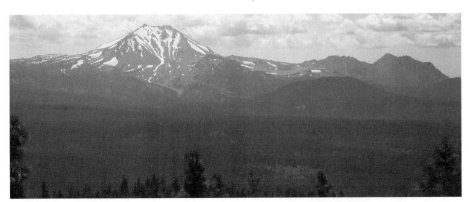

View from Prospect Peak

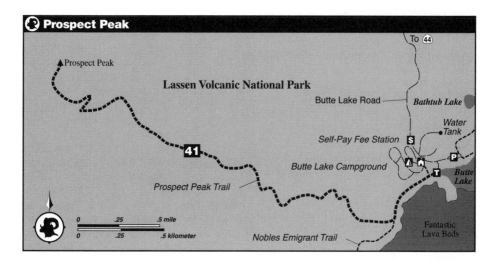

Prospect Peak

To (44)

▲ Prospect Peak

Lassen Volcanic National Park

Butte Lake Road — Bathtub Lake

Water Tank

Self-Pay Fee Station S

41

Butte Lake Campground

Butte Lake

Prospect Peak Trail

0 .25 .5 mile
0 .25 .5 kilometer

Nobles Emigrant Trail

Fantastic Lava Beds

Just above 8000 feet, the trail switch-backs northeast up the south flank of Prospect Peak's summit cinder cone. Views start to open up as red firs yield to Jeffrey pines and shrubs, both of which are able to tolerate the drier and rockier soils found near the top of the peak. Common shrubs at this elevation include sagebrush, gold-enbush, rabbitbrush, bitterbrush, cream bush, and alpine prickly currant. Upon gaining the crest of the ridge, the trail circles clockwise along the rim of the cinder cone through scattered western white pines. Continuing on the arcing path, mountain hemlocks appear along the cold, shady, and windswept north-facing slope—condi-tions that foster lingering snowfields well into the summer. Reach the end of the trail near the site of the old lookout. The cinder cone's depression harbors snow and a shal-low pond that usually lasts until mid-July, and the vegetation reflects this increase in groundwater, with water-tolerant lodgepole pines the primary conifer.

Views are not as easy to come by as they were during the heyday of the fire lookout, as conifers have grown to heights that obscure the line of sight in places; you may have to move around to take full advantage of the lofty heights. On a clear day, the vista extends as far north as Oregon's pyra-midal Mt. McLoughlin (140 miles away) and the Crater Lake rim (165 miles away);

snow-capped Mt. Shasta (70 miles away) is to the northwest. Much closer at hand, West Prospect Peak is 2 miles northwest, with a small cinder cone on its lower east slopes. On the northwest skyline, the high summits of Magee, Crater, and Fredonyer peaks lie just left of West Prospect Peak, with Burney Mountain between it and Mt. Shasta. Sugarloaf Peak is the mountain above and just left of Shasta.

Walking clockwise along the rim, you should easily recognize L-shaped Butte Lake, Cinder Cone, and the bleak and dark Fantastic Lava Beds, with Snag Lake imme-diately to the south. Red Cinder Cone is the high point on the southeast horizon, stand-ing roughly above the east base of Cinder Cone. Lower, Mt. Hoffman rises from Snag Lake's eastern shore, barely reaching the skyline, while Mt. Harkness rises in the dis-tance beyond and to the right of Snag Lake's western shore. Lassen Peak is obviously the most dominant peak, flanked on the east by Reading Peak and on the north by Chaos Crags. A rolling forest lies between Prospect Peak and Lassen Volcanic, containing more than two dozen significant lakes hidden from view. However, Rainbow Lake, due south and lying at the southwest base of Fairfield Peak, is clearly visible.

Ⓡ Fires are prohibited.

Trip **42**

Cinder Cone Nature Trail

 DH

DISTANCE: 7 miles semiloop

ELEVATIONS: 6075/6900, +1015/-1015

SEASON: Late May to October

USE: Moderate

MAP: *Prospect Peak*

INTRODUCTION: As its name suggests, many of the features of Lassen Volcanic National Park are centered on the geologic processes of volcanism. The Cinder Cone Nature Trail celebrates this theme, with stark black chunks of lava, volcanic bombs, vast cin- der and ash fields, and lava-scorched tree snags providing the setting for the primary feature of the trail, the 700-foot Cinder Cone. The self-guided trail—described in a brochure available at the trailhead—leads through a devastated landscape of recent volcanic activity. The 14 numbered posts on the route are keyed to information in the brochure about the geologic, cultural, and natural history of the area. Initially, the path, which wanders through a pine forest to the edge of a massive lava flow, follows in the footsteps of early pioneers on the Nobles Emigrant Trail. Then it leaves the pioneer route to attack the steep slopes on the way to Cinder Cone's rim and a pan- oramic view of the surrounding terrain and nearby features such as Fantastic Lava Beds, Painted Dunes, and Snag and Butte lakes. Fittingly, the park's most prominent feature, Lassen Peak, dominates the view.

The round-trip takes about three or four hours. Those not interested in the full trip

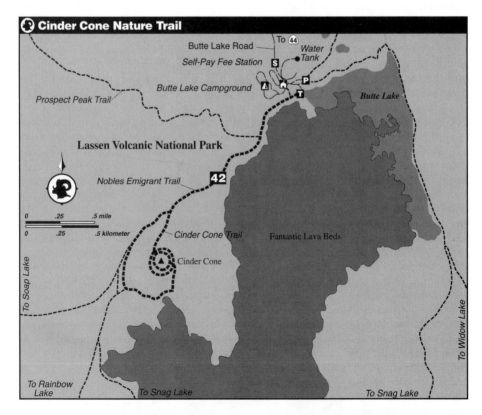

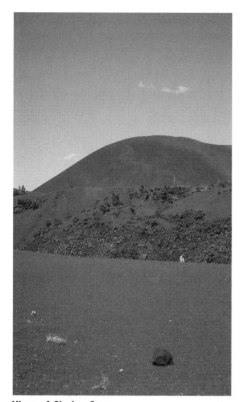

View of Cinder Cone

should at least plan on the gently graded, mile-plus hike to the view of Cinder Cone. Normal daytime temperatures are usually quite warm—if not downright hot—in the summer, and water is not available at any point on the journey. Plan on wearing a hat and sunglasses, and carry plenty of water. Wearing sturdy footwear is also advisable, as small pebbles are almost certain to work their way into all but the highest of boots during the steep ascent and descent of Cinder Cone's loose slopes. Equestrians should note that horses are prohibited on the section of the Cinder Cone Trail that does not coincide with the Nobles Emigrant Trail. Nonequestrians should obey all signs requesting that visitors remain on the trail.

DIRECTIONS TO TRAILHEAD: Leave Highway 44 about 11 miles east of the Highway 89 junction and 16.8 miles west of the junction of County Road A21, and head south on well-graded gravel Forest Road 32N21, signed for Butte Lake. Pass a turnoff for the primitive Butte Creek Campground and proceed to the Butte Lake area. After stopping at the self-pay registration station, continue past the campground to the right-hand turn to the Cinder Cone Trailhead at the end of the road.

DESCRIPTION: A number of signs providing interesting tidbits about the geology and history of the area greet hikers at the beginning of the Cinder Cone Trail. For more information about this historical and geologically interesting spot, you can also pick up the $0.50 Cinder Cone Nature Trail pamphlet, which is keyed to the numbered posts along the route. Gently rising tread leads southwest through Jeffrey and ponderosa pines past a junction with an unmarked path from the campground. Proceed ahead to a junction with the Prospect Peak Trail at 0.5 mile.

From that junction, continue straight ahead through loose, volcanic soil along the edge of the Fantastic Lava Beds until the trail veers slightly southwest and the grade increases. Near a sign warning visitors to stay off the cinder field, the pine forest nearly disappears, allowing the dark hulk of Cinder Cone to burst into full view. Proceed across the bleak and open terrain to a signed junction at 1.4 miles.

Turn left (south), following signed directions to the top of the Cinder Cone. Shortly, reach the base, where a very steep ascent over extremely loose cinders begins. By placing your feet in the tracks of previous

PAINTED DUNES

From about 1567 to 1851, after the Painted Dunes lava flow spread out, Cinder Cone erupted at least three times, spraying cinders for miles around. Cinders falling on the hot lava were oxidized and thereby colored by the intense heat, producing the vivid hues visible today.

hikers, you may be able to minimize the slippage common on such steep (30 to 35 degrees) and loose slopes. Fortunately, this section of trail is only about a quarter mile in length—but it sill gains about 700 feet in the process, leaving mere mortals winded by the time they find easier going at the rim of the cone.

Twin concentric paths ring the lip of the cone and the inside of the crater, offering differing perspectives of this geological wonder. The view from the rim is remarkable, with several landmarks clearly visible, including Lassen Peak, Brokeoff Mountain, Prospect Peak, Chaos Crags, and Reading Peak. Closer at hand, Snag Lake and Butte Lake bookend the dark expanse of the Fantastic Lava Beds, formed by a series of Cinder Cone basalt eruptions that occurred within the last 500 years. The colorful Painted Dunes lie near the southeast base of the cone.

After spending the time to fully appreciate the views of and from the crater, you have the option of following a short loop around the south side of Cinder Cone, as described next, or simply retracing your steps to the trailhead.

For the extended loop section, descend the trail that leaves the west side of the rim near a grove of stunted pines, and drop steeply away from the rim toward a minor ridge. Beyond the rim, the trail follows a descending traverse around the south base of the cone, past the multicolored Painted Dunes before bottoming out just before reaching a junction with a connector trail. Turn right (north) and make a moderate climb to a junction with the Nobles Emigrant Trail. From there, turn right (northeast) and follow the pioneer trail back to the trailhead.

[R] Fires are prohibited, and camping is prohibited within a quarter mile of Cinder Cone and Painted Dunes. Equestrians are not allowed on Cinder Cone.

BUTTE LAKE TRAILHEADS

Trip **43**

Lower Twin-Horseshoe-Snag Lakes Loop

Ⓜ ↻ DH, BP

DISTANCE: 18.1 miles loop

ELEVATIONS: 6075/6710/6075, +1825/-1825

SEASON: Late June to October

USE: Light

MAPS: *Prospect Peak, Mount Harkness*

INTRODUCTION: This lightly traveled loop offers a wide variety of features that includes open forests, interesting geology, and several of the park's largest lakes. Energetic hikers will want to take advantage of a 1.2-mile side trip for fantastic views from the top of Cinder Cone. The terrain is fairly mellow, which makes for easy travel for backpackers (as well as exceptionally strong hikers capable of knocking off the 18.1 in one day), and Rainbow, Lower Twin, Swan, Horseshoe, and Snag lakes all offer secluded camping and refreshing swimming. Although fishing is rarely considered excellent within the park, fishing is not bad for some species of trout in Rainbow, Horseshoe, and Snag lakes. A number of connecting trails are available for extending the trip to a variety of additional destinations.

Water is virtually nonexistent, except near the lakes and ponds en route, so plan accordingly. Despite the arid nature of the area, mosquitoes can be problematic near bodies of water until mid- or late July. The open cinder fields surrounding Cinder Cone can be extremely hot on sunny days—if possible, arrange to cross these areas during the cooler parts of the day.

DIRECTIONS TO TRAILHEAD: Leave Highway 44 about 11 miles east of the Highway

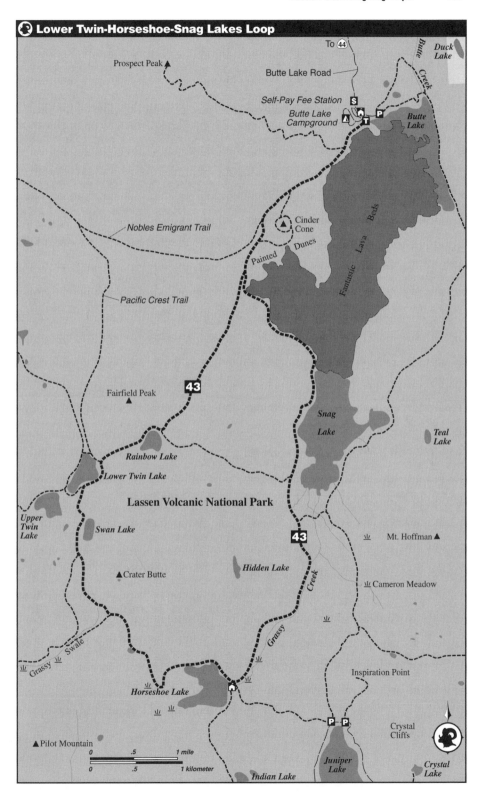

Lower Twin-Horseshoe-Snag Lakes Loop

To 44
Duck Lake
Butte Creek
Prospect Peak ▲
Butte Lake Road
Self-Pay Fee Station S
Butte Lake Campground
Butte Lake
Nobles Emigrant Trail
Cinder Cone
Fantastic Lava Beds
Painted Dunes
Pacific Crest Trail
Fairfield Peak ▲
43
Snag Lake
Teal Lake
Rainbow Lake
Lower Twin Lake
Lassen Volcanic National Park
Upper Twin Lake
Swan Lake
43
Mt. Hoffman ▲
▲ Crater Butte
Hidden Lake
Cameron Meadow
Grassy Creek
Inspiration Point
Grassy Swale
Grassy
Horseshoe Lake
P P
Crystal Cliffs
▲ Pilot Mountain
0   .5   1 mile
0   .5   1 kilometer
Juniper Lake
Crystal Lake
Indian Lake

89 junction and 16.8 miles west of the County Road A21 junction, and head south on well-graded gravel Forest Road 32N21, signed for Butte Lake. Pass a turnoff for the primitive Butte Creek Campground and proceed to the Butte Lake area. After stopping at the self-pay registration station, continue past the campground to the right-hand turn to the Cinder Cone Trailhead at the end of the road.

DESCRIPTION: A number of signs providing interesting tidbits about the geology and history of the area greet hikers at the beginning of the Cinder Cone Trail. For more information about this historical and geologically interesting spot, you can also pick up the $0.50 Cinder Cone Nature Trail pamphlet, which is keyed to the numbered posts along the route. Gently rising tread leads southwest through Jeffrey and ponderosa pines past a junction with an unmarked path from the campground. Proceed ahead to a junction with the Prospect Peak Trail at 0.5 mile.

From that junction, continue straight ahead through loose, volcanic soil along the edge of the Fantastic Lava Beds until the trail veers slightly southwest and the grade increases. Near a sign warning visitors to stay off the cinder field, the pine forest nearly disappears, allowing the dark hulk of Cinder Cone to burst into full view. Proceed across the bleak and open terrain to a signed junction at 1.4 miles.

⑤ **SIDE TRIP TO CINDER CONE:** Drop your backpack at the junction and turn left (south), following signed directions to the top of the Cinder Cone. Shortly, reach the base, where a very steep ascent over extremely loose cinders begins. By placing your feet in the tracks of previous hikers, you may be able to minimize the slippage common on such steep (30 to 35 degrees) and loose slopes. Fortunately, this section of trail is only about a quarter mile in length—but it sill gains about 700 feet in the process, leaving mere mortals winded by the time they find easier going at the rim of the cone.

Twin concentric paths ring the lip of the cone and the inside of the crater, offering differing perspectives of this geological wonder. The view from the rim is remarkable, with several landmarks clearly visible, including Lassen Peak, Brokeoff Mountain, Prospect Peak, Chaos Crags, and Reading Peak. Closer at hand, Snag Lake and Butte Lake bookend the dark expanse of the Fantastic Lava Beds, formed by a series of Cinder Cone basalt eruptions that occurred within the last 500 years. The colorful Painted Dunes lie near the southeast base of the cone. After enjoying the view, retrace your steps to the trail junction. **END OF SIDE TRIP**

Proceed ahead (southwest) from the junction in the shadow of Cinder Cone on mildly rising and then mildly descending tread for a total of 0.5 mile to the next junction, where the Nobles Emigrant Trail veers to the right.

Turn left at the junction and make a moderate descent around the shoulder of Cinder Cone to the south junction of the trail to the top of the cone. Here, the top of Lassen Peak pops into view. Continue the descent on loose cinder tread past an unmarked but well-defined trail (not on USGS map) angling from behind and to the right. At the bottom of the descent, a swath of vegetation stands in stark contrast to the otherwise bleak volcanic slopes. A short climb away from this miniature oasis leads to a signed junction at 2.5 miles.

Veer ahead on the right-hand trail, following signed directions for Lower Twin Lake, crossing a thin drainage swale lined with a row of lodgepole pines. Here, you leave the cinder fields for a lightly charred forest of lodgepole pines, Jeffrey pines, and white firs, with western white pines eventually joining the mix ahead. The patchy groundcover includes currant and pinemat manzanita. Mildly ascending trail continues through the trees for the next couple of uneventful miles, until a brief descent leads to a junction with a connector to Snag Lake near the north shore of forest-

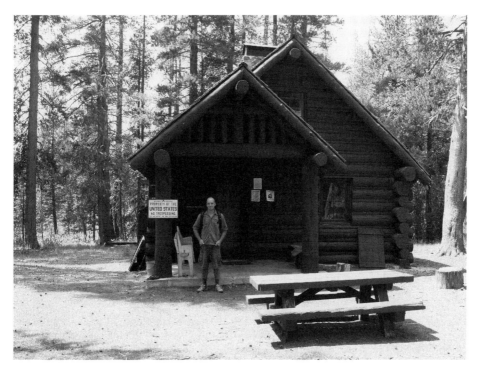

Ranger Station near Horseshoe Lake

rimmed Rainbow Lake, 2.7 miles from the trailhead.

Veer right at the junction and follow the trail well above the north shore of Rainbow Lake, along the base of Fairfield Peak, the 7162-foot cinder cone directly northwest, until the path drops alongside the shoreline. The straightforward, 650-foot optional climb to the summit of Fairfield Peak begins from the west corner of the lake, near a fair-ly large campsite nestled beneath the trees, and heads cross-country north-northwest to the top. Additional campsites may be available on the east side, accessible from a use trail. The lake offers decent swimming, at least until the customary wind whips up, usually in mid-afternoon.

A brief climb heads away from Rainbow Lake on a wildflower-lined path, followed by a mild descent to the northeast side of Lower Twin Lake, where you meet the Pacific Crest Trail from Soap Lake and Badger Flat. Turn left and proceed around the east side of the large but relatively shal-

low lake, past several lodgepole-shaded campsites. The water temperature is usually warm enough to provide refreshing swimming by mid- or late July. Expect vociferous Steller's jays throughout the season, and voracious mosquitoes before late July.

At another junction about halfway around the east shore, where a trail heads west toward Upper Twin Lake and beyond, proceed ahead to the left on the PCT. A short, moderate climb incorporating a single switchback leads over a hump and then down a flower-lined path to Swan Lake, 0.5 mile from the junction. The quiet, forest-rimmed lake sees fewer visitors than its more popular neighbors, and, as a result, its campsites are less developed and fewer in number—leave the trail to look for a site above the south shore or on a bench above the east shore.

Climb out of Swan Lake's basin for a quarter mile to a junction, where the PCT travels southwest toward Grassy Swale. Veer left here and continue on gently graded, flower-lined trail toward Horseshoe Lake, arcing around the west flank of Crater Butte, another of the park's many cinder cones. Plan on an hour round-trip if you're interested in the 500-foot climb to the summit of Crater Butte and the small body of water that seasonally occupies its crater. Soon, a moderate descent takes you through a seasonal stream gully filled with lush vegetation. Rather than descending straight to the floor of Grassy Swale, the trail crosses the gully and makes a short climb to a junction with a trail heading southwest down Grassy Swale to the PCT.

Turn left at the junction and climb up a side canyon, through a swath of lush plants and flowers, and then follow a gentle descent past a pair of seasonal ponds/meadows and a much larger pond on the way toward Horseshoe Lake.

Upon reaching the northwest shore of Horseshoe Lake, a sign and map indicates that camping is not allowed for the next mile of trail, which traverses the north end of the lake close to the shoreline. The north half of the lake offers a very attractive, if oversized, swimming hole, as the lake's pebbly bottom quickly drops away from shore to level off at about 10 to 15 feet, without rocks, snags, and other submerged obstacles for swimmers to fret about. Since the middle of the lake is relatively shallow—less than 5 feet deep in places—colder water from the deeper southern half is effectively kept out of the north end, where water temperatures become relatively warm by midsummer. Proceed to the northwest end of the lake and continue above aptly named Grassy Creek, a crystalline stream flowing out of the lake and gurgling downstream through some of the most verdant meadowlands in Lassen Volcanic. Soon reach a junction, at 9.75 miles, where backpackers should head across a bridge of halved log rounds and continue past the Horseshoe Lake ranger station to legal campsites along the east shore.

When you are ready to move on, proceed ahead from the junction and follow the west bank of picturesque Grassy Creek on gently graded trail for nearly a mile to a junction with a trail providing access to Cameron Meadow and Jakey Lake. Beyond this junction, the canyon grows narrow and steep, as the trail clings tightly to the hillside above the creek. The terrain becomes so confining at one point that the trail is forced to make two bridged crossings of the creek, one right after the other. Shrubs replace the meadows beyond the bridges and threaten to overgrow the path before the trail climbs above the creek through drier vegetation. Eventually, the trail leaves the creek for good and drops toward a junction to the south of Snag Lake, 12 miles from the trailhead.

Angle left at the junction and proceed through lodgepole pines and a few white firs, with the lake out of sight ahead and to the right. Reach the edge of an extensive burned area just as the lake comes into view.

Head north along the west shore of the lake to a signed junction with a trail heading west to Rainbow Lake. Backpackers

SNAG LAKE

Although the name of the lake corresponds quite well with the presence of numerous charred snags carpeting the landscape above the west shore, the lake owes its appellation to a prior event. Scientists estimate an outpouring of lava around 1630 dammed Grassy Creek, which previously flowed through a wide, flat, glaciated valley to Butte Lake, creating the lake and drowning the surrounding forest. Early settlers saw many snags still standing after this event, which resulted in the name. None of the snags that are here today were left over from the era of the lake's birth; rather, they are the result of a more recent forest fire and bark beetle infestation. Interestingly, the waters of Snag Lake still drain north into Butte Lake, albeit underground beneath the Fantastic Lava Beds.

may find the best campsites down a use trail on the right that leads to a small peninsula near the southwest shore (fortunately, the fire didn't touch the lodgepole-shaded peninsula). By mid-July, the lake is warm enough for pleasant swimming, particularly in the south and east lobes, where the average depth is a mere 5 to 10 feet. By late summer, the lake level drops a few feet, and these two areas decrease noticeably in size.

Continue north through open terrain, as the trail draws closer to the shoreline. A grove of intact forest near the north end of Snag Lake provides some welcome shade and a fine place to camp, picnic, or rest before the climb ahead. You may share this spot with a spotted sandpiper, killdeer, or California gull, or a variety of forest-edge birds. Although Snag Lake is the park's second largest body of water, the lake is uncommonly shallow for its size, only 20 to 25 feet deep along the south margin of the Fantastic Lava Beds.

From the northwest tip of Snag Lake, the trail leaves the lake behind and climbs along the southwest edge of the bleak and dark Fantastic Lava Beds with a scattered to light forest on the left. The route climbs across slopes laden with pumice, which appear to be as difficult to negotiate as sand dunes. The grade eventually eases just before a short drop brings you to the open expanse of cinder fields surrounding Cinder Cone, which cuts a stunning profile in the near distance. If possible, time your arrival for the cooler part of the day, as crossing the open cinder field under the scorching afternoon sun can be exceedingly unpleasant. At 15.5 miles, you close the loop southwest of Cinder Cone, turn right (northeast), and then retrace your steps to the trailhead.

R Wilderness permits are required for overnight stays, and fires are prohibited.

BUTTE LAKE TRAILHEADS

Trip **44**

Widow-Jakey-Snag Lakes Loop

Ⓜ ↻ DH, BP

DISTANCE: 19.3 miles loop

ELEVATIONS: 6070/7670/6070, +2450/-2450

SEASON: Late June to October

USE: Light

MAPS: *Prospect Peak, Mount Harkness*

INTRODUCTION: You won't have much company on this loop, as the few backpackers who set out for Widow Lake generally go no farther. Those who do will be treated to two of the park's most remote lakes, Widow and Jakey, and wildflower-laden Cameron Meadows. Additionally, peakbaggers can scramble up Red Cinder for the wide-ranging view, or take a more difficult route up nearby Red Cinder Cone for an even better vista.

DIRECTIONS TO TRAILHEAD: Leave Highway 44 about 11 miles east of the Highway 89 junction and 16.8 miles west of the County Road A21 junction, and head south on well-graded gravel Forest Road 32N21, signed for Butte Lake. Pass a turnoff for the primitive Butte Creek Campground and proceed to the Butte Lake area. After stopping at the self-pay registration station, continue to the left-hand turn into the day-use parking area, equipped with restrooms and a nearby picnic area.

DESCRIPTION: From the day-use parking area, head east above the cottonwood-lined north shore of Butte Lake and past the picnic area. Proceed through a mature forest of ponderosa and Jeffrey pines and climb to a spectacular viewpoint at the south end

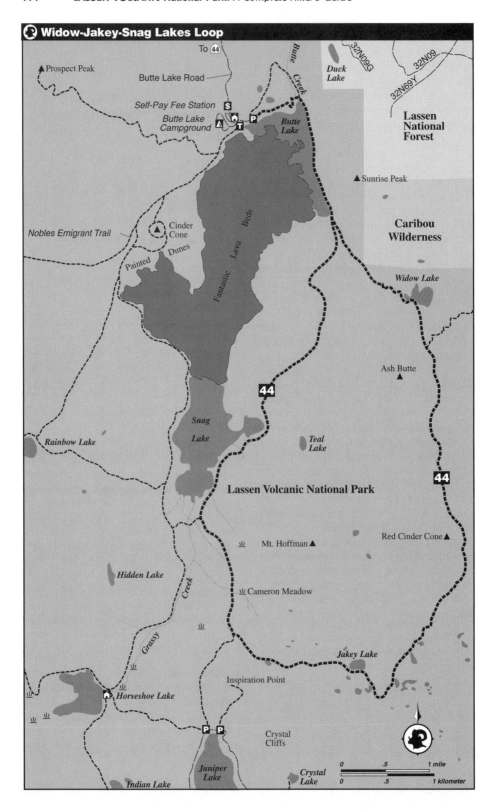

Widow-Jakey-Snag Lakes Loop

THE FORMATION OF SNAG LAKE

Geologists theorize that three events caused Butte Lake to evolve into its current configuration. First, land gradually subsided along one or more faults, creating a primordial Butte Lake and the east-shore escarpment. Second, glaciers (which may have preceded this faulting and were likely active for long periods during the faulting) subsequently scraped and enlarged the faulted basin, leaving behind a larger and deeper lake. Finally, during the eruption of Cinder Cone, a number of lava flows moved south and east, forming the present-day Fantastic Lava Beds, which dammed Grassy Creek and thereby created Snag Lake. These flows pushed eastward, reducing the size of Butte Lake. The last flow barely reached the lake's western shore. Assuming no more lava flows for the near future—a risky assumption—the Fantastic Lava Beds may one day be covered with a pine forest—in about 2000 years.

of a narrow ridge, among some mountain mahoganies, where you may note Butte Lake's asymmetrical configuration: a nearly straight, forested east shore (although charred by a recent forest fire) versus a highly lobed, nonvegetated west shore.

Some of the landmarks seen from the shrubby ridge crest viewpoint include a quartet of cinder cones: Sunrise Peak, an eroded cinder cone atop Butte Lake's eastern escarpment; Ash Butte, rising beyond the lake's southeast tip; and Red Cinder and Red Cinder Cone, partly hidden behind Ash Butte's west and east flanks. Mt. Hoffman, a deeply eroded andesitic stratovolcano, stands beyond the lake's west shore.

To avoid descending the steep rock slopes down to Butte Lake's outlet, this route climbs momentarily north before plunging via switchbacks to the west bank

of Butte Creek, just below the outlet. Travel several yards upstream and then cross the outlet on a tangle of driftwood logs to pick up the single-track trail at a three-way junction on the far side. The crossing is usually uneventful, except at high water during early summer, when you may have to wade the stream.

Veer right (south-southeast) at the junction and traverse along the east shore of Butte Lake; in a half mile, pass a miniature island harboring several conifers that beautifully frame Cinder Cone, 2 miles to the southwest. Farther on, the trail offers unobstructed views of the Fantastic Lava Beds and Prospect Peak. Pass clumps of willows and aspens near the south end of the lake on the way to a junction at 2.25 miles.

Proceed ahead (southeast) from the junction toward Widow Lake (the right-hand trail will be your return route) along Widow Lake's ephemeral outlet stream, which more or less descends along Butte Lake's east-shore fault. Cross the usually dry creek about 0.4 mile from the junction—the first of several fords—and soon shift gears as the easy climb becomes moderate. Pines and firs that shade the way provide ideal low-light conditions for snow plant, pinedrops, and other parasites. The moderate climb leads to a glade abounding in corn lilies and bracken ferns, beyond which the grade increases to a steep ascent beside a boulder-filled talus slope up to a glacial moraine damming Widow Lake.

Widow Lake actually drains through the moraine, rather than over the surface, first appearing above ground near the base of the talus slope. Widow Lake, at about 6800 feet, is bordered by the usual complement of willows and lodgepole pines common to this elevation, along with a few black cottonwoods that are somewhat rare at this altitude. The lake appears small at first, but what you see initially is merely the lake's forebay, which usually becomes separated from the main body of the lake by a thin strip of land covered with grasses and pines as the water level drops late in the season. More than enough fine campsites spread around the shoreline accommodate the light use Widow Lake receives.

Climb south from Widow Lake, soon leaving behind all of the white firs and most of the Jeffrey pines, as the forest transitions to red firs, western white pines, and lodgepole pines—the most prevalent forest grouping in the park. A half mile from Widow Lake, you reach a T-junction with a trail heading east to Triangle Lake in Caribou Wilderness. Proceed straight ahead, continuing the climb toward a saddle between Red Cinder and Red Cinder Cone. About halfway between Widow Lake and the saddle, a fair-size pond offers refreshing swimming and one of the limited opportunities to acquire water before Jakey Lake, at least through midseason. Pass a tiny pond a half mile farther, and then spot the first mountain hemlocks—harbingers of long-lasting snowfields. Snow may cover the upper part of the trail to the saddle until mid-July, although the funnel-like terrain would make the route clearly obvious even in the dead of winter.

[S] SIDE TRIP TO RED CINDER CONE: From the 7600-foot saddle, Red Cinder Cone stands a quarter mile west, tempting peakbaggers to scramble over boulders and through brush to the summit, but an easier approach would be to briefly descend south and then climb up a gully to the north side of a knoll, a quarter mile south of Red Cinder Cone. From there, walk west to views from a rocky bench about 250 feet below the summit. A far superior view awaits at the top of the north summit of twin-coned Red Cinder Cone, where the Fantastic Lava Beds, Cinder Cone, Butte Lake, and Prospect Peak dominate the scene. Additional points of interest include snowy Lassen Peak, finlike Bonte Peak, and spreading Mt. Harkness. **END OF SIDE TRIP**

[S] SIDE TRIP TO RED CINDER: Reaching the top of Red Cinder from the saddle involves a hardy struggle east up steep, brushy slopes for 700 feet—a route only the most ardent of peakbaggers will find enjoyable. However, at 8374 feet, Red Cinder is the highest summit for miles around, providing an unobstructed vista of a vast area of Lassen Volcanic, Caribou Wilderness, and numerous features beyond. To the south, Lake Almanor is clearly obvious, but a Forest Service map would be handy in helping to identify the numerous summits to the northeast. Fourteen miles to the west, Crater Mountain is the foremost peak, a shield volcano similar to Prospect Peak and Mt. Harkness. This youthful volcano rose out of the middle of a large valley, mostly obliterating it in the process. The summit eventually collapsed into a caldera, which subsequently filled with water to form Crater Lake. **END OF SIDE TRIP**

From the saddle between Red Cinder and Red Cinder Cone, the trail descends 2.5 miles to the east shore of Jakey Lake. Only the first 0.75-mile is moderately steep, followed by a gently rolling descent past ponds and small lakes to the south shore of forest-rimmed Jakey Lake. The shallow lake is good for swimming in early and mid-August, after the height of mosquito season. Due to the infrequent use, campsites are few and far between—look around the outlet for the best one.

Away from Jakey Lake, the seldom-traveled trail follows Jakey Lake creek (which does not appear on the USGS map) downstream (west) through nearly continuous forest, interrupted only by a seasonal pond/swamp about a mile from the lake and just prior to a crossing of the creek. Continue downstream, bidding farewell to Jakey Lake creek after a quarter mile and then crossing a seasonal stream on the way to a junction with the trail between Juniper Lake and Cameron Meadow.

Turn right (northwest) at the junction, headed toward Cameron Meadow, which lies an easy half mile away. About midway, you pass a junction with a shortcut trail trending west-southwest to the Grassy Creek Trail, and then follow gently descending trail to the meadow, reaching a cabin site on the west edge after several minutes. Through July, a shallow pond fills the northwest corner of the meadow, with the remainder not much drier, creating an ideal environment for mosquito heaven—or hell, depending on your perspective. Such conditions are common for mountain meadows, with the peak of insect season corresponding to the peak of flower season. Although a highly unpleasant nuisance to hikers and backpackers, mosquitoes are important pollinators in the grand scheme of wildflower ecology.

Boggy conditions persist along the next stretch of trail, as you plow past corn lilies, alders, willows, and lodgepole pines, crossing over Jakey Lake creek twice on the way to a snowmelt pond at the northeast edge of a low, nearby ridge. From there, a moderate, 15-minute descent along glacial sediments leads to a junction above unseen Snag Lake.

Proceed ahead (north) from the junction to the southeast shore, the shallowest part of Snag Lake, which dries up by late summer. Hop over a pair of rivulets and pass several campsites on the trek along the shoreline toward the northeast lobe.

Beyond a grove of aspens, leave the lake and begin a stiff, mile-long climb to the top of a low divide directly east of Point 6379, followed by a viewless, 1.75-mile descent to the close of the loop at the junction with the trail to Widow Lake just south of Butte Lake.

From there, turn left and retrace your steps 2.3 miles to the trailhead.

R Wilderness permits are required for overnight stays, and fires are prohibited.

CONE LAKE TRAILHEAD

Trip **45**

Widow Lake

Ⓜ ⁄ DH, BP

DISTANCE: 10 miles out and back

ELEVATIONS: 6775/7100/6825, +600/-600

SEASON: Mid-June to late October

USE: Light

MAPS: *Bogard Buttes, Prospect Peak*

INTRODUCTION: Of the relative few who visit Widow Lake during the course of the season, most do so via the shorter 3.6-mile trail from Lassen Volcanic's Butte Lake Trailhead. This 5-mile route, from the Cone Lake Trailhead on the outskirts of Caribou Wilderness, is definitely the road less traveled, offering hikers and backpackers an almost ironclad guarantee of solitude and serenity. The trail passes through gently rolling forest for most of the way to the lake, which makes for easy and straightforward hiking. Well-suited for an overnight trip, Widow Lake offers quiet camping along with temperate swimming by midsummer. However, anglers should leave their poles at home, as the lake is devoid of fish.

DIRECTIONS TO TRAILHEAD: Near the Bogard Rest Area on Highway 44 (4.75 miles west of the County Road A21 junction, and 23 miles eastbound of the Highway 89 junction), head west on Forest Road 10, following signs for Silver Lake. At 5.9 miles, where Road 10 bends sharply south toward Silver Lake, turn right onto Forest Road 32N09A, signed CONE LAKE 3, BOGARD WORK CENTER 6. After 1.1 miles, veer left at a junction, remaining on Road 32N09A. Proceed for 1 mile to another junction, and turn right to continue on Road 32N09A 0.8 mile to the Cone Lake Trailhead, 8.8 miles from Highway 44. Primitive camping

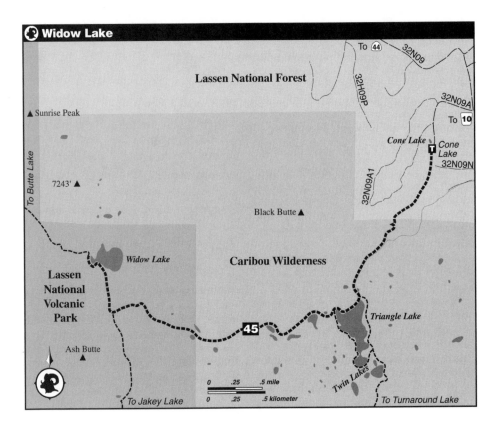

is available at nearby Cone Lake, which is usually waist deep after winter's snowmelt but merely a wet meadow by autumn. The mosquito-infested water is uninviting for either swimming or drinking, so make sure you fill your water containers before reaching the trailhead. There are no improvements at the trailhead.

DESCRIPTION: Begin climbing mildly south on the Cone Lake Trail through a scattered forest of lodgepole pines, Jeffrey pines, and white firs, with clumps of manzanita and currant sprinkled across the forest floor. At the 0.75-mile mark, step into the signed Caribou Wilderness and continue the ascent for another mile to a junction near the north shore of Triangle Lake, which is irregularly shaped but bears little resemblance to its geometric namesake.

Turn right (southwest) and proceed along the north shore of the lodgepole-rimmed lake to a junction on its far side. Continue west, following signs for Lassen National Park and Widow Lake. A very brief climb leads past a small pond, followed shortly by a fairly large pond to the left of the trail. Continue on loose, sandy, gently graded trail past additional ponds, as western white pines start to join the mixed forest. At 3.5 miles from the trailhead, near yet another pond of fair size, you enter Lassen Volcanic National Park.

Just beyond the boundary, the trail drops to a seasonal pond/meadow and then continues on gently graded trail. The outline of Ash Butte is vaguely discernible through the trees to the southwest before mildly descending tread leads to a junction, 4.5 miles from the trailhead.

Turn right (north) and make a half-mile, moderate descent to the wooded and grassy shore of Widow Lake. Widow Lake, at about 6800 feet, is bordered by the willows and lodgepole pines common to this elevation, along with a few black cottonwoods that are somewhat rare at this altitude. If you're visiting in late season, you may notice a forebay at the far side of the lake that forms when the water level drops and a thin strip of land covered with grasses and pines is revealed. More than enough fine campsites are spread around the shoreline to accommodate the light use Widow Lake receives.

R Wilderness permits are required for overnight stays, and fires are prohibited.

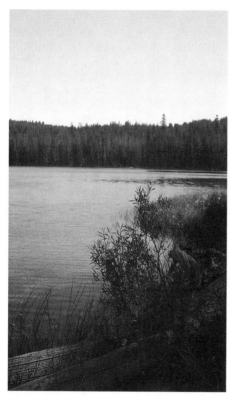
Widow Lake

CONE LAKE TRAILHEAD

Trip **46**

Triangle, Twin, and Turnaround Lakes

Ⓔ / DH, BP

DISTANCE: 7.4 miles out and back

ELEVATIONS: 6775/7065, +430/-430

SEASON: Mid-June to late October

USE: Light

MAP: *Bogard Buttes*

INTRODUCTION: There are two chief attractions of a hike from the Cone Lake Trailhead into the northern part of Caribou Wilderness: easy hiking and scenic lakes. Backpackers searching for a short and gently graded walk to good campsites will not be disappointed with this 2-mile hike to Triangle Lake, which has minimal elevation gain They may, however, may be disappointed with the mosquitoes, which can be problematic until midsummer.

DIRECTIONS TO TRAILHEAD: Near the Bogard Rest Area on Highway 44 (4.75 miles west of the County Road A21 junction, and 23 miles eastbound of the Highway 89 junction), head west on Forest Road 10, following signs for Silver Lake. At 5.9 miles, where Road 10 bends sharply south toward Silver Lake, turn right onto Forest Road 32N09A, signed CONE LAKE 3, BOGARD WORK CENTER 6. After 1.1 miles, veer left at a junction, remaining on Road 32N09A. Proceed for 1 mile to another junction, and turn right to continue on Road 32N09A 0.8 mile to the Cone Lake Trailhead, 8.8 miles from Highway 44. Primitive camping is available at nearby Cone Lake, which is usually waist deep after winter's snowmelt but merely a wet meadow by autumn. The mosquito-infested water is uninviting for either swimming or drinking, so make sure you fill your water containers

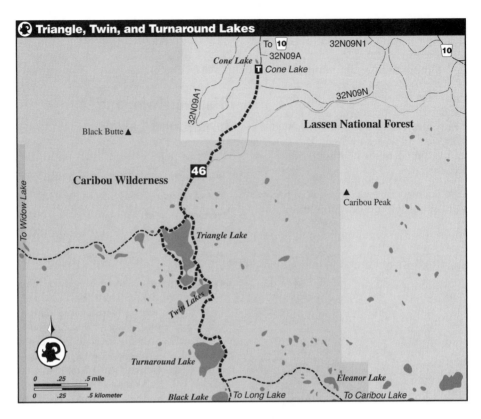

Triangle, Twin, and Turnaround Lakes

before reaching the trailhead. There are no improvements at the trailhead.

DESCRIPTION: Begin climbing mildly south on the Cone Lake Trail through a scattered forest of lodgepole pines, Jeffrey pines, and white firs, with clumps of manzanita and currant sprinkled across the forest floor. At the 0.75-mile mark, step into the signed Caribou Wilderness and continue the ascent for another mile to a junction near the north shore of Triangle Lake, which is irregularly shaped but bears little resemblance to its geometric namesake.

Backpackers should turn right, as the most desirable campsites are found on the west side of the lake. Proceed along the north shore of the lodgepole-rimmed lake to a junction on the far side and then turn left (south) to follow the west shore trail. About halfway along the lakeshore, a small, grassy peninsula juts into the azure water, where a pair of campsites near the trail may tempt

overnighters. However, a rocky, tree-shaded bench offers perhaps the best camping in the whole wilderness—away from the trail with good views of the lake. Swimmers will find the water temperature warm enough for refreshing swimming, and anglers can ply the waters in search of the resident brook and rainbow trout. Continue down the west shore trail to the southern arms of Triangle Lake, which are quite shallow and visually less pleasing, especially as the water level drops later in the season. At the south end, the trail moves away from the lakeshore and rejoins the east shore trail.

Turn right to pass a shallow pond on the way to the easternmost Twin Lake. The other "twin" is shallow and undesirable. The only campsites are too close to the water and far inferior to sites at Triangle Lake.

The trail makes a brief climb away from Twin Lakes before dropping to the north shore of Turnaround Lake and a T-junction

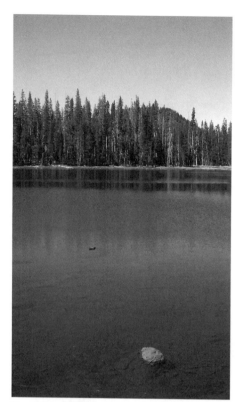

One of the Twin lakes

with a lesser-used path on the right to campsites along the west side. Most of the campsites here are too close to the water. One campsite has a particularly unsightly crude rock wall that should be destroyed. The best spots for camping are found back at Triangle Lake.

The trail continues away from Turnaround Lake for 0.1 mile or so to a junction with the trail heading west from the Caribou Lake Trailhead. Retrace your steps back to the junction with the east shore trail around Triangle Lake. For variety, you can follow the more direct route along the east shore of the lake back to the junction at the north end and then retrace your steps northwest back to the trailhead.

O From the junction with the trail from the Caribou Lake Trailhead, additional routes to several other lakes in Caribou Wilderness are possible.

Trip **47**

Middle Caribou Lakes Loop

E ◯ DH, BP

DISTANCE: 7.2 miles loop

ELEVATIONS: 6550/7120/6550, +570/-570

SEASON: Mid-June to late October

USE: Light

MAPS: *Bogard Buttes, Red Cinder*

INTRODUCTION: This 7-mile-plus loop is probably the most popular hike in Caribou Wilderness. However, such popularity is relative, as the area sees very light traffic, even in the most heavily traveled parts. Of those who do set out from the Caribou Lake Trailhead, most don't complete the entire loop, preferring to stop at the closest lakes to the trailhead. While the distance is short enough for a comfortable dayhike, backpackers will find good campsites at several locations. The mostly forested loop visits numerous lakes and ponds, some of which offer fine swimming and angling. Adding a side trip to Emerald, Rim, and Cypress lakes provides even more desirable locations, as well as sweeping views that are lacking along the loop route (see Trip 48).

DIRECTIONS TO TRAILHEAD: County Road A21 provides a shortcut between Highway 36 in Westwood to Highway 44. From A21, about 14 miles north of Highway 36 and 4.5 miles southwest of Highway 44, turn west onto Silver Lake Road (County Road 110) and proceed 5 miles to a junction with Forest Road 10. Following signed directions for Caribou Wilderness, turn right and travel on Road 10 for 0.4 mile to another junction. Remaining on Road 10, continue 0.2 mile, and then turn left at a road marked CARIBOU WILDERNESS EAST TRAILHEAD, CARIBOU LAKE. Follow this single-lane road for 0.1 mile to a fork, where the left-hand road leads shortly to a

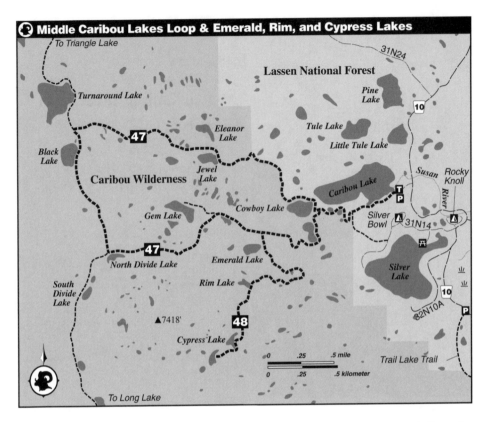

Middle Caribou Lakes Loop & Emerald, Rim, and Cypress Lakes

large parking area for backpackers, and the right-hand road leads just as shortly to the day-use trailhead above the Caribou Lake dam. The day-use trailhead has a trash can and a pit toilet.

DESCRIPTION: From the backpacker parking lot, make a short climb up a hillside to the trailhead above heavily fished Caribou Lake. From there, proceed west through a forest of lodgepole pines, Jeffrey pines, and firs above the lake. At 0.4 mile, pass a feeder trail from the private homes around Silver Lake, and then reach the signed boundary of Caribou Wilderness shortly afterward. The trail skirts a fair-size pond covered with lily pads and then passes a smaller pond before reaching a junction, 0.7 mile from the trailhead, where the loop section of the trip begins.

Take the right-hand trail, which very shortly brings you to the east shore of

Cowboy Lake, which is too shallow for decent swimming. However, the shoreline does provide a scenic spot from which to enjoy a view of the picturesque lake and its backdrop of low cliffs on the far side. The trail travels around the north shore of the lake to the west end.

From the lake's west end, turn sharply north-northwest on a moderate, switch-backing climb up an escarpment into a dry, open forest, where pinemat and greenleaf manzanita flourish and a few western junipers take root. Soon, the trail heads into deeper forest cover, and at the top of the climb, you reach Jewel Lake at 1.8 miles. Good and legal campsites may be found above the lake's north shore, as well as near the southwest shore of nearby Eleanor Lake, accessible from the main trail by a pair of use trails. Both of these shallow lakes possess their own charm—Jewel has a scenic setting and greater depth, and

Eleanor provides a sense of isolation and seclusion. Despite appearing on USGS and USFS maps, the connecting trail from the east end of Jewel Lake that heads south to the trail from Gem Lake no longer exists.

From Jewel Lake, the trail winds through an open forest past some small ponds before climbing moderately along the base of a brushy escarpment. Where the grade eases again, you pass more ponds, some seasonal in nature, before gently descending to a three-way junction, 3.2 miles from the trailhead. The trail north goes to Turnaround Lake, and the southern trail leads to Black Lake.

Turn left (south) and walk about 200 yards to the north shore of Black Lake, a pleasant body of water rimmed by forest with a rock cliff above the far shore. Fair campsites may be found along the south shore on either side of the usually dry outlet. The lake offers passable swimming and angling.

From Black Lake, the gently graded trail follows the outlet downstream through a forest primarily composed of lodgepole pines. Nearing the north shore of North Divide Lake, 4.2 miles from the trailhead, you reach a junction with the continuation of trail ahead to the string of lakes accessible primarily from the Hay Meadow Trailhead, and your trail east back toward the Caribou Lake Trailhead. Knee-to-waist-deep North Divide Lake offers marginal campsites. However, much better campsites exist above the west shore of deeper, though still shallow, South Divide Lake, just 0.3 mile to the south, across a stretch of flower-covered meadow and a small pocket of pine forest.

As you head east from the junction, the route passes above the north shore of North Divide Lake, crosses the usually dry and rocky channel of the outlet, and then crosses back over the channel to the north bank. Gently descending tread veers northeast and leads past a small pond on the way to a three-way junction at 5.2 miles.

S **SIDE TRIP TO GEM LAKE:** To visit Gem Lake, turn left at the three-way junction and head west up a gully for 0.2 miles, and over the lip of the lake's basin to the northeast shore. The lake is hemmed in on all sides by the topography, limiting potential campsites to a few small level areas away from the deteriorating tread of a use trail above the north shore. The scenic lake offers refreshing swimming and fair fishing. **END OF SIDE TRIP.**

Head southeast from the Gem Lake junction and stroll past a seasonal pond/meadow to a junction with the trail to Emerald, Rim, and Cypress lakes, 5.6 miles from the trailhead. Continue east-southeast on a moderate descent through mixed forest, interrupted briefly by a gently graded stretch of trail. Where the descent resumes, a series of switchbacks leads down the steep wall of an escarpment until the trail bottoms out near the base of a slope covered with large, blocky talus. Soon, the trail turns north and passes to the right of a large, unnamed pond before intersecting the main trail from Caribou Lake at the close of the loop section. From there, turn right (west) and retrace your steps 0.7 mile to the trailhead.

O Adding a side trip to Emerald, Rim, or Cypress lakes is a straightforward trip extension (see the description in Trip 48).

Trip **48**

Emerald, Rim, and Cypress Lakes

Ⓜ / DH, BP

DISTANCE:	7 miles out and back
ELEVATIONS:	6550/7155, +585/-585
SEASON:	Mid-June to late October
USE:	Light
MAPS:	*Bogard Buttes, Red Cinder*

INTRODUCTION: This out and back trip to a trio of lakes offers some of the best scenery in Caribou Wilderness. Each lake is picturesque in its own right, but the trail's sweeping views provide further attractions, and backpackers will find good campsites and fine swimming at each of the lakes. Most of the elevation gain occurs during the last 2.25 miles, which seems to deter the masses, as these lakes—especially Rim and Cypress—receive light use. From Cypress Lake, the straightforward cross-country route to the top of 7793-foot North Caribou Mountain provides another potentially rewarding endeavor.

DIRECTIONS TO TRAILHEAD: County Road A21 provides a shortcut between Highway 36 in Westwood to Highway 44. From A21, about 14 miles north of Highway 36 and 4.5 miles southwest of Highway 44, turn west onto Silver Lake Road (County Road 110) and proceed 5 miles to a junction with Forest Road 10. Following signed directions for Caribou Wilderness, turn right and travel on Road 10 for 0.4 mile to another junction. Remaining on Road 10, continue 0.2 mile, and then turn left at a road marked CARIBOU WILDERNESS EAST TRAILHEAD, CARIBOU LAKE. Follow this single-lane road for 0.1 mile to a fork, where the left-hand road leads shortly to a

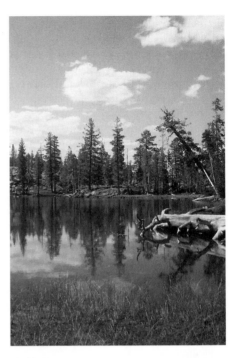

Rim Lake

large parking area for backpackers, and the right-hand road leads just as shortly to the day-use trailhead above the Caribou Lake dam. The day-use trailhead has a trash can and a pit toilet.

DESCRIPTION: From the backpacker parking lot, make a short climb up a hillside to the trailhead above heavily fished Caribou Lake. From there, proceed west through a forest of lodgepole pines, Jeffrey pines, and firs above the lake. At 0.4 mile, pass a feeder trail from the private homes around Silver Lake, and then reach the signed boundary of Caribou Wilderness shortly afterward. The trail skirts a fair-size pond covered with lily pads and then passes a smaller pond before reaching a junction, 0.7 mile from the trailhead.

Turn left (south) at the junction and pass a large, unnamed pond before the trail angles west and then attacks the wall of a steep escarpment via a set of switchbacks. The grade eases at the top to a gentle ascent through mixed forest on the way to a junction at 1.6 miles.

Veer left (south) and make a brief climb through open forest with pinemat manzanita covering the forest floor to the northeast shore of Emerald Lake, one of the deepest lakes in Caribou Wilderness. The low, rocky bench above the north shore has several good campsites and sunny perches for lounging. Anglers should find the fishing to be fair to good. Because of the lake's depth, swimming is refreshing throughout the summer season.

Beyond the steep-sided bowl of Emerald Lake, the trail winds through mostly open terrain past a seasonal pond/meadow to the edge of an escarpment with a good view of Caribou and Silver lakes and the surrounding terrain. The trail then courses through sparsely forested bedrock slabs toward Rim Lake. Because of the slabs, the trail may be hard to discern at times, but a preponderance of ducks should keep you on track. If you do happen to lose the route, simply proceed upslope toward the west for about 0.5 mile, and you're almost certain to run into Rim Lake. On a hot day, pleasant Rim Lake is inviting for swimmers; look for deeper waters and diving rocks midway along the south shore. Spartan campsites are available between rock slabs without much shade, but the sweeping views from the edge of the escarpment make camping here worthwhile. The persistent breeze helps keep the mosquitoes at bay in midseason.

A winding, rocky trail climbs away from Rim Lake for 0.5 mile to an unnamed lake back-dropped by a prominent escarpment. The trail swings around the lake's south arm, which is also at the brink of an escarpment, and then rolls over a low divide to Cypress Lake.

Rockbound and scenic Cypress Lake was named for the few western junipers in the vicinity—true cypress trees are nonexistent in these parts. Secluded campsites may be found among the small slabs and gravel flats tucked around the lakeshore.

From the low divide near Cypress Lake, the cross-country route south up to the summit of North Caribou Mountain takes about an hour.

Trip **49**

Trail Lake from Silver Lake

E / DH

DISTANCE: 1.8 miles out and back
ELEVATIONS: 6520/6535, Negligible
SEASON: Late May to late October
USE: Light
MAP: *Red Cinder*

INTRODUCTION: Just south of the summer resort area Silver Lake, a little-used path offers a gently graded stroll to shallow, forest-rimmed Trail Lake, a classic example of the numerous lakes that dot this part of Lassen National Forest. Although this description ends at the lake, the trail continues another 3-plus miles to a trailhead near Echo Lake (see Trip 50). Be aware that this is a designated mountain bike route, but chances are slim that you'll encounter anyone, whether on a bike, on foot, or on a horse. Parking is extremely limited at the Silver Lake Trailhead but appears to be more than adequate for the extremely limited amount of use the trail receives.

DIRECTIONS TO TRAILHEAD: County Road A21 provides a shortcut between Highway 36 in Westwood to Highway 44. From A21, about 14 miles north of Highway 36 and 4.5 miles southwest of Highway 44, turn west onto Silver Lake Road (County Road 110) and proceed 5 miles to a junction of Forest Road 10. Turn left and remain on Road 10 at all junctions. After 0.9 mile, reach the signed trailhead on the right side of the road, 5.8 miles from Road A21. Park in the limited space along the opposite shoulder.

DESCRIPTION: Start climbing south, away from the road, up a hillside amid a scattered to light mixed forest of lodgepole, ponderosa, western white pines, and firs,

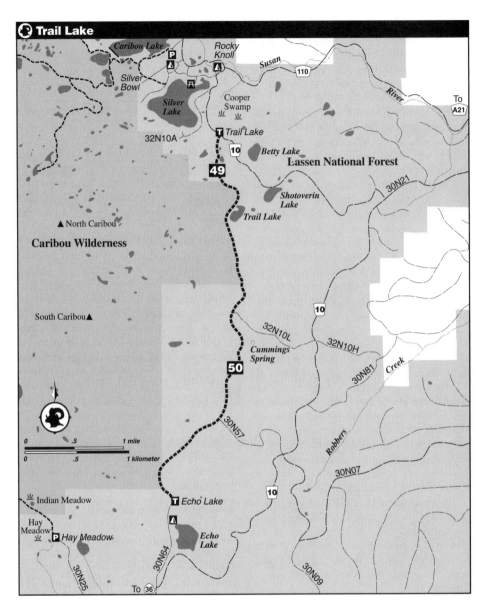

where logging has left an unsightly mark on the area. Fortunately, the ugly logging scar is soon behind you, as gently graded trail leads through intact forest. Pass a rocky depression on the left that doubles as a pond early in season before drying up into a grassy meadow by midsummer. Farther on, pass by a couple of meadows, as the trail comes alongside and then follows the boundary of Caribou Wilderness, which is immediately to the west. Soon reach the tree- and grass-rimmed lake to the left of the trail, which then continues onward to a trailhead near Echo Lake.

ECHO LAKE TRAILHEAD

Trip **50**

see
map on
p.156

Trail Lake
from Echo Lake

E ↗ DH

DISTANCE: 7.4 miles out and back

ELEVATIONS: 6510/6540, +810/-810

SEASON: Late May to late October

USE: Light

MAP: *Red Cinder*

INTRODUCTION: This trip takes the long way to Trail Lake from a trailhead near Echo Lake. The route to shallow, forest-rimmed Trail Lake is fairly uneventful, passing through a mixed forest typical of the many lakes and ponds in this part of Lassen National Forest. Even fewer souls elect to take this route to the lake than the ones who start at the Silver Lake Trailhead. This trail may be more than five times as long, but it guarantees solitude.

DIRECTIONS TO TRAILHEAD: From Highway 36, opposite County Road A13 (about 5 miles east of Chester and 8 miles west of County Road A21 in Westwood), turn north onto Forest Road 10, which bends left at a T-junction very soon after leaving the highway. At 0.6 mile from Highway 36, Road 10 bends sharply right (north).

After 9 miles, the paved surface gives way to gravel, and at 10.5 miles from Highway 36, Road 10 bends to the right at a junction. Now continue straight ahead on Forest Road 30N64, signed ECHO LAKE. Follow Road 30N64 past a turnoff into the primitive Echo Lake Campground and proceed to the turnaround at the end of the road, 11.5 miles from Highway 36. The trail begins a short walk back down the road, but there is no room to park right at the trailhead.

DESCRIPTION: A mild to moderate climb north leads through a mixed forest of firs, lodgepole pines, and western white pines until the grade eases after 0.3 mile. Pinemat manzanita, interspersed with some wildflowers in early season, is the principal groundcover. Near the 0.75-mile mark, the trail begins a general descent, and at 1.2 miles, crosses an old road. You reach the bottom of the descent just before 2 miles and then climb moderately through more open forest with an understory of tobacco brush, pinemat manzanita, greenleaf manzanita, and chinquapin. A very brief descent leads to a survey monument in a pile of rocks with blue paint around the base. From here to the lake, the trail follows the eastern boundary of Caribou Wilderness.

Another stretch of mild to moderate climbing is followed by a moderately steep descent into the lake's basin. Through thicker forest, you then follow gently graded trail past a seasonal pond/meadow to the south shore of Trail Lake. As described in Trip 49, it is possible to continue north on this trail to the Silver Lake Trailhead.

Trip **51**

Beauty, Evelyn, Long, and Hidden Lakes Loop

(M) (Q) DH, BP

DISTANCE: 7.2 miles loop

ELEVATIONS: 6940/7040/6940, +700/-700

SEASON: Mid-June to late October

USE: Light

MAP: *Red Cinder*

INTRODUCTION: Gentle terrain and a host of lakes make this loop trip from the Hay Meadow Trailhead a pleasant experience. Similar to just about anywhere in Caribou Wilderness, this area is not heavily used,

despite the high number of desirable places to camp, fish, and swim, and the relative ease of getting around. Following the loop in a clockwise direction, as described here, avoids the only steep section on the circuit, a quarter-mile stretch of trail below Hidden Lakes. If you have extra time, take one of the connecting trails to additional lakes farther north in the wilderness.

DIRECTIONS TO TRAILHEAD: From Highway 36, opposite County Road A13 (about 5 miles east of Chester and 8 miles west of County Road A21 in Westwood), turn north onto Forest Road 10, which bends left at a T-junction very soon after leaving the highway. At 0.6 mile from Highway 36, Road 10 bends sharply right (north). Around the 9-mile mark, the paved surface gives way to gravel. At 10 miles, turn left onto Forest Road 30N25 and proceed 1.4 miles to a junction with Forest Road 30N72 on the left. Proceed straight ahead at the junction

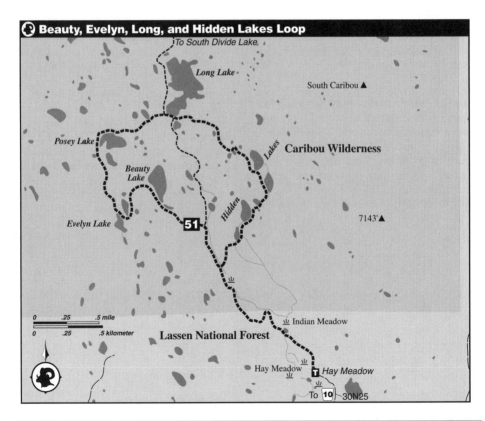

Beauty, Evelyn, Long, and Hidden Lakes Loop

To South Divide Lake

Long Lake

South Caribou ▲

Posey Lake

Caribou Wilderness

Beauty Lake

Evelyn Lake

Hidden Lakes

7143'▲

51

Lassen National Forest

Indian Meadow

Hay Meadow ᵀ Hay Meadow

To 10 30N25

for 0.2 mile to the wide turnaround at the Hay Meadow Trailhead, 11.6 miles from Highway 36. The trailhead is equipped with a modern vault toilet.

DESCRIPTION: The trail begins on a lodgepole-shaded path that skirts the northeast edge of expansive Hay Meadow, filled with grasses, sedges, and pockets of willow. Past the meadow, you cross the wilderness boundary and follow gently graded trail beneath a shady forest of lodgepole and western white pines to the south end of Indian Meadow, which sports a shallow pond through midsummer. Pass around the meadow's southwest edge and hop across the stream that drains it. In early season, the trail is lined with a fine assortment of corn lily, buttercup, gentian, lupine, and aster. Farther on, a steady climb leads alongside and then follows a flower-lined seasonal stream to a junction with the trail to Hidden Lakes at the start of the loop section, 1.3 miles from the trailhead.

Veer left and continue along the stream's channel until the trail ascends an open, pinemat manzanita-covered hillside. At 1.6 miles, reach a junction, where the right-hand trail provides a direct shortcut to the south shore of Long Lake in just over a mile.

For the scenic route, follow the left-hand trail northwest on a half-mile, moderate climb to Beauty Lake. Though it's a good-sized lake in surface area, Beauty Lake is fairly shallow, providing warm and enjoyable swimming, at least before the typical afternoon windchill takes effect. Overnighters should search for campsites along the west shore just north of where the trail leaves the lakeshore.

Beyond Beauty Lake, the trail arcs around a small, linear lake on the way to Evelyn Lake. Good campsites may be found on high ground to the north of Evelyn Lake, and anglers should find the fishing to be fair.

Beyond Evelyn Lake, the trail ascends north to top a low ridge, the high point of the route, and then drops toward Posey Lake's west shore. Except in early season, the lake is composed of a southern, large, neck-deep wading pond barely separated from a northern, larger, shallow lake. Campsites may be found on the southwest peninsula, or above the north shore.

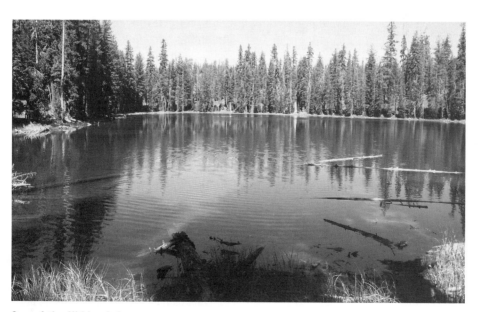

One of the Hidden Lakes

Rolling trail leads away from Evelyn Lake to the vicinity of a bilobed pond. Stroll across a grassy swale and then follow gently descending trail through the trees to a junction, 3.8 miles from the trailhead, near the southwest shore of Long Lake, one of the largest lakes in Caribou Wilderness. To visit or camp at Long Lake, head north from the junction along the west shore. Some of the campsites afford views of North Caribou and South Caribou mountains. Beyond the lake, this trail continues north to South and North Divide lakes and the rest of the lakes in the midsection of Caribou Wilderness (see Trip 47).

To continue the loop, proceed ahead from the junction a short distance to another three-way junction, this one with a shortcut between Long Lake and the Hay Meadow Trailhead. Continue ahead (east) past a rocky depression that holds early-season overflow from Long Lake and a use trail to campsites along the east shore. After 0.3 mile, the trail bends south, passes a shallow pond, and, near a hillside of blocky talus, enters a more open stretch of forest with an understory of manzanita. Pass more shallow ponds on the way to the first of the five Hidden Lakes, Hidden Lake 5. Fair campsites will entice overnighters on the flat divide between Lake 5 and Lake 4. These are the deepest of the Hidden Lakes, and offer the best scenery as well.

Beyond Lake 4, the trail follows the usually dry outlet down to Lake 3, a shallow, warm, and fairly uninteresting body of water. A short drop then leads to Lake 2, which is fair-size and offers the best swimming conditions of all the Hidden Lakes. From there, a short stroll brings you to Lake 1, a small, shallow lake rimmed by grasses and lodgepole pines. Past the Hidden Lakes, a moderate to moderately steep descent winds down a hillside before bottoming out near some pocket meadows on the way to the close of the loop at the junction. Turn south to retrace your steps 1.3 miles to the trailhead.

Introduction to the Greater Susanville-Chester Area

Somewhat overlooked as a recreational area in the greater Lassen region, the lands around the communities of Susanville and Chester do offer a few opportunities for trail users. Eagle Lake, north of Susanville, has a paved recreation trail that runs nearly 5 miles along the south shore of California's second largest natural lake. A second, shorter trail offers a chance to see an osprey nest and enjoy sweeping views across the lake. From the center of Susanville, the Bizz Johnson Trail follows the grade of the old Fernley & Lassen Branch Line of the Southern Pacific Railroad 30 miles to Westwood. Similar to the Eagle Lake Recreation Trail, an 11-mile paved trail runs along the south shore of Lake Almanor.

Access

State highways 36, 44, and 89 provide the principal access to this area. County Road A1 leads to the south shore of Eagle Lake from Highway 36.

Amenities

Both Susanville and Chester are full-service communities offering motels, bed-and-breakfast inns, restaurants, gas stations, and stores. Chester also has a couple sporting goods stores where hikers can find a limited selection of gear.

Ranger Stations and Visitor Information

Lassen National Forest headquarters is located in Susanville, the Almanor Ranger District office is in Chester, and the Eagle Lake Ranger District office is near the County Road A1 and Highway 36 junction.

Good to Know Before You Go

During the height of summer, reservations (if available) are recommended for popular campgrounds in this area.

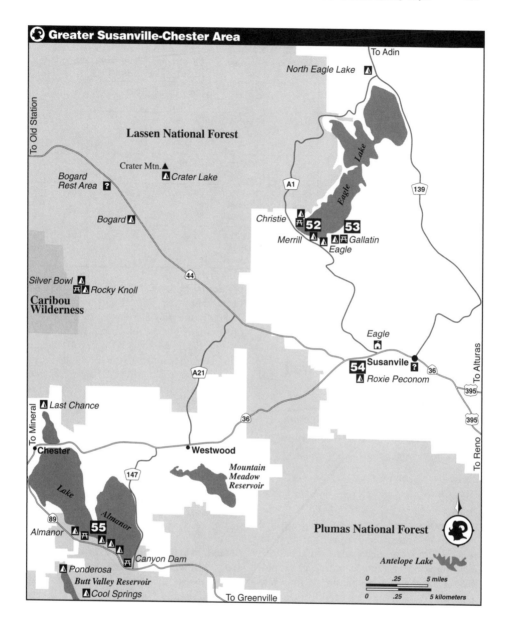

Greater Susanville-Chester Area

To Adin

North Eagle Lake

Lassen National Forest

To Old Station

Crater Mtn.

Bogard
Rest Area

Crater Lake

A1

139

Bogard

Christie

52 53

Merrill   Gallatin
Eagle

Silver Bowl
Rocky Knoll

Caribou
Wilderness

44

Eagle

A21

54 Susanvile

Roxie Peconom

36

To Alturas

395

To Mineral

Last Chance

395

To Reno

36

Chester   Westwood

147

Mountain
Meadow
Reservoir

Lake

89

Almanor   55

Almanor

Plumas National Forest

Canyon Dam

Ponderosa
Butt Valley Reservoir
Cool Springs

To Greenville

Antelope Lake

0   .25   5 miles

0   .25   5 kilometers

Campgrounds

Campground	Fee	Elevation	Season	Restrooms	Running Water	Bear Boxes
Goumaz (30N03, 7 miles NW of 36)	$10	5200′	May to October	Vault	No	No
Roxie Penconom (29N03, 2.3 miles S of 36)	No fee	4800′	May to October	Vault	Yes	No
Almanor (Lake Almanor)	$18	4500′	May to October	Vault	Yes	No
Rocky Point (PG&E) (Lake Almanor)	$18	4500′	Mid-May to mid-October	Flush	Yes	No
Last Chance (PG&E) (2 miles N of 36)	$18	4500′	Mid-May to mid-October	Flush	Yes	No

EAGLE LAKE TRAILHEADS

Trip **52**

Eagle Lake Recreation Trail

E / DH

DISTANCE: 4.5 miles point to point

ELEVATIONS: 5145/5140, Negligible

SEASON: May to late October

USE: Light

MAP: *Pikes Point*

INTRODUCTION: The nearly 5-mile, paved Eagle Lake Recreation Trail runs around the south shore of its namesake lake, connecting campgrounds, picnic areas, an amphitheater, a swimming beach, boat ramps, and a marina. A diverse group of visitors use the path during the summer months, including dog walkers, hikers, joggers, bicyclists, in-line skaters, skateboarders, anglers, boaters, photographers, and bird-watchers. All of this activity is a far cry from the serenity found on a backcountry trail, but the lake's sweeping scenery and wildlife-viewing opportunities are fine rewards in and of themselves. Don't forget to pack a picnic lunch and a swimsuit.

DIRECTIONS TO TRAILHEAD: START: Leave Highway 36, about 3 miles west of Susanville and 3 miles east of the junction with Highway 44, and head north on County Road A1 for 13.3 miles. At a junction near the south shore of Eagle Lake, remain on A1, and travel 2.5 more miles to the Christie day-use parking area (equipped with a modern vault toilet and picnic tables) along the southwest shore.

END: From the junction near the south shore of Eagle Lake, head northeast on County Road 231, past turnoffs for Eagle Campground, Gallatin Marina, and Aspen Grove Campground, to a left turn on the access road for Gallatin Beach. Park in the day-use area at the end of the road.

DESCRIPTION: From the Christie day-use area, follow either paved trail or closed road toward the lakeshore to the Eagle Lake Recreation Trail, coming from Christie Campground. Head right (southeast) on the wide, paved trail that skirts the south shoreline of giant Eagle Lake along the fringe of a mixed forest of Jeffrey pines, incense cedars, and firs. The usually abundant waterfowl bobbing on the surface and gliding through the sky complements the sweeping views of the lake from the trail. Depending on the season, the path may be lined with bright dashes of color from lupines in early

EAGLE LAKE

At 37,013 acres, Eagle Lake is California's second largest natural lake. The massive Brockman Flat Lava Flow on the west side blocked the lake's outlet, creating a closed basin that subsequently raised the alkalinity of the water. Eagle Lake trout, a subspecies of rainbow trout, have adapted to the higher alkalinity, allowing anglers the opportunity to fish for 3- 5-pound specimens. The lake is also home to a vast number of waterfowl, including Canada geese, western grebes, white pelicans, herons, and bald eagles.

the highway. Cross the access road and proceed to the east end of the campground, where a bridge spans Merrill Creek. Shortly, you walk across the road to the amphitheater.

Beyond Merrill Campground, the trail stays a good distance away from the shoreline. Past a handful of private residences, it takes you closer to the lake on the way past West Eagle Group Campground. Shortly afterward, as the path arcs northwest to match the shoreline's curve toward Pikes Point, you reach a signed T-junction, 3.6 miles from the parking area. The left-hand trail follows the lakeshore to a marina, which also has a small store, laundry, showers, and restrooms.

Take the right-hand trail toward Gallatin Beach, through a previously logged forest of Jeffrey pines. After 0.3 mile, cross the marina's access road and immediately reach a T-junction with the left-hand path that parallels the access road to the marina.

summer and yellow flowers of rabbitbrush in late summer and early fall.

Approaching Merrill Campground, the trail heads inland to squeeze through a thin strip of fenced land between campsites and

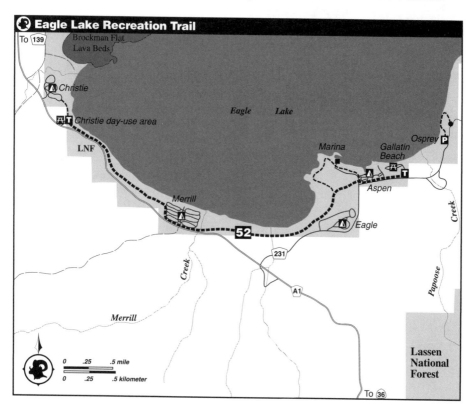

Turn right and follow Gallatin Road past a day-use parking area and across the access road into Aspen Group Campground before reaching the end of the trail at the road to Gallatin Beach. A short walk down the road leads to a parking area with restrooms, picnic tables, and barbecues just above the swimming beach.

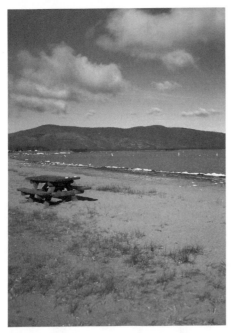

Gallatin Beach

Trip **53**

Osprey Overlook Trail

E ✓ DH

DISTANCE: 1.2 miles out and back

ELEVATIONS: 5200/5295, +255/-255

SEASON: May to late October

USE: Light

MAP: *Pikes Point*

INTRODUCTION: Any casual observation of Eagle Lake reveals a vast number of waterfowl floating on or flying above the surface. One of the more interesting members of the lake's avian community is the osprey, a black and white hawk that feeds almost exclusively on fish. Some time ago, wildlife biologists hoping to lure ospreys placed an osprey nest on the top of a Jeffrey pine snag near the southeast shore of the lake, which visitors can glimpse from this short and easy trail. With a little more energy, you can continue along the shoreline and then up a steep hillside to an overlook for excellent views across the large lake. The overlook, which is equipped for telescopes and has a picnic table nearby, is wheelchair accessible.

DIRECTIONS TO TRAILHEAD: Leave Highway 36 about 3 miles west of Susanville and 3 miles east of the junction with Highway 44, and head north on County Road A1 for 13.3 miles to a junction near the south shore of Eagle Lake. Turn right and follow Gallatin Road (County Road 231) 1.5 miles to a junction with the Forest Road 31N79 to the marina. Turn right again, this time following signs for Ronald McDonald Camp, and continue ahead at a junction with a road to Gallatin Beach in 0.5 mile. Pass Ronald McDonald Camp and soon reach the marked Osprey Overlook Trailhead on the left, 2.6 miles from Road A1. The main road on the right, which is now Forest Road

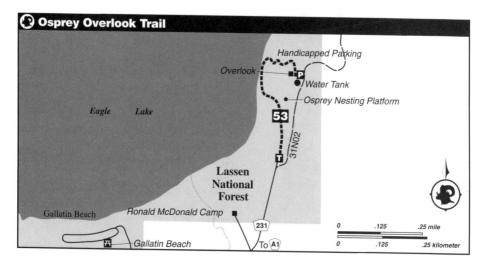

Osprey Overlook Trail

Handicapped Parking

Overlook

Water Tank

Osprey Nesting Platform

Eagle   Lake

53

31N02

Lassen
National
Forest

Gallatin Beach   Ronald McDonald Camp

231

Gallatin Beach

To A1

0   .125   .25 mile

0   .125   .25 kilometer

31N02, continues up a hillside a quarter mile to a handicapped parking area (two spaces) for access to the overlook at the upper end of the trail.

DESCRIPTION: Grab a pamphlet from the trailhead signboard and follow single-track trail north, immediately intersecting a path from the Ronald McDonald Camp and then merging with the wide track of an old road through Jeffrey pine forest, with an understory of sagebrush and rabbitbrush. A wood-pole fence heralds your arrival at the site of the osprey nest atop a Jeffrey pine. Wildlife biologists hoping to lure ospreys placed the nest here, and occasionally the birds comply. When the nest is occupied, please limit your noise and activity.

Away from the nesting area, the trail turns west and descends toward the shoreline. Most visitors go no farther than the nesting area, so the continuation of the trail

north along the edge of the lake may be hard to locate. The trail traverses across the hillside just above the shore, passing through a deeper forest of Jeffrey pines, mountain mahoganies, incense cedars, western junipers, white firs, and ponderosa pines. Along the way, you have good views of the lake. All too soon, the grade increased as the trail attacks the hillside via a switchbacking climb toward the lookout.

At the top, a short, paved path leads to the overlook, which provides sweeping views across Eagle Lake to the west shore. Three interpretive signs here provide information about bald eagles and ospreys; bring binoculars for bird-watching. A picnic table and trash can are located near the handicapped parking area, and a nearby water tank has a mural painted on the side that depicts the natural environment around Eagle Lake. After fully absorbing the view, retrace your steps to the trailhead.

SUSANVILLE TRAILHEAD

Trip 54

Bizz Johnson Trail

ⓔ / DH

DISTANCE: 6.5 miles point to point

ELEVATIONS: 4225/4675, +450

SEASON: March to late December

USE: Moderate

MAPS: *Susanville, Roop Mountain*

INTRODUCTION: The Bizz Johnson Trail follows the historic route of the Fernley Lassen Railroad between the communities of Susanville and Westwood. The railroad was built in 1914 primarily to carry logs from a mill in Westwood to Fernley,

Nevada, where lumber products were then shipped around the country and also to foreign markets. The mill's eventual decline in 1956 signaled the end of the railroad. In 1978, Southern Pacific Railroad abandoned the line, and eventually, 30 miles of the route was converted to recreational trail. The trail is named for Harold T. "Bizz" Johnson, a California congressman who championed the cause of the trail in the U.S. House of Representatives.

The gently graded trail, with a maximum 3-percent grade, is open to hikers, equestrians, mountain bikers, and cross-country skiers (when snow cover is adequate) from Susanville to Devils Corral. Beyond Devils Corral, snowmobiles are allowed to use the trail in winter, and motor vehicles have access to the trail 2.4 miles west of the Goumaz Trailhead (15.1 miles from Susanville). Therefore, the section of trail from the train depot in Susanville to

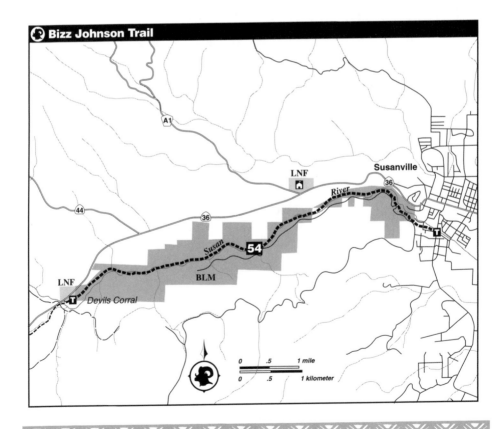

Bizz Johnson Trail

the Devils Corral Trailhead will be the most attractive to those on foot. Once past the development of Susanville, the trail follows the Susan River through a volcanic canyon beneath mixed forest and alongside riparian vegetation. Between the two trailheads, hikers pass through two tunnels and over seven bridges.

DIRECTIONS TO TRAILHEAD: START: From Main Street (Highway 36) in the old downtown district of Susanville, head south-southwest on Weatherlow Street, which becomes Richmond Road after 0.2 mile. Continue on Richmond Road to the historic Susanville railroad depot (about a half mile from Main Street), which is equipped with a visitor center and interpretive displays.

END: From Susanville, head west on Highway 36 to the turnoff to Devils Corral Trailhead, about 7 miles from town. Take the paved access road 0.2 mile to the parking area, which features a vault toilet, picnic tables, and an information board.

DESCRIPTION: Follow the trail northwest, along the Susan River through the outskirts of Susanville, for the first 0.7 mile before you leave civilization behind for a more pristine section of the canyon. Swimmers and anglers can take various paths to the river on the way to a pair of bridges—one at 1.4 miles, and another just after it. A ponderosa pine shaded log bench offers a fine place to rest and enjoy the river scene a half mile farther. A pair of tunnels at 4.7 and 5 miles are carved out of the volcanic basalt that comprises the canyon walls. Proceed upstream, crossing the river on four bridges on the way to Devils Corral Trailhead.

O The trail's main users are mountain bikers. Every weekday throughout the year and on limited weekends from June to mid-October, a shuttle bus serves four stops along the 30-mile route. Check out the website at www.bizzjohnsontrail.com or call (530) 257-4323 for more information.

Trip 55

Lake Almanor Recreation Trail

E ⁄ DH

DISTANCE:	9.5 mile point to point
ELEVATIONS:	4580/4540, Negligible
SEASON:	March to late October
USE:	Heavy
MAPS:	*Almanor, Canyon Dam*

INTRODUCTION: A hike along the Lake Almanor Recreation Trail is far from a wilderness experience, but this paved path provides a pleasant tour along the southwest side of the lake through campgrounds, picnic areas, and summer homes. Several access points allow trail users to shorten the journey, which provides plenty of good lake views, as well as sights of Lassen Peak and other summits within the park, and Dyer Mountain to the northeast. Pack a picnic lunch, swimsuit, or fishing pole for added fun.

DIRECTIONS TO TRAILHEAD: From Highway 36 just west of Chester, head south on State Highway 89 about 4.4 miles to a dirt road opposite the Humbug/Humboldt Road. The northernmost parking area is just a short drive northeast. The trail can also be accessed from parking areas for the Almanor boat ramp, Dyer View day-use area, and three PG&E campgrounds on the southwest shore.

DESCRIPTION: From the parking area, head southeast. The Lake Almanor Recreation Trail is the most civilized path in this guidebook, a 10-foot wide, paved path that winds along the southwest shore of the lake. Joggers, inline skaters, dog walkers, bicyclists, anglers, and naturalists commonly use portions of the trail. The 9.5-mile trail passes through stands of mixed forest, mountain meadow, and developed

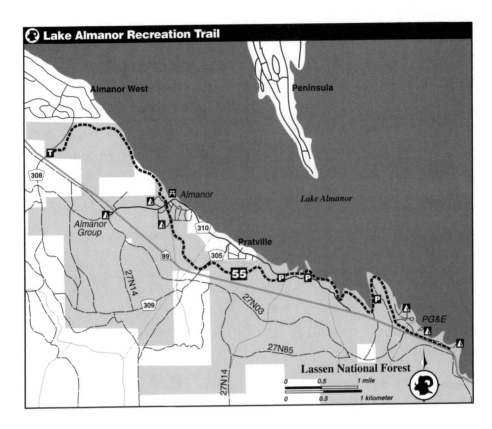

areas. Views along the way include Dyer Mountain to the northeast and peaks within Lassen National Park. Along with a wide variety of waterfowl, you should watch for osprey and bald eagles.

Introduction to Juniper Lake

Located in the southeast corner of Lassen Volcanic, Juniper Lake is the park's least-crowded camping, fishing, and hiking area. The small campground near the lake's south end is rarely full, and the miles of backcountry trails that depart from here are blissfully lonely. The lack of visitors is not surprising, for although the scenery rivals that of any other part of the park, the trailheads around Juniper Lake are the most difficult to reach, near the end of a dirt road that is much rougher in spots and more poorly graded than those to Butte Lake and Drakesbad. However, this minor annoyance has some benefits, as unspoiled wilderness is preserved for those who are willing to make the journey.

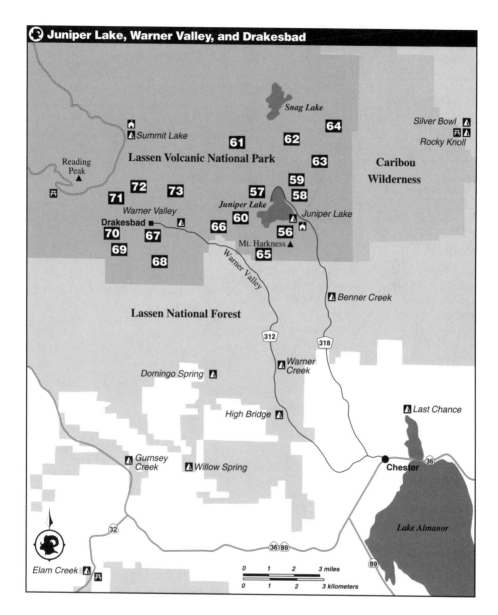

Juniper Lake, Warner Valley, and Drakesbad

Snag Lake

64

Silver Bowl

Rocky Knoll

Summit Lake

61

62

Reading Peak

Lassen Volcanic National Park

63

Caribou Wilderness

72   73

59

58

71

57

Warner Valley

Juniper Lake

Juniper Lake

Drakesbad

60

70   67

66

56

Mt. Harkness

69

68

65

Warner Valley

Benner Creek

Lassen National Forest

312

318

Warner Creek

Domingo Spring

Last Chance

High Bridge

Gurnsey Creek

Willow Spring

Chester

36

32

36 89

89

Lake Almanor

Elam Creek

0   1   2   3 miles

0   1   2   3 kilometers

The first trail climbs the area's most prominent peak, Mt. Harkness, offering one of the best park views from the summit lookout. Next comes the loop around Juniper Lake, combining stretches of little-used, single-track trail and a section of dirt road for a circumnavigation of the lakeshore. Short treks to Crystal Lake and Inspiration Point involve straightforward hikes to a fine swimming hole and an excellent vista. Four out of the next five trips are loops through the seldom-visited backcountry—great options for backpackers with plenty of time to enjoy the wilderness, or for dayhikers in excellent condition. The other hike is a short journey to remote Jakey Lake.

Campgrounds

Campground	Fee	Elevation	Season	Restrooms	Running Water	Bear Boxes
Benner Creek (Juniper Lake Road)	$11	5500'	May to October	Vault	No	No
Juniper Lake	$10	6790'	Early July to late September	Vault	Yes	Yes
High Bridge (Warner Valley Road)	$13	5200'	May to October	Vault	Yes	No
Warner Creek (Warner Valley Road)	$11	5500'	May to October	Vault	No	No
Warner Valley	$14	5650'	Early June to late September	Vault	Yes	Yes

Access

From Highway 36 in Chester, the Feather River Road leads to a junction of County Roads 318 and 312. Road 318 becomes the Juniper Lake Road, which leads to Juniper Lake, and Road 312 becomes the Warner Valley Road, which leads to Warner Valley and Drakesbad. Both roads eventually turn to a dirt surface, and trailers are not advised on the Juniper Lake Road.

Amenities

Heading west on Highway 36 from the junction of Highway 44, you pass through the tiny community of Westwood, with a gas station, store, and motel, on the way to Chester, the commercial hub for the greater Lake Almanor area. Chester does have a couple of sporting goods stores along with an array of restaurants, motels, bed and breakfast inns, gas stations, golf courses, and stores. From Chester, County Road 312 (Warner Valley Road) leads 17 miles to Drakesbad Guest Ranch, which is open from June to early October (for reservations call 530-529-1512 or visit the website at www.drakesbad.com). Highway 36 continues 10 miles west from Chester to St. Bernard Lodge, complete with restaurant, tavern, stables, and seven guest rooms. Call 530-258-3382 for reservations or for restaurant hours, as the restaurant is generally not open every day of the week.

Ranger Stations and Visitor Information

Within Lassen Volcanic, the seasonal Juniper Lake Ranger Station is located near the road just south of the lake. The nearest year-round Forest Service ranger station is in Chester, toward the west end of town.

Good to Know Before You Go

Since the Juniper Lake Road is not suited for trailers, the seldom-full Juniper Lake Campground provides a fine basecamp for dayhiking the surrounding trails.

JUNIPER LAKE TRAILHEADS

Trip 56

Mount Harkness

MS ⟋ ⟲ DH

DISTANCE: 3.8 miles out and back; 5.6 miles loop

ELEVATIONS: 6800/8646, +1846/-1846 out and back; +1925/-1925 loop

SEASON: Early July to October

USE: Light

MAP: *Mount Harkness*

INTRODUCTION: From the lookout atop Mt. Harkness, snow-capped Lassen Peak and the rest of the peaks along ancient Mt.

Tehama's rim seem close enough to touch. The impressive vista extends far beyond the park boundary, encompassing an expansive section of the northern Sierra and southern Cascades. Although the climb is stiff, the trip is short enough that just about anyone in reasonable condition can manage it. Unlike most fire lookouts today, the Mt. Harkness lookout is still staffed, so plan on a friendly welcome from the resident park employee. As with all high peaks, avoid the upper slopes when lightning threatens. Thanks to the fine network of connecting trails within the park, hikers with extra time and energy can alter their return by following a loop along the south shore of Juniper Lake back to the trailhead.

DIRECTIONS TO TRAILHEAD: From Highway 36 in Chester, take Feather River Road west-northwest for just over a half mile and veer right on County Road 318, following signed directions for Juniper Lake. Cross

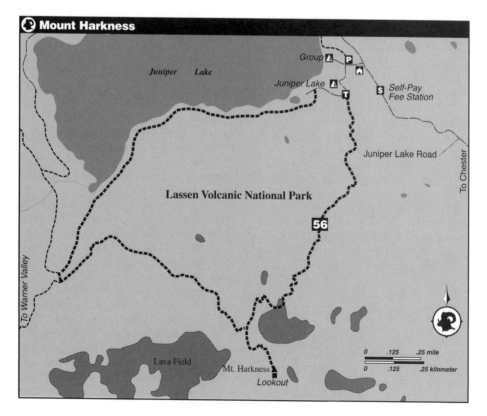

into national park land at 8.8 miles from Highway 36, and proceed to the self-pay registration station across from the ranger station at 11.1 miles. Continue a short distance to a signed, left turn into Juniper Lake Campground. Follow the campground access road a short distance to a dirt trailhead parking area on the right. From the parking area, walk west to a fork, veer left, and continue to the Mt. Harkness Trailhead near Campsite #5.

DESCRIPTION: The trail begins with a mild climb south that quickly increases to moderate through a viewless forest of red firs, western white pines, and lodgepole pines. Switchbacks take you farther up the hillside to where mountain hemlocks first appear. The grade increases on the approach to more open slopes around 7500 feet, where a prominent cliff of gray rock appears on the left, a ridge of similar rock is to the right, and slopes of rubblelike red cinders are ahead.

A 500-foot climb awaits from the base of the cinder cone to the fire lookout on the rim of the peak. Start west, climbing steeply through a grove of hemlocks to a nearby volcanic ridge, where you have a fine view of the cinder cone. The northern third of the cone was removed by various erosive processes, leaving behind a conspicuous bowl. The trail climbs another 130 yards along the west rim of the bowl to a junction with a trail from Warner Valley (see Trip 65).

The raucous sound of Clark's nutcrackers among the few remaining whitebark pines may accompany you on a climb across gravely slopes, bedecked with acres of silver-leaved lupine and Bloomer's goldenbush through midseason. The trail crosses a lightning ground wire from the lookout and signs advise passersby that touching it is unwise. A few last switchbacks take you to the crater rim, where the lookout springs into view.

An easy stroll leads to the base, followed by a short climb of the stairs to the deck that runs around the perimeter of the fire lookout. Unlike most fire lookouts today, the one atop Mt. Harkness is still staffed,

---

GEOLOGY OF MOUNT HARKNESS

By geological standards, Mt. Harkness is considered an andesitic shield volcano, which means it has a post-glacial cinder cone summit. The gray rock outcrops are composed of lava flows that oozed from the summit during the peak's more recent geologic history. After these flows, the summit area was either eroded away, blown out by a new eruption, or a combination of the two, and then it was replaced by a cinder cone after the last glacial period.

During this last icy period, small glaciers descended outward from Mt. Harkness, particularly on the north side, mildly eroding the mountain. Most of the glaciers united with a large ice cap that spilled south from the ridge north of Juniper Lake, flowing partly into Warner Valley but mostly down the Benner Creek drainage, through which is now the road to Juniper Lake.

---

and a park employee will most likely welcome you into his or her summer residence. The lookout is equipped with a stove, and fuel and supplies are flown in by helicopter at the beginning of the season. The park employee makes once-a-week trips to Chester to acquire additional supplies, such as fresh produce.

The view from the lookout is stunning. With Lassen Peak as a reference point, most of the park's prominent features are easy to identify. The long, sometimes snowy ridge extending south from Lassen Peak is composed of the northwest flank of ancient Mt. Tehama, an ice age volcano heavily eroded by glaciers. The highest remnant is Brokeoff Mountain, at the apex of the ridge's south end, and the high point just north of Brokeoff is Mt. Diller. Clockwise from Lassen Peak, the relatively close peak is Saddle Mountain, sloping down into Warner Valley. In the distance, Chaos Crags

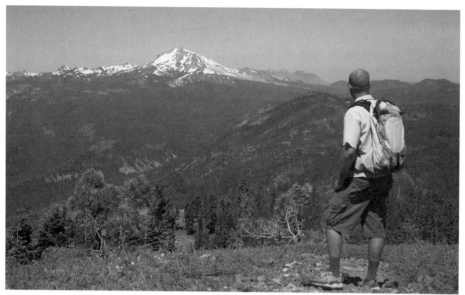

Lassen Peak from Mt. Harkness

stand above and mostly left of Saddle Mountain. Hat Mountain is the conspicuous, flat-topped cinder cone breaking the horizon just right of Saddle Mountain, while above and beyond the west shore of Juniper Lake lies Fairfield Peak. Rising just right and behind Fairfield is West Prospect Peak, connected to slightly higher Prospect Peak. At the base of Prospect Peak, famous Cinder Cone barely peeks over the ridge above the north corner of Juniper Lake. Mt. Hoffman, with steep southwest-facing slopes breaks the skyline just east of Juniper Lake, while to the east stand two higher peaks, Red Cinder Cone and Red Cinder. Bonte Peak, 2 miles east-northeast of the lookout, is easily recognizable by its finlike appearance. Black Cinder Rock is the high point immediately behind Bonte Peak, standing on a ridge in western Caribou Wilderness that runs 3 miles north to Red Cinder. North and South Caribou are the two distant peaks behind Black Cinder Rock. To the south and southeast, long ridges, principally glacial moraines, extend toward the large blue mass of Lake Almanor.

⊙ **LOOP TRIP TO JUNIPER LAKE:** Return to the junction with the trail from Warner

Valley, and turn left (west) to descend along a sometimes steep and rocky trail that sees much less use than the ascent route. Very soon, you leave the open slopes and return to light forest with patches of pinemat manzanita; fair views of Lassen Peak accompany the winding descent. Reach a four-way junction in thicker forest, 1.7 miles from the top.

From the junction, follow the right-hand trail north-northeast on a gently graded stroll toward the outlet of Juniper Lake. Eventually, the large blue lake springs into view where the trail follows closely along the south shoreline. Thicker forest greets you on the approach to the Juniper Lake Campground. Immediately before the campground, pass a meadow near the lakeshore that is lined with willows, and another meadow farther inland composed of grasses and corn lilies. The trail terminates at the campground access road near Campsites #9 and #10. From there, take the road back to the day-use parking lot.

ℝ Fires and camping are prohibited on Mt. Harkness.

Trip 57

Juniper Lake Loop

E 🔄 **DH**

DISTANCE: 6.3 miles loop

ELEVATIONS: 6800/6880/6800, +350/-350

SEASON: Mid-June to October

USE: Light

MAP: *Mount Harkness*

INTRODUCTION: The loop around Juniper Lake won't make anyone's top-10 list of must-do trips, but the 6.3-mile circuit is a fine alternative for those seeking a relatively easy morning or afternoon hike, especially for those staying at Juniper

Lake Campground. The route incorporates stretches of little-used trail and a section of dirt road to circumnavigate the lake, with plenty of opportunities along the way for a refreshing swim or for dropping a line in hopes of hooking a rainbow trout or two.

Good views across the lake feature a variety of highlights, including Lassen Peak, which is visible from the shoreline only near Juniper Lake Campground. Photographers looking to capture the peak reflected in the lake's still waters should arrive early in the morning. Saddle Mountain is the spreading mass to the left of Lassen Peak. Mt. Hoffman, when viewed from the lake's outlet forebay, is the unimpressive looking, asymmetrical mountain whose summit reaches directly above Inspiration Point (see Trip 59). This "point" is composed of a pair of small knolls on a nearly level, forested ridge above Juniper Lake's north shore. The best views of Mt. Harkness and the cinder

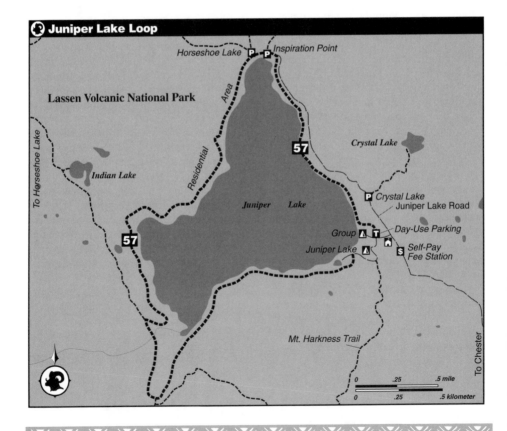

cone comprising the upper part of the peak are from the lake's north end.

DIRECTIONS TO TRAILHEAD: From Highway 36 in Chester, take Feather River Road west-northwest for just over a half mile and veer right on County Road 318, following signed directions for Juniper Lake. Cross into national park land at 8.8 miles from Highway 36, and proceed to the self-pay registration station across from the ranger station at 11.1 miles. Continue a short distance to a signed, left turn into Juniper Lake Campground. Follow the campground access road a short distance to a dirt trailhead parking area on the right.

DESCRIPTION: Head north from the dirt parking area through mixed forest on faint, single-track tread that immediately bends toward Juniper Lake and passes around the group campground. After merging with a path from the group area, the trail approaches the shoreline and then proceeds toward the north end of the lake, roughly paralleling Juniper Lake Road. This lonely stretch of trail (with the occasional angler or two) provides good views of Saddle Mountain across the lake's surface. In 2006, there were a number of deadfalls covering the trail, and the tread almost disappeared completely before it reached the road just shy of the Inspiration Point Trailhead. Although the tread may be hard to follow in places, the constant presence of the lake to your left should be enough to keep you pointed in the right direction.

From there, follow the road around the north shore past the Inspiration Point and Horseshoe Lake trailheads, and then continue south for a little over a mile along a road that accesses the rustic private cabins along the west shore. The single-track resumes near some trail signs at 2.5 miles from the parking area.

Beyond the road and cabins, the mixed forest casts a wilder ambiance, and the trail travels well above the southwest shore of the lake. Soon after a boulder hop of a seasonal stream, you draw close to the shoreline again and skirt a passable campsite about a half mile from the resumption of single-track. Soon, the trail veers away from the lakeshore once more and proceeds south-southeast through forest before bending west across a slope above the lake's outlet, a tributary of Kings Creek. A brief walk leads to a junction with a trail northwest to Indian Lake, 3.8 miles from the parking area.

Follow the left-hand trail down to a ford of the outlet stream, and then make a half-mile climb through the trees to a four-way junction with the trail to Mt. Harkness from Warner Valley.

Turn left here and veer northeast on a gently graded trail back toward the outlet of Juniper Lake. Eventually, the large blue lake springs into view where the trail follows closely along the south shoreline. Thicker forest greets you on the approach to the Juniper Lake Campground. Immediately before the campground, pass a meadow near the lakeshore that is lined with willows, and another farther inland with grasses and corn lilies. The trail terminates at the campground access road near Campsites #9 and #10. From there, take the road back to the day-use parking lot.

R Fires are prohibited.

JUNIPER LAKE TRAILHEADS

Trip **58**

Crystal Lake

E / DH

DISTANCE: 0.8 mile out and back

ELEVATIONS: 6835/7215, +380/-380

SEASON: Mid-June to October

USE: Light

MAP: *Mount Harkness*

INTRODUCTION: Usually, the combination of a scenic destination and a short trail is prescription for overuse, especially within the boundaries of a national park. Fortunately, Crystal Lake is located in one of the more remote areas of Lassen Volcanic, so the scenic lake and its simple 0.4-mile trail are relatively quiet. Despite its short length, the path is moderate to moderately steep almost the entire way. Crystal Lake is a favorite among swimmers searching for a refreshing dip and anglers hoping to hook a good-size trout. Fair to good views of nearby Juniper Lake, Mt. Harkness, and Lassen Peak provide an added bonus.

DIRECTIONS TO TRAILHEAD: From Highway 36 in Chester, take Feather River Road west-northwest for just over a half mile and veer right on County Road 318, following signed directions for Juniper Lake. Cross into national park land at 8.8 miles from Highway 36, and proceed to the self-pay registration station across from the ranger station at 11.1 miles. From there, head past the turnoff to Juniper Lake Campground on the left and proceed 0.3 mile to a small parking area on the left-hand shoulder directly across from the trailhead.

DESCRIPTION: Upon reaching Crystal Lake, many hikers question the accuracy of the 0.4-mile distance posted on the sign near the trailhead, as the 15 to 20 percent grade makes the trail seem much longer. Despite this, most hikers arrive at the lakeshore in a mere 15 minutes, strong hikers even faster. The trail, which heads northeast, climbs right from the start, up a hillside cloaked with red firs, lodgepole pines, and some western white pines higher up the slope. Near the top of the climb, the forest opens up a tad, allowing enough sunlight to support an assortment of shrubs, including chinquapin, manzanita, and squaw carpet, a matted ceanothus that sprouts clusters of tiny lavender flowers in early and mid-July. Normally flourishing between 3000 and

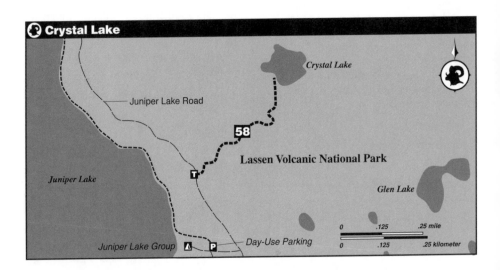

Crystal Lake

Crystal Lake

Juniper Lake Road

58

Lassen Volcanic National Park

Juniper Lake

T

Glen Lake

Juniper Lake Group ⛺ **P** — Day-Use Parking

| 0 | .125 | .25 mile |
| 0 | .125 | .25 kilometer |

MOUNTAIN HEMLOCKS

Mountain hemlocks typically reside at elevations above 7500 feet, appearing at this elevation only on cooler, north-facing slopes. However, the variable topography of Crystal Lake's south-facing basin creates microclimates conducive to a diverse assortment of plants. Normally distant neighbors, squaw carpet and mountain hemlocks thrive here in totally different environments a mere 100 yards apart, both growing beyond their normal elevation limits.

6500 feet in the Lassen area, this ankle-high evergreen is at its upper elevation limit here at 7200 feet. A set of short switchbacks finishes the ascent, with good views of Juniper Lake and Mt. Harkness along the way. Reach the shore of Crystal Lake near the seasonal outlet.

Without the usually monotonous ring of dense lodgepole pines, Crystal Lake is one of the park's most beautiful lakes. The varying topography around the shoreline is blessed with an open, pleasing assortment of red firs, western white pines, lodgepoles, and even a few mountain hemlocks.

A use trail leads to the top of a low knoll just west of the lake's outlet, offering an unobstructed view of Juniper Lake, Mt. Harkness, and Lassen Peak. Most visitors come to Crystal Lake to swim, as the water temperature ranges from the mid-60s to the low 70s during the summer months. Fishing is also possible, as the lake, unlike many in the park, harbors a healthy population of rainbow trout.

R Fires and camping are prohibited at Crystal Lake.

JUNIPER LAKE TRAILHEADS

Trip **59**

Inspiration Point

E ✓ DH

DISTANCE: 1.4 miles out and back

ELEVATIONS: 6760/7190, +430/-430

SEASON: Mid-June to October

USE: Light

MAP: *Mount Harkness*

INTRODUCTION: Not as inspirational as it used to be (thanks to maturing forest) and not the best overall view from a Juniper Lake area summit (Mt. Harkness takes that honor), the easily obtained vista from Inspiration Point is nevertheless a fine reward for the little effort required. A somewhat steep but relatively short climb gets hikers to the viewpoint, where a number of noteworthy landmarks can be seen, including Lassen Peak and several other summits and lakes.

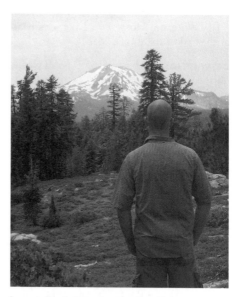

Lassen Peak from Inspiration Point

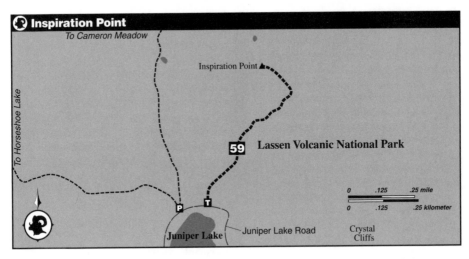

DIRECTIONS TO TRAILHEAD: From Highway 36 in Chester, take Feather River Road west-northwest for just over a half mile and veer right on County Road 318, following signed directions for Juniper Lake. Cross into national park land at 8.8 miles from Highway 36, and proceed to the self-pay registration station across from the ranger station at 11.1 miles. From there, head past the turnoff to Juniper Lake Campground and the Crystal Lake Trailhead to the signed Inspiration Point Trailhead on the right side of the road at the north end of Juniper Lake (just before the Horseshoe Lake Trailhead at the end of the public road).

DESCRIPTION: Gently rising tread leads northeast from the trailhead before a moderate to steep climb ensues through red firs, lodgepole pines, and western white pines to a low ridge. Briefly climb along the ridge northwest to the top of the low knoll known as Inspiration Point. On top of the knoll, scattered forest allows chinquapin and greenleaf and pinemat manzanita to carpet the ground. In days gone by, the view from the rocky knoll must have been inspiring, but nowadays mature white firs and Jeffrey pines have somewhat obscured the vista. White firs and Jeffrey pines normally grow below the red firs and western white pines seen during the ascent, but the temperatures on the knoll are warmer than

those around Juniper Lake, and the winters are less severe as well, which creates a more hospitable environment than one would usually expect at this elevation. A use trail running northwest along the rocky ridge to a second, lower knoll has evolved over the years, beaten into the soil from the boots of previous hikers searching for the most impressive viewpoints.

Considering the low elevation of the two knolls, the views are indeed remarkable. Visible from the second knoll are Snag Lake, Fantastic Lava Beds, and Cinder Cone, along with Prospect Peak and West Prospect Peak. To the west, Lassen Peak and the modern-day summits along the rim of ancient Mt. Tehama poke up through the trees, while Mt. Harkness and Juniper Lake are seen to the south. Closer to the southeast are the Crystal Cliffs. An unbroken sea of green forest lies to the northeast, bounded by Mt. Hoffman and Red Cinder Cone on the north, and a ridge extending south from Red Cinder on the east. The eastern boundary of Lassen Volcanic National Park is just over a half mile west of the ridge. Toward the northwest end of the ridge, the snow-capped summit of Mt. Shasta can be seen to the northwest, providing the sky is clear of summer haze.

R Fires are prohibited.

JUNIPER LAKE TRAILHEADS

Trip **60**

Horseshoe and Indian Lakes Loop

E ♀ DH, BP

DISTANCE: 6.5 miles loop

ELEVATIONS: 6760/7125/6760, +850/-850

SEASON: Mid-June to October

USE: Light

MAP: *Mount Harkness*

INTRODUCTION: This loop trip, well-suited for a dayhike or an easy overnight, visits a trio of lakes—Horseshoe, Indian, and Juniper—that offer plenty of opportunities to swim, fish, or camp.

DIRECTIONS TO TRAILHEAD: From Highway 36 in Chester, take Feather River Road west-northwest for just over a half mile and veer right on County Road 318, following signed directions for Juniper Lake. Cross into national park land at 8.8 miles from Highway 36, and proceed to the self-pay registration station across from the ranger station at 11.1 miles. From there, head past the turnoff to Juniper Lake Campground and the Crystal Lake and Inspiration Point trailheads to the north end of Juniper Lake and the Horseshoe Lake Trailhead on the right, about 50 yards before the end of the public road.

DESCRIPTION: Walk northwest 50 yards to a junction with a trail on the right to Cameron Meadow and Jakey Lake. Veer left (west-northwest) and make a mild climb through a light forest of red firs, western white pines, and lodgepole pines, along the course of an old road to the top of a

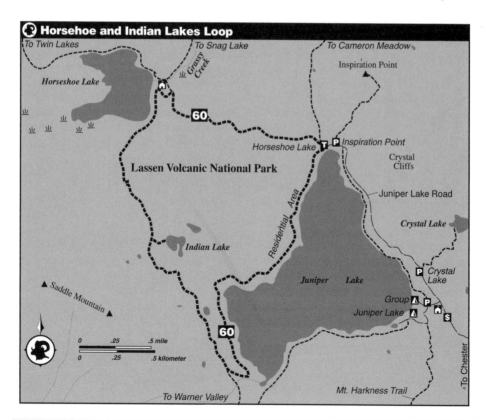

Horsehoe and Indian Lakes Loop

forested rise. After a short bit of nearly level grade, the trail begins a nearly mile-long descent toward Horseshoe Lake's eastern shore. With the faint sound of trickling Grassy Creek ahead, you spy the log cabin of the Juniper Lake ranger station through the trees and reach a junction, 1.4 miles from the trailhead.

The ranger station lies a mere 100 feet ahead, and the grounds are well worth a quick visit—if you arrive during the middle of the day, the seasonal ranger will more than likely be out on patrol. Just past the ranger station is the verdant swale of Grassy Creek and a junction on the far side with trails northeast to Snag Lake and northwest to Twin Lakes.

From the first junction (before the ranger station), turn left, following signed directions south for Indian Lake, and skirt the east side of Horseshoe Lake, although you'd never guess the lake was on your right, thanks to the thick wall of trees. Backpackers should look for campsites 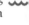 along the west shore (camping is banned along the north shore). Farther south, you catch a brief glimpse of the water and pass a lush meadow before the trail starts a moderate climb away from Horseshoe Lake.

During the ascent, a more open forest allows extensive patches of pinemat manzanita to flourish on the sun-drenched slopes. A few small but welcome pockets of shade provide brief respite from the sunny climb before you gain gentler terrain near the crest of the broad ridge that separates Horseshoe and Juniper lakes. From the top of the ridge,

mildly descending trail drops to a T-junction with a lateral heading east to shady Indian Lake, 2.9 miles from the trailhead.

To visit the lake, head down the lateral across open slopes carpeted with pinemat manzanita past a murky seasonal pond, and then come under forest cover just before reaching the tree-rimmed shore. Camping is allowed at Indian Lake and at the smaller, semiclear, unnamed lake to the northeast, providing you can find a spot more than 100 feet from the water that's level enough to pitch your tent. Both lakes are better suited for day use, with the best swimming area and fewest mosquitoes located near a rocky point on Indian Lake's north shore.

From the Indian Lake junction, gently graded trail wanders through the trees past several seasonal ponds and an open area carpeted with manzanita before a moderate descent drops toward Juniper Lake's outlet. Once the creek is within earshot, you reach a junction, 4.1 miles from the trailhead.

Turn left (east) and swing around above the southwest shore of Juniper Lake, now visible through the trees to the right. Continue along the shoreline trail past a campsite near the westernmost bay of the 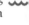 lake; shortly, your single-track trail merges with the access road for the private cabins along the west shore. From there, follow the road for 1.3 miles to the close of the loop at the Horseshoe Lake Trailhead.

R Wilderness permits are required for overnight stays, and fires are prohibited.

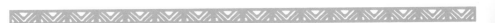

JUNIPER LAKE TRAILHEADS

Trip 61

Horseshoe, Snag, and Swan Lakes Loop

Ⓜ Ⓠ DH, BP

DISTANCE: 13 miles loop

ELEVATIONS: 6760/6085/6760, +1725/-1725

SEASON: Mid-June to October

USE: Light

MAPS: *Mount Harkness, Prospect Peak*

INTRODUCTION: Sampling several lakes in the heart of Lassen Volcanic's backcountry, this loop trip will delight strong dayhikers and backpackers alike. The moderate route does have its share of ups and downs, the majority of which occur during the last 3.5 miles of the trip, but the elevation gain and loss is worth it. Along with the numerous lakes, travelers will visit the verdant swale of Grassy Creek and have a couple of opportunities to bag Crater and Fairfield peaks via short and straightforward cross-country routes. Most of the lakes offer secluded camping, refreshing swimming, and fair to good fishing.

DIRECTIONS TO TRAILHEAD: From Highway 36 in Chester, take Feather River Road west-northwest for just over a half mile and veer right on County Road 318, following signed directions for Juniper Lake. Cross into national park land at 8.8 miles from Highway 36, and proceed to the self-pay registration station across from the ranger station at 11.1 miles. From there, head past the turnoff to Juniper Lake Campground

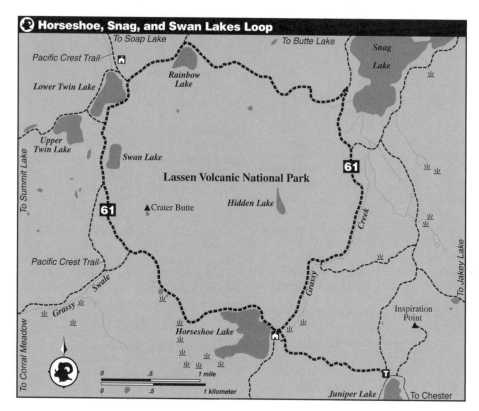

Horseshoe, Snag, and Swan Lakes Loop

HORSESHOE LAKE

The view across Horseshoe Lake from the peninsula may be plain, but what lies below the surface is far from ordinary. By placing an imaginary line southwest to the north shore of the lake's southwestern arm, you effectively divide the shallow part of the lake on the right from a much deeper part on the left. The north part has an average depth of 10 feet or less, with the lone exception being a 20-foot deep spot near the west end of the northwest arm. (Strangely, yellow pond lilies, which usually prefer shallow water, cover the surface of this deep part.) The north part is generally so shallow that one could almost wade from the tip of the peninsula halfway across the lake.

The south part can be further divided into two basins: the southwest arm, which drops to about 40 feet, and a larger area to the east, which achieves a depth of 75 feet. Most of Lassen's smaller lakes were created by glaciers scouring out shallow depressions that later filled with water. But Lassen's larger lakes, such as Juniper, Snag, Butte, and Horseshoe, owe their origin to volcanism. Successive eruptions of lava led to the creation of Horseshoe's three basins, which were subsequently modified by a glacier flowing north from the ridge above the lake.

and the Crystal Lake and Inspiration Point trailheads to the north end of Juniper Lake and the Horseshoe Lake Trailhead on the right, about 50 yards before the end of the public road.

DESCRIPTION: Walk northwest 50 yards to a junction with a trail on the right to Cameron Meadow and Jakey Lake. Veer left (west-northwest) and make a mild climb through a light forest of red firs, western white pines, and lodgepole pines, along the course of an old road to the top of a forested rise. After a short bit of nearly level grade, the trail begins a nearly mile-long descent toward Horseshoe Lake's eastern shore. With the faint sound of trickling Grassy Creek ahead, you spy the log cabin of the Juniper Lake ranger station through the trees and reach a junction, 1.4 miles from the trailhead. The ranger station lies a mere 100 feet ahead, and the grounds are well worth a quick visit—if you arrive during the middle of the day, the seasonal ranger will more than likely be out on patrol. Continue past the ranger station to the verdant, willow-lined swale of Grassy Creek, cross a wood-plank bridge, and immediately reach a junction on the far side.

Turn left and travel upstream along the bank of Grassy Creek to the outlet of Horseshoe Lake, which, with a view across the water of Lassen Peak, is a fine setting for a lunch or rest stop. A sign and map indicate that camping along the north shore of the lake is not permitted (backpackers intending to camp at Horseshoe Lake should backtrack to the junction east of the ranger station and head south to the camping area on the east shore). Proceed along the north shore past a small peninsula that affords a good, although rather plain, view across the lake.

The north half of the lake offers an attractive, if oversized, swimming hole, as the lake's pebbly bottom quickly drops away from shore to level off at about 10 to 15 feet, without rocks, snags, and other submerged obstacles for swimmers to fret about. Since the middle of the lake is relatively shallow—less than 5 feet deep in places—colder water from the deeper southern half is effectively kept out of the north end, where water temperatures become relatively warm by midsummer.

Beyond Horseshoe Lake, the trail follows a nearly level course for nearly 1.5 miles through the forest and past a handful of seasonal ponds to a junction with a trail down Grassy Swale at 3.6 miles.

Proceed ahead (west) from the junction on the right-hand trail, dipping across a verdant swale lined with vibrant wildflowers and lush plants. Make a moderately steep ascent up a side canyon that is nearly as verdant. A mosaic of wildflowers includes Applegate's paintbrush, Christine's lupine, California stickseed, coyote mint, and mountain violet. Where the grade eventually eases, you may notice silver-leaved lupine and pumice paintbrush monopolizing the gravelly forest floor on the way around the western base of Crater Butte to a junction with the Pacific Crest Trail, 4.5 miles from the trailhead.

[S] **SIDE TRIP TO CRATER BUTTE:** A 0.6-mile, 500-foot ascent southeast to the summit of Crater Butte is a straightforward enterprise from the vicinity of the PCT junction and takes about an hour, round-trip. Similar to nearby Fairfield Peak, Crater Butte is composed mostly of lava flows instead of cinders, although both peaks are technically referred to as cinder cones. **END SIDE TRIP**

Proceed north on the PCT for about 250 yards to the crest of a low divide and then drop into the Butte Creek drainage on the way to forest-rimmed Swan Lake. Backpackers who plan to overnight at this typical Lassen lake should find passable campsites above the south shore, or along an east shore bench. The trail draws near to the lake at the northwest corner, then immediately crosses the barely discernible outlet before leaving Swan Lake.

After surmounting a low rise north of Swan Lake, a mild descent on the lupine-lined PCT leads to a junction near the southeast shore of lodgepole-fringed Lower Twin Lake. Westward, a 4-plus-mile route skirts along Lower Twin Lake's south shore, then climbs past Upper Twin and Echo lakes to campgrounds at Summit Lake. Continuing ahead on the PCT, you arc around the east side of Lower Twin Lake, passing a campsite or two, to another junction, 5.7 miles from the trailhead.

At the junction, turn right to leave the PCT and travel northeast on a gentle climb to crescent-shaped Rainbow Lake. Peakbaggers interested in adding Fairfield Peak to their list of ascents can leave the trail just before the lake and take a 0.4-mile cross-country trip north to the summit. Fairfield Peak may be responsible for damming Rainbow Lake in a similar fashion to the formation of Horseshoe Lake, when lava flows dammed the creek. Steep terrain surrounding the lake limits the number of available campsites. However, a use trail at the south end heads around the lake to a few small campsites with filtered views of Lassen Peak. Above the northeast shore is a junction with a trail northeast toward Cinder Cone, 6.6 miles from the trailhead.

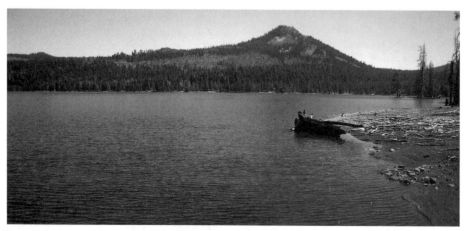

Snag Lake

Follow the right-hand trail on a brief climb southeast to the crest of a low ridge, and then drop to a nearby gully. A protracted traverse leads across rolling, open terrain on deep and loose tread that will remind you of walking on a sandy beach. A profusion of Bloomer's goldenbush attempts to stabilize the loose soil, as this late-blooming sunflower thrives on dry, gravely flats. Midway between Rainbow and Snag lakes, the trail begins a steep descent that may be accompanied by more gravel-loving wildflowers, including cycladenia, with tubular rose flowers and broad, smooth-edged leaves, and Lobb's nama, with tubular magenta flowers and narrower, shallow-toothed leaves. Less attractive is the increasing evidence of a forest fire that devastated acres of lodgepole pines. About a quarter mile before Snag Lake, you cross a rivulet and proceed to a junction a good distance away from its southwest shore, 8.6 miles from the trailhead.

Due to the fire, campsites along Snag Lake's northwest shore have lost much of their appeal. However, the peninsula just north of the junction has an intact grove of trees that shades several good campsites. The water around the peninsula is fairly shallow—5 to 10 feet in most places—and therefore is relatively warm, luring weary backpackers with the prospect of a refreshing swim. Anglers can ply the waters in search of good-size rainbow trout.

To continue the loop trip, turn south at the junction and soon leave Snag Lake on the way to another junction with a trail that travels along the east side of the lake. Continue ahead (south) at this junction and follow the Grassy Creek Trail on a 2-plus-mile, gentle to moderate ascent to Horseshoe Lake. Initially, the trail crosses moist to dry soils characterized by spreading phlox, coyote mint, dwarf lousewort, California stickseed, and California butterweed.

After a half mile, the trail draws alongside the creek, where July visitors will be presented with a lush, wildflower extravaganza that includes several dozen species.

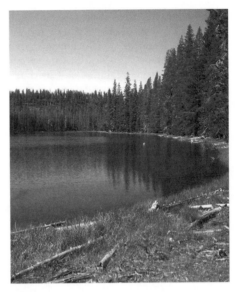

Rainbow Lake

Look for corn lily, marsh marigold, alpine shooting star, Nuttall's larkspur, crimson columbine, wandering daisy, common dandelion, yarrow, and many, many others. Fortunate botanists may find all three of the park's stickseeds, all six of the violets, and many representatives of the figwort and buttercup families. Follow the charming creek through thick shrubs that threaten to overgrow the trail beneath a forest of western white pines and firs. About halfway to Horseshoe Lake, the narrowing canyon forces the trail to make a couple crossings of Grassy Creek over a set of log rounds. Beyond the crossings, the origin of the creek's name becomes even more apparent, as lush grasses line the banks all the way to the verdant swale near the Horseshoe Lake ranger station. Reach a junction with a trail around the north shore of Horseshoe Lake, 11.6 miles from the trailhead. From there, turn left to retrace your steps 1.4 miles to the trailhead.

R Wilderness permits are required for overnight stays. Fires are prohibited, and camping is prohibited along the north shore of Horseshoe Lake.

Trip **62**

Cameron Meadow-Grassy Creek Loop

Ⓜ ↻ DH, BP

DISTANCE: 7.2 miles loop

ELEVATIONS: 6760/6085/6760, +1160/-1160

SEASON: Mid-June to October

USE: Light

MAPS: *Mount Harkness, Prospect Peak*

INTRODUCTION: The Cameron Meadow-Grassy Creek loop, with a profusion of showy wildflowers and lush plants filling the meadow and lining the banks of the creek, is a delight for botanists. July is the best month to observe the spectacular wildflower display, but be prepared for the hordes of mosquitoes that accompany the peak of flower season. Along with the vegetation, the loop visits two of the more magnificent lakes in the Lassen backcountry, Horseshoe and Snag, offering plenty of opportunities to camp, swim, fish, or simply enjoy the scenery.

DIRECTIONS TO TRAILHEAD: From Highway 36 in Chester, take Feather River Road west-northwest for just over a half mile and veer right on County Road 318, following signed directions for Juniper Lake. Cross into national park land at 8.8 miles from Highway 36, and proceed to the self-pay registration station across from the ranger station at 11.1 miles. From there, head past the turnoff to Juniper Lake Campground and the Crystal Lake and Inspiration Point

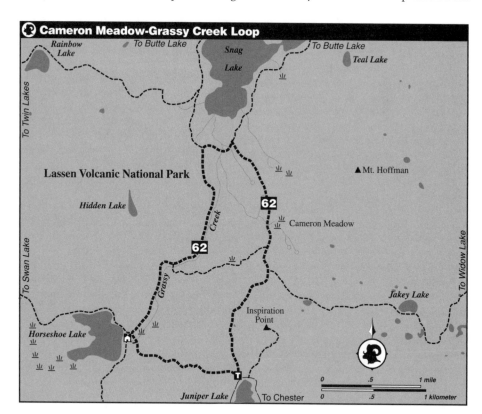

trailheads to the north end of Juniper Lake and the Horseshoe Lake Trailhead on the right, about 50 yards before the end of the public road.

DESCRIPTION: Walk 50 yards northwest from the trailhead to a junction with a trail on the left to Horseshoe Lake. Veer right (north) and climb moderately through Lassen's predominant forest type, composed of red firs, western white pines, and lodgepole pines, along with an understory primarily of pinemat manzanita. After a half-mile, viewless climb to a crest, drop north a short distance to a rumpled bench and head north to a brink, where you have tree-filtered views of Prospect Peak, Cinder Cone, Fantastic Lava Beds, and Snag Lake. This is followed by a half-mile, knee-knocking descent that may be marked with lingering snowfields well into July. The grade eases on an approach to and descent down a tributary of Jakey Lake Creek. Cross the creek, which may be a wet ford in early season, and reach a junction near a small meadow with a trail east to Jakey Lake, 1.4 miles from the trailhead.

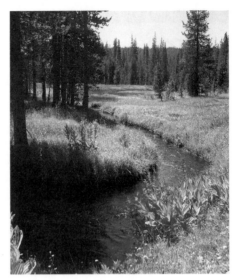

Grassy Creek

Continue north, arriving at Jakey Lake Creek in about 110 yards, a good spot to filter water, take a break, and perhaps identify some streamside flowers. The corn lily, which is the most common species in wet, open, mountain environments, is present, as is the large-leaved lupine, the park's only water-loving lupine. Marsh marigolds grow in the wettest soils, while plantain-leaved buttercup, bud saxifrage, and western spring beauty thrive in slightly drier soils. Along the creek and ahead to Cameron Meadow, you may be fortunate enough to spot up to five species of violet—all of the park's species except for water-shunning mountain violet.

Gently graded trail leads to a junction halfway to Cameron Meadow, where a shortcut heads west 1.2 miles to the Grassy Creek Trail, about a mile north of the Horseshoe Lake ranger station. Gently descend north to Cameron Meadow, where, through July, a shallow pond fills the northwest corner of the meadow. The remainder of the flower-carpeted meadow is quite boggy, which produces a mosquito heaven, or hell, depending on the point of view. Unfortunately, since mosquitoes are important pollinators, the peak of mosquito season coincides with the peak of wildflower season.

On the boggy trail, you plow north past corn lilies, alders, willows, and lodgepole pines, soon making a pair of crossings over Jakey Lake Creek. Proceed north to a snowmelt pond at the northeast edge of a low ridge, and then begin a moderate descent along glacial sediments to a junction south of unseen Snag Lake, 2.9 miles from the trailhead.

Turn left (southwest) and stroll easily to a sizeable bridge spanning lushly lined Grassy Creek, another excellent spot from which to botanize. Beyond the bridge, the trail arcs around to a junction with the Grassy Creek Trail at 3.3 miles. Backpackers who wish to camp at Snag Lake should turn right (north) at this junction and proceed 0.7 mile to a peninsula, where a grove of trees shades several good campsites. The water around the peninsula is fairly shallow—5 to 10 feet in most places—and therefore is relatively warm, luring weary backpackers with the prospect of a refreshing swim. Anglers can ply the waters in search of good-size rainbow trout.

To continue on this route, turn left (south) and follow the Grassy Creek Trail on a 2-plus-mile gentle to moderate ascent to Horseshoe Lake. Initially, the trail crosses moist to dry soils characterized by spreading phlox, coyote mint, dwarf lousewort, California stickseed, and California butterweed. After a half mile, the trail draws alongside the creek, where July visitors will be presented with a lush, wildflower extravaganza that includes several dozen species. Look for corn lily, marsh marigold, alpine shooting star, Nuttall's larkspur, crimson columbine, wandering daisy, common dandelion, yarrow, and many, many others. Fortunate botanists may find all three of the park's stickseeds, all six of the violets, and many representatives of the figwort and buttercup families.

Follow the charming creek through thick shrubs that threaten to overgrow the trail beneath a forest of western white pines and firs. About halfway to Horseshoe Lake, the narrowing canyon forces the trail to make a couple crossings of Grassy Creek over a set of log rounds. Beyond the crossings, the origin of the creek's name becomes even more apparent, as lush grasses line the banks all the way to the verdant swale near the Horseshoe Lake ranger station. Reach a junction with a trail around the north shore of Horseshoe Lake, 5.6 miles from the trailhead. Before continuing on the loop route, take a few minutes to walk west to the lake and take in the view of Lassen Peak.

From the junction, head southeast across the bridge over Grassy Creek and pass by the ranger station before embarking on a nearly mile-long ascent to the crest of a forested ridge. Beyond the crest, a mild to moderate descent leads back to the close of the loop at the junction with the trail to Cameron Meadow. From there, retrace your steps on an easy, 50-yard stroll to the trailhead.

R Wilderness permits are required for overnight stays, and fires are prohibited.

JUNIPER LAKE TRAILHEADS

Trip 63

Jakey Lake

E ∕ DH, BP

DISTANCE:	5.8 miles out and back
ELEVATIONS:	6760/6960, +1200/-1200
SEASON:	Mid-June to October
USE:	Light
MAPS:	*Mount Harkness, Prospect Peak*

INTRODUCTION: Forest-rimmed Jakey Lake is definitely off the beaten path and, despite the trip's short distance, there's a high probability of finding solitude.

DIRECTIONS TO TRAILHEAD: From Highway 36 in Chester, take Feather River Road west-northwest for just over a half mile and veer right on County Road 318, following signed directions for Juniper Lake. Cross into national park land at 8.8 miles from Highway 36, and proceed to the self-pay registration station across from the ranger station at 11.1 miles. From there, head past the turnoff to Juniper Lake Campground and the Crystal Lake and Inspiration Point trailheads to the north end of Juniper Lake and the Horseshoe Lake Trailhead on the right, about 50 yards before the end of the public road.

DESCRIPTION: Walk 50 yards northwest from the trailhead to a junction with a trail on the left to Horseshoe Lake. Veer right (north) and climb moderately through Lassen's predominant forest type, composed of red firs, western white pines, and lodgepole pines, along with an understory primarily of pinemat manzanita. After a half-mile, viewless climb to a crest, drop north a short distance to a rumpled bench and head north to a brink, where you have

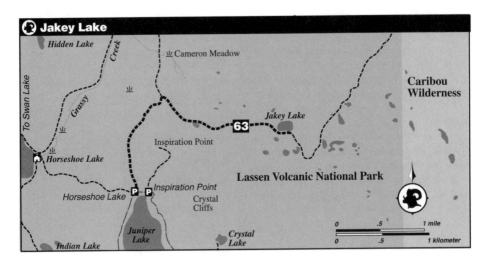

Jakey Lake

Hidden Lake

Creek

Cameron Meadow

To Swan Lake

Grassy

Jakey Lake

63

Caribou Wilderness

Inspiration Point

Horseshoe Lake

Lassen Volcanic National Park

Inspiration Point

Horseshoe Lake

P P

Crystal Cliffs

Juniper Lake

Indian Lake

Crystal Lake

| 0 | .5 | 1 mile |
| 0 | .5 | 1 kilometer |

tree-filtered views of Prospect Peak, Cinder Cone, Fantastic Lava Beds, and Snag Lake. This is followed by a half-mile, knee-knocking descent that may be marked with lingering snowfields well into July. The grade eases on an approach to and descent down a tributary of Jakey Lake Creek. Cross the creek, which may be a wet ford in early season, and reach a junction near a small meadow with your trail east to Jakey Lake, 1.4 miles from the trailhead.

Turn right at the junction and follow Jakey Lake Creek (not shown on USGS maps) on a half-mile climb to the northwest edge of a swampy area holding a knee-deep pond. The pond is one of several dozen in the area, left behind by a glacier. The abundance of standing water assures an equally abundant population of mosquitoes through midsummer. The swampy area is home to thousands of frogs that feast on the mosquitoes—but invariably, mosquito-bitten hikers will wish there were even more of these princely amphibians.

About 0.2 mile past the swamp, the trail passes one of the largest western white pines in the park, a two-trunked specimen, the larger of which is near 6 feet in diameter. Gently rising trail approaches the creek again and follows alongside the waterway for just over a half mile to the west end of Jakey Lake. The shallow lake is best suited for swimming in early and mid-August, after most of the mosquitoes have disappeared. Campsites are somewhat limited, but the number seems adequate for the low use the area receives.

R Wilderness permits are required for overnight stays, and fires are prohibited.

JUNIPER LAKE TRAILHEADS

Trip 64

Jakey Lake-Widow Lake Loop

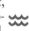 DH, BP

DISTANCE: 18.7 miles loop

ELEVATIONS: 6760/7660/6065/6955/6760,
+2700/-2700

SEASON: Mid-June to October

USE: Light

MAP: *Mount Harkness*

INTRODUCTION: Lakes, streams, views, and flowers—fine attributes for any backpack. Only one thing is blessedly lacking on this loop through the easternmost backcountry of Lassen Volcanic—people.

DIRECTIONS TO TRAILHEAD: From Highway 36 in Chester, take Feather River Road west-northwest for just over a half mile and veer right on County Road 318, following signed directions for Juniper Lake. Cross into national park land at 8.8 miles from Highway 36, and proceed to the self-pay registration station across from the ranger station at 11.1 miles. From there, head past the turnoff to Juniper Lake Campground and the Crystal Lake and Inspiration Point trailheads to the north end of Juniper Lake and the Horseshoe Lake Trailhead on the right, about 50 yards before the end of the public road.

DESCRIPTION: Walk 50 yards northwest from the trailhead to a junction with a trail on the left to Horseshoe Lake. Veer right (north) and climb moderately through Lassen's predominant forest type, composed of red firs, western white pines, and lodgepole pines, along with an understory primarily of pinemat manzanita. After a half-mile, viewless climb to a crest, drop north a short distance to a rumpled bench and head north to a brink, where you have tree-filtered views of Prospect Peak, Cinder

Cone, Fantastic Lava Beds, and Snag Lake. This is followed by a half-mile, knee-knocking descent that may be marked with lingering snowfields well into July. The grade eases on an approach to and descent down a tributary of Jakey Lake Creek. Cross the creek, which may be a wet ford in early season, and reach a junction near a small meadow with your trail east to Jakey Lake, 1.4 miles from the trailhead.

Turn right at the junction and follow Jakey Lake Creek (not shown on USGS maps) on a half-mile climb to the northwest edge of a swampy area holding a knee-deep pond. The pond is one of several dozen in the area, left behind by a glacier. The abundance of standing water assures an equally abundant population of mosquitoes through midsummer. The swampy area is home to thousands of frogs that feast on the mosquitoes—but invariably, mosquito-bitten hikers will wish there were even more of these princely amphibians.

About 0.2 mile past the swamp, the trail passes one of the largest western white pines in the park, a two-trunked specimen, the larger of which is near 6 feet in diameter. Gently rising trail approaches the creek again and follows alongside the waterway for just over a half mile to the west end of Jakey Lake. The shallow lake is best suited for swimming in early and mid-August, after most of the mosquitoes have disappeared. Campsites are somewhat limited, but the number seems adequate for the low use the area receives.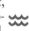

The trail continues east, barely staying above Jakey Lake on a shoreline traverse. Cross the seasonal inlet stream and turn south for an easy climb to a nearby pond, which has a rocky west shore peninsula that is a perfect spot for you to bask in the sun after a dip in the relatively warm swimming hole. During summer, tiny wildflowers flourish along the seasonally wet trail; flowers here might include long-horned steershead (scarcely an inch tall) and western spring beauty (several inches tall). Later in the season, as the area's bodies of water begin to drop, the equally small prim-

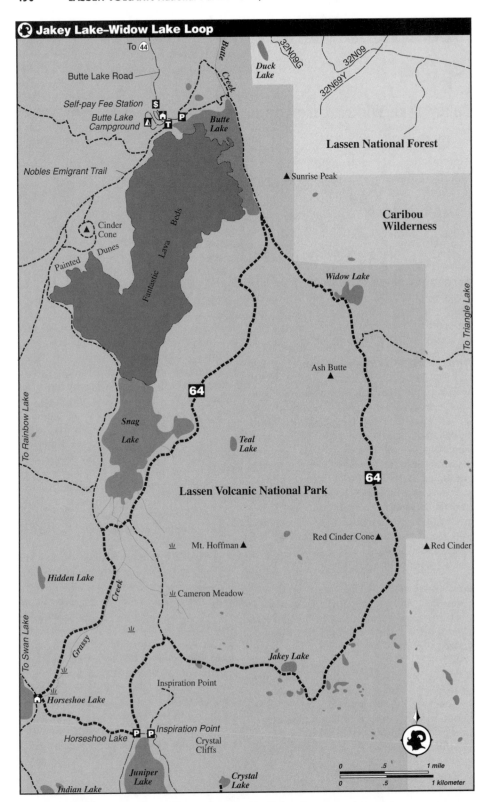

rose monkeyflower forms a ring of yellow around some of their perimeters.

From the pond, the trail swings north to a second pond, which shrivels to a shallow pool by the time the mosquitoes abate in mid- to late summer. Just ahead is a fine pond with an unseen, curved lake immediately to the east. Flat ground near these two swimming holes could be used for a campsite. Since you left Jakey Lake, all the ponds have been to the right of the trail, but soon a triangular pond with semiclear water appears on the left; unfortunately, camping and swimming opportunities here are poor. Beyond the triangular pond, the trail cuts through a linear seasonal pond/meadow, and then, after about 50 yards, it passes the seasonal western arm of a small lake. Although abounding with dead snags, the small lake has some swimming and camping potential, which is more than one can say about the next pond that appears shortly on the left.

Leaving the ponds and lakes behind, the route remains dry on the way to the Red Cinder-Red Cinder Cone saddle. The first half mile is gently rising, followed by a steep 300-foot climb to where the trail almost levels out near a low, open knoll.

S SIDE TRIP TO RED CINDER CONE & RED CINDER: Leave the trail near the low, open knoll and traverse north cross-country to a rocky bench with sweeping but somewhat disappointing views. A better vista is available from the twin summits of Red Cinder Cone, especially the northern one, where the Fantastic Lava Beds, Cinder Cone, Butte Lake, and Prospect Peak dominate the scene. Additional points of interest include snowy Lassen Peak, finlike Bonte Peak, and spreading Mt. Harkness.

Reaching the top of Red Cinder from the saddle involves a hardy off-trail struggle east up steep, brushy slopes for 700 feet—a route only the most ardent peakbaggers will find enjoyable. However, at 8374 feet, Red Cinder is the highest summit for miles around, providing an unobstructed vista of a vast area of Lassen Volcanic, Caribou Wilderness, and numerous features beyond.

To the south, Lake Almanor is obvious, but a Forest Service map would be handy in helping to identify the numerous summits to the northeast. Fourteen miles to the west, Crater Mountain—a shield volcano similar to Prospect Peak and Mt. Harkness—is the foremost peak. This youthful volcano rose out of the middle of a large valley, mostly obliterating it in the process. The summit eventually collapsed into a caldera, which subsequently filled with water to form Crater Lake. **END SIDE TRIP**

A very brief climb leads to a saddle before you begin a nearly 5-mile descent toward Butte Lake. Along this extended drop, the trail passes through a number of forest zones. The north slope of the saddle may be cloaked with snow until mid-July, as you descend through droopy-tipped mountain hemlocks. Farther below the trail, you see red firs, western white pines, and lodgepole pines, the park's most common forest belt. Pass a tiny pond and a sizeable swimming hole a half mile farther, about midway between the saddle and Widow Lake.

A half mile before the lake is a junction with a trail east to Triangle Lake in neighboring Caribou Wilderness. From there, follow a moderate descent to the wooded and grassy shore of Widow Lake. At about 6800 feet, Widow Lake is bordered by the usual complement of willows and lodgepole pines common to this elevation, along with a few black cottonwoods that are somewhat rare at this height. As the water level drops in late season, a forebay at the far side of the lake becomes separated from the lake's main body by a thin strip of land covered with grasses and pines. More than enough fine campsites spread around the shoreline can accommodate the light use Widow Lake receives.

Beyond Widow Lake, steeply descending trail, augmented by short switchbacks, follows a boulder-covered talus slope for about 0.75 mile until the grade eases near a glade abounding in corn lilies and bracken ferns. Beyond this glade, a gentler descent follows the course of Widow Lake's usually dry outlet, crossing the stream several times before the trail reaches a junction south of Butte Lake, 10.3 miles from the trailhead.

Turn left (south) and make a 1.75-mile, viewless but not unpleasant climb to a shallow divide, and then drop a mile on a rather steep descent to the northeast lobe of Snag Lake. A glade of giant aspens highlights the clockwise route around the east lobe, where a number of campsites may lure overnighters; unfortunately, most of them are within 100 feet of the lake and therefore are not legal sites. The best (and legal) campsites around Snag Lake may be found just west of a creek that drops to the wide mouth of the east lobe, part of a recessional moraine that runs across to the prominent west shore peninsula. On the approach to the very shallow end of Snag Lake, which usually dries up by mid- to late summer, the trail veers away from the shore, climbing briefly and crossing a pair of streams, before reaching a junction between a trail to Cameron Meadow on the left and the route up Grassy Creek to Horseshoe Lake on the right.

Follow the right-hand trail west from the junction about 300 yards to a bridge across Grassy Creek and proceed to a junction with Snag Lake's west shore trail. Turn left (south) and follow the Grassy Creek Trail on a 2-plus-mile gentle to moderate ascent to Horseshoe Lake. Initially, the trail crosses moist to dry soils characterized by spreading phlox, coyote mint, dwarf lousewort, California stickseed, and California butterweed. After a half mile, the trail draws alongside the creek, where July visitors will be presented with a lush, wildflower extravaganza that includes several dozen species. Look for corn lily, marsh marigold, alpine

shooting star, Nuttall's larkspur, crimson columbine, wandering daisy, common dandelion, yarrow, and many, many others. Fortunate botanists may find all three of the park's stickseeds, all six of the violets, and many representatives of the figwort and buttercup families. Follow the charming creek through thick shrubs that threaten to overgrow the trail beneath a forest of western white pines and firs.

About halfway to Horseshoe Lake, the narrowing canyon forces the trail to make a couple of crossings of Grassy Creek over a set of log rounds. Beyond the crossings, the origin of the creek's name becomes even more apparent, as lush grasses line the banks all the way to the verdant swale near the Horseshoe Lake ranger station. Reach a junction with a trail around the north shore of Horseshoe Lake, 5.6 miles from the trailhead. Before continuing on the loop route, take a few minutes to walk west to the lake and enjoy the view of Lassen Peak. Backpackers wishing to spend one more night out in the backcountry will find good campsites on the west shore.

From the junction, head southeast across the bridge over Grassy Creek and pass the ranger station before embarking on a nearly mile-long ascent to the crest of a forested ridge. Beyond the crest, a mild to moderate descent leads back to the close of the loop at the junction with the trail to Cameron Meadow. From there, retrace your steps 50 yards to the trailhead.

R Wilderness permits are required for overnight stays. Fires are prohibited, and camping is prohibited along the north shore of Horseshoe Lake.

Introduction to Warner Valley and Drakesbad

see map on p.169

For many, the Drakesbad and Warner Valley area is a magical place. Generations of families have made an annual pilgrimage to the Drakesbad Guest Ranch, a remote getaway over a century old, for a week or more of rest and relaxation. Drakesbad has the unhurried ambiance of a bygone era, where the pace of life slows and guests enjoy some of life's simple pleasures, like soaking in the thermal pool, enjoying a fine meal in the rustic dining room, or strolling along one of the area's many trails.

Fortunately, you don't have to be a guest at the ranch to enjoy the stunning terrain around Drakesbad near the head of verdant Warner Valley. The trails, although occasionally steep, are generally short and packed with outstanding scenery. With sufficient moisture, the meadows surrounding the resort harbor prolific wildflower displays, and nearby hydrothermal features provide dazzling examples of the park's volcanic origins, without the crush of tourists who frequent similar features along the main park road. Due to the relatively low elevations, the summers can be hot, but some of the trails lead to lakes that are perfect for a refreshing afternoon swim. Other activities include watching the beavers at Dream Lake, strolling through the flower-filled meadows and observing the grazing deer and busy marmots, or simply listening to the chorus of songbirds feeding in foliage near Hot Springs Creek.

The first trail in this section takes the long route to the stunning views atop Mt. Harkness, with a strenuous, 3.8-mile climb from Warner Valley to the 8046-foot summit. Next is a very infrequently used trail that follows a lonely stretch of Kings Creek to Corral Meadow. More popular trails emanating from Drakesbad include trips to the area's most interesting hydrothermal features (Boiling Springs Lake, Terminal Geyser, and Devils Kitchen) and most interesting lakes (Little Willow, Drake, Dream, and Sifford). The section closes with longer journeys to Kings Creek Falls and Corral Meadow.

Access

From State Highway 36 in Chester, take Feather River Road just over a half mile to a junction with County Road 312 (Warner Valley Road), which proceeds another 5.5 miles to a junction with County Road 311. From there, follow Warner Valley Road past Warner Creek Campground and the cabins of Warner Valley. The road, which turns to gravel just before a bridge over Warner Creek, continues into Lassen Volcanic, past Warner Valley Campground, before ending at Drakesbad Guest Ranch. The road into the park is generally closed from mid-October through early May.

Campgrounds						
Campground	Fee	Elevation	Season	Restrooms	Running Water	Bear Boxes
High Bridge (Warner Valley Road)	$13	5200′	May to October	Vault	Yes	No
Warner Creek (Warner Valley Road)	$11	5500′	May to October	Vault	No	No
Warner Valley	$14	5650′	Early June to late September	Vault	Yes	Yes

Amenities

Heading west on Highway 36 from the junction of Highway 44, you pass through the tiny community of Westwood, with a gas station, store, and motel, on the way to Chester, the commercial hub for the greater Lake Almanor area. Chester has a couple sporting goods stores, as well as an array of restaurants, motels, bed-and-breakfast inns, gas stations, golf courses, and stores. From Chester, Warner Valley Road leads 17 miles to Drakesbad Guest Ranch, which is open from June to early October; for reservations call 530-529-1512 or visit the website at www.drakesbad.com.

Ranger Stations and Visitor Information

The seasonal Warner Valley ranger station is located a mile before the entrance to Warner Valley Campground. The nearest all-year Forest Service ranger station is in Chester.

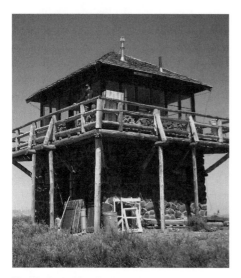

Mt. Harkness Lookout

Trip **65**

Warner Valley to Mount Harkness

S ✓ DH

DISTANCE: 7.6 miles out and back

ELEVATIONS: 5265/8046, +2781/-2781

SEASON: Mid-June to October

USE: Light

MAP: *Mount Harkness*

INTRODUCTION: This route is definitely the road less traveled to the lookout on top of Mt. Harkness. Twice as long as and gaining almost a thousand feet more than the standard trail from Juniper Lake Campground, at first glance this trip would seem to hold little, if any, interest for most hikers. However, upon further inspection, the route is not that difficult in terms of overall length and elevation gain. For those who don't mind the extra effort, the trail from Warner Valley to the top of Mt. Harkness is a fine experience with even less company than the standard route. No matter how you get to the lookout on top, the view is one of the best in the park.

DIRECTIONS TO TRAILHEAD: From Highway 36 in Chester, follow Feather River Road for just over a half mile to a junction and veer left on County Road 312, following signs for Drakesbad. Pass the turnoff to High Bridge Campground on the way to a junction, 6.1 miles from Highway 36, where County Road 311 veers left toward Domingo Springs Campground. Proceed on Road 312 past the entrance to Warner Valley Campground and through the residential community of Warner Valley. Cross a bridge over Warner Creek and travel another 3.4 miles to the somewhat indistinct trailhead on the right-hand side of the road, 12.5 miles from Highway 36 (if

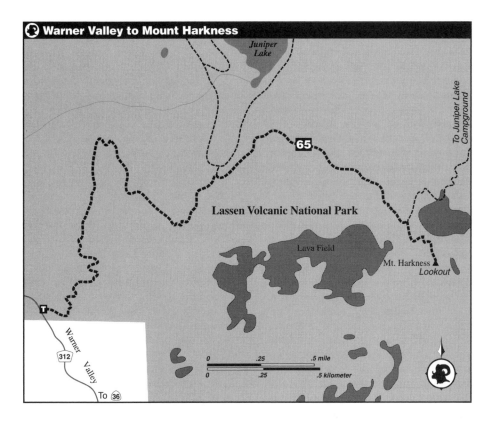

Warner Valley to Mount Harkness

you reach a prominent fork in the road, the trailhead is 0.8 mile back down the road). Park on the narrow shoulder opposite the trailhead.

DESCRIPTION: Beneath moderate forest cover, the trail heads east, beginning an unrelenting climb (albeit with switchbacks) right from the start. Although the bottom section of the trail is shaded, the relatively low elevation means that the ascent will be hot in all but the coolest parts of the day. Farther on, the forest lightens a bit and eventually gives way to shrub-covered slopes, where greenleaf and pinemat manzanita, tobacco brush, and chinquapin flourish. Good views of Warner Valley and over-the-shoulder views of Lassen Peak will spur you on toward the much better views at the lookout. Heading southeast, a steep, upward traverse across shrubby slopes leads beneath some rock bands before the trail turns northeast. Farther on, the grade tem-

porarily abates in a light forest of lodgepole pines, western white pines, and red firs. Cresting a low rise, you reach a junction with trails from Juniper Lake, 2.4 miles from the trailhead.

Turn right (east) to follow directions to Mt. Harkness lookout. The ascent soon resumes on a winding course through open forest with patches of pinemat manzanita and plenty of rock carpeting the slopes. Lassen Peak is visible almost constantly, but unless you have eyes on the back of your head, you won't enjoy the view. Higher up the slope, mountain hemlocks and then whitebark pines join the forest as you approach the next junction with the more popular route to the summit from Juniper Lake Campground, 3.5 miles from the trailhead.

Turn right (south), and climb among the few remaining whitebark pines across gravely slopes bedecked with acres of silver-leaved lupine and Bloomer's goldenbush through midseason. The trail crosses a lightning ground wire, and signs advise passersby that touching it would be unwise. A few last switchbacks lead to the crater rim, where the lookout springs into view.

Stroll easily to the base and climb the short stairs to the deck that runs around the perimeter of the fire lookout. Unlike most fire lookouts today, the one atop Mt. Harkness is still staffed, and a ranger will most likely welcome you into his or her summer residence. The lookout is equipped with a stove, and fuel and supplies are flown in by helicopter at the beginning of the season. The ranger makes once-a-week trips to Chester to acquire additional supplies, such as fresh produce.

The view from the lookout is stunning. With Lassen Peak as a reference point, most of the park's prominent features are easy to identify. The long, sometimes snowy ridge extending south from Lassen Peak is the remains of the northwest flank of ancient Mt. Tehama, an ice age volcano heavily eroded by glaciers. The highest remnant is Brokeoff Mountain, at the apex of the south end of the ridge, and the high point just north of Brokeoff is Mt. Diller. Clockwise from Lassen Peak is the relatively close Saddle Mountain, sloping into Warner Valley. In the distance, Chaos Crags stand above and mostly left of Saddle Mountain. Hat Mountain is the conspicuous, flat-topped cinder cone breaking the horizon adjacent to Saddle Mountain, while above and beyond the west shore of Juniper Lake lies Fairfield Peak. Rising just to the right of and behind Fairfield is West Prospect Peak, connected to slightly higher Prospect Peak. At the base of Prospect Peak, famous Cinder Cone barely peeks over the ridge above the north corner of Juniper Lake. Mt. Hoffman, with its steep, southwest-facing slopes, breaks the skyline just east of Juniper Lake; to the east are two higher peaks, Red Cinder Cone and Red Cinder. Bonte Peak, 2 miles east-northeast of the lookout, is easily recognizable by its finlike appearance. Black Cinder Rock, the high point immediately behind Bonte Peak, is on a ridge in western Caribou Wilderness that runs 3 miles north to Red Cinder. North and South Caribou are the two distant peaks behind Black Cinder Rock. To the south and southeast, long ridges, principally glacial moraines, extend toward the large blue mass of Lake Almanor.

R Fires and camping are prohibited.

WARNER VALLEY TRAILHEAD

Trip **66**

Lower Kings Creek to Corral Meadow

Ⓜ ↗ DH, BP

DISTANCE: 8 miles out and back

ELEVATIONS: 5330/6000, +780/-780

SEASON: Mid-May to November

USE: Light

MAPS: *Mount Harkness, Reading Peak*

INTRODUCTION: Solitude is the primary lure for hikers on the lower section of the Kings Creek Trail. So few walk this path that the Forest Service has not even bothered to mark

the trailhead (although, to be fair, most of the route travels through Lassen Volcanic National Park). This 4-mile section of trail goes to the vicinity of Corral Meadow, which, with the encroaching forest, is not as dramatic as it once was. However, there are many other virtues to this route, including Kings Creek, a fine mountain stream. Once at Corral Meadows, connecting trails offer further hiking opportunities.

DIRECTIONS TO TRAILHEAD: From Highway 36 in Chester, follow Feather River Road for just over a half mile to a junction and veer left on County Road 312, following signs for Drakesbad. Pass the turnoff to High Bridge Campground on the way to a junction, 6.1 miles from Highway 36, where County Road 311 veers left toward Domingo Springs Campground. Proceed on Road 312 past the entrance to Warner Valley Campground and through the residential community of Warner Valley. Cross a bridge

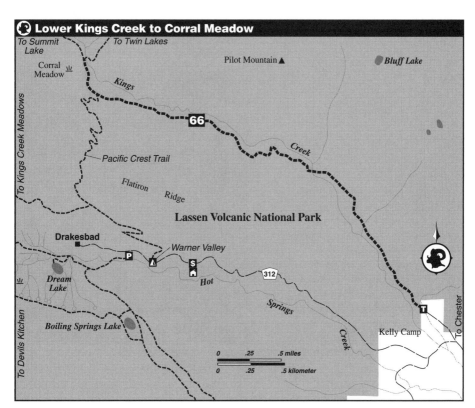

Lower Kings Creek to Corral Meadow

over Warner Creek and travel 4.2 miles to a major fork, where Road 312 bends sharply to the left to cross Kings Creek and then continues to Drakesbad. Proceed ahead at the fork on a much less-traveled dirt road across a spring-fed rivulet and past the last residence to the inauspicious end of the road. Park your vehicle as conditions allow. No signs mark the trailhead.

DESCRIPTION: The most difficult part of the trip will more than likely be locating the start of the trail, which has very indistinct tread and no signs to aid your search. Head northwest on the left side of the usually dry and boulder-strewn overflow channel of Kings Creek. The path becomes more distinct after a short bit, and two signs mark your location—one with mileages to Corral Meadow and Summit Lake and one national park sign.

Beyond the boundary, the trail is much more obvious, if seldom used. The trail follows a slightly undulating course across the east wall of Kings Creek canyon, sometimes right alongside it and sometimes high above the creek. The trail crosses a trio of small, lushly lined side streams and a washed-out seasonal swale on the way to a log crossing of Kings Creek, 1.4 miles from the trailhead. During the peak flows of early summer, the crossing may feel a bit daunting, as the log is perched high above the swift and turbulent waters of Kings Creek.

Once you're safely on the west bank, climb briefly up a washed-out swale to the top of the bank, where good tread resumes and heads upstream on a moderate climb. Lassen Peak makes a very brief appearance as you head up the canyon, but the route is primarily through shady forest, sometimes near the creek and sometimes out of sight but always within earshot. Reach a junction with the Pacific Crest Trail at 3.7 miles.

Proceed ahead (northwest) on the PCT a fair distance from the creek, and follow more gently graded trail across a usually dry swale filled with tall wildflowers and plants, and then walk on the boardwalk over a boggy patch of meadow filled with alders, willows, and other tall plants along the right-hand edge of Corral Meadow. Eventually, the trail draws near to Kings Creek again on the way to the next junction, where the PCT crosses the creek and heads northeast up Grassy Swale. Near this junction, several passable campsites offer possible overnight shelter for backpackers.

[O] Options are many for those looking to extend their trip, with trails headed to virtually every corner of the park.

[R] Wilderness permits are required for overnight stays, and fires are prohibited.

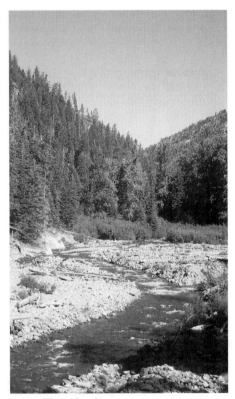

Lower Kings Creek

DRAKESBAD TRAILHEADS

Trip **67**

Boiling Springs Lake

Ⓜ 𝒫 DH

DISTANCE: 2.4 miles semiloop

ELEVATIONS: 5640/6020/5640, +385/-385

SEASON: Late May to mid-October

USE: Moderate

MAP: *Reading Peak*

INTRODUCTION: Similar to the trail to Bumpass Hell, this trip leads to one of the most active hydrothermal areas of the park, where heat and water meet below ground to emerge from the earth's surface in a variety of interesting manifestations. Unlike

Bumpass Hell, however, the trail to Boiling Springs Lake has one principal advantage—far fewer tourists, due to a location in a more remote part of Lassen Volcanic, accessed via a sometimes steep gravel road. Despite its remote location, don't expect to be totally alone, as vacationers from the Drakesbad Guest Ranch frequent the area's trails. Another advantage of Boiling Springs Lake is its lower elevation, which results in warmer temperatures and a much earlier hiking season. Also, the meadows of Warner Valley are blessed with many more species of wildflowers.

DIRECTIONS TO TRAILHEAD: From Highway 36 in Chester, follow Feather River Road for just over a half mile to a junction and veer left on County Road 312, following signs for Drakesbad. Pass the turnoff to High Bridge Campground on the way to a junction, 6.1 miles from Highway 36, where County Road 311 veers left toward

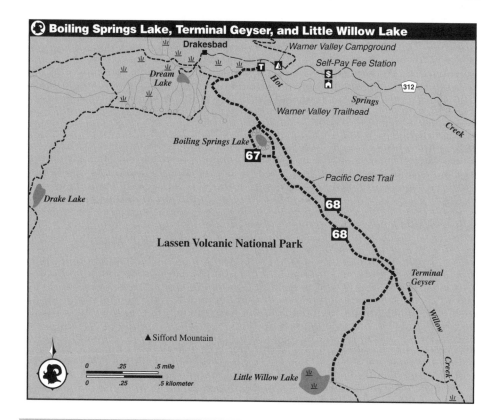

Boiling Springs Lake, Terminal Geyser, and Little Willow Lake

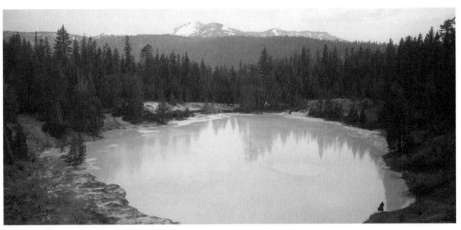

Boiling Springs Lake

Domingo Springs Campground. Proceed on Road 312 past the entrance to Warner Valley Campground and through the residential community of Warner Valley. Cross a bridge over Warner Creek and travel 4.2 miles to a major fork, where Road 312 bends sharply to the left to cross Kings Creek and then continues toward Drakesbad. Enter national park land at 14 miles and continue another mile to the self-pay entrance station near the Warner Valley ranger station. Another mile leads to the entrance into Warner Valley Campground and the northbound Pacific Crest Trail trailhead. Continue ahead a short distance to the left-hand turn into the parking area for the Warner Valley Trailhead, 16.3 miles from Highway 36. The trailhead is equipped with a modern vault toilet, bear-proof trash cans, and picnic tables.

DESCRIPTION: Follow the Pacific Crest Trail southwest through open forest near the fringe of the extensive and lush meadows of the Drakesbad area, and continue along the north bank of spring-fed Hot Springs Creek. Along with such notable thermal features as Boiling Springs Lake and Devils Kitchen (as well as several unnamed hot springs), Hot Springs Creek is also fed by a number of cold springs trickling down the sides of Warner Valley, which keeps the summertime water temperature somewhere between 50 and 55 degrees. Watch for the dipper, a small, chunky, bobbing gray bird that feeds in the fast-flowing water. Mountain alder lines the creek and springs, with extensive patches growing in the meadows as well. Numerous species of water-loving wildflowers carpet the slopes before late July: white- or cream-colored flowers include Brewer's bittercress, white brodiaea, corn lily, Gray's lovage, long-stalked starwort, Brewer's thistle, naked star tulip, and yarrow; yellow flowers include sticky cinquefoil, common dandelion, common large, and monkeyflower; pink flowers are most likely Oregon checker; red-violet flowers could be California blue-eyed grass or meadow penstemon; and blue-violet flowers might be alpine brookline or large-leaved lupine. Boardwalks span some of the boggy sections of meadow on the way to a wood-plank bridge across the creek.

Proceed across the hillside above the south bank, passing above the inviting-looking hot springs pool of the Drakesbad resort. At a Y-junction with a trail accessing Dream Lake, Devils Kitchen, and the horse trail from the resort's stables, follow signs for Boiling Springs Lake and veer left. Proceed on a steady climb along the PCT through a scattered to light forest of firs, incense cedars, ponderosa pines, and lodgepole pines, reaching another Y-junction at 0.9 mile.

BOILING SPRINGS LAKE

The thumping sound you hear is created from the bubbling mud pots. The temperature of the water in the lake is usually between 120°F and 125°F in the summer, and around 110°F in the winter. Pools near the shore can be even hotter—about 190°F to 200°F, which is near the boiling point of water at this elevation.

Lying along a young fault, the lake is heated by steam and fumes rising through underground vents and fissures. On cool days, water vapor may be seen rising from the surface. During the course of the summer, the water level drops about a foot, exposing clay mud around the edge of the lake that dries and cracks.

The lake is approximately 630 feet in length, and has a shoreline perimeter of about 2000 feet. The yellow-tan color comes from a composition of clay, opal, and iron-oxide particles suspended in the water. The green color seen in shallow water and wet mud is from algae—microscopic plants that have adapted to the hot-water environment.

Turn right at the junction and follow the Boiling Springs Lake circuit on a mild climb toward the lake. Soon come to the crossing of a seasonal stream that carries the geothermal outflow from the lake. A red warning sign nearby encourages visitors to stay on the trail and away from unstable ground for their own safety. After the crossing, you emerge from the forest and make a short uphill walk to where steamy Boiling Springs Lake is visible. You'll probably smell the lake before you see it; the characteristic rotten egg odor is from hydrogen sulfide produced from sulfur in oxygen-poor rising gases.

At the south end of the lake, the trail veers away from the edge and climbs a bit into the trees in order to avoid steep and unstable slopes above the south shore. Reach a three-way junction southeast of the lake and head left to complete the circuit. Eventually, the lake returns to view, backdropped by majestic Lassen Peak. Continue around the east shore and head back into forest on the way to a junction, where you turn left and proceed shortly to the close of the loop above the northwest shore. From there, retrace your steps northeast to the trailhead.

R Fires are prohibited, and camping is prohibited within a quarter mile of Boiling Springs Lake.

DRAKESBAD TRAILHEADS

Trip **68**

see map on p.199

Terminal Geyser and Little Willow Lake

M **℞** DH

DISTANCE:	5.8 miles semiloop
ELEVATIONS:	5640/6250/5735; +1185/-1185
SEASON:	Late May to mid-October
USE:	Moderate
MAP:	*Reading Peak*

INTRODUCTION: On this trip, hikers can sample some of the park's more interesting hydrothermal features while avoiding the hordes of tourists found in similar areas near the main park road, like Sulphur Works and Bumpass Hell. After visiting the flower-covered meadows around Drakesbad, hikers arc around the west side of geologically fascinating Boiling Springs Lake. From there, 2 miles of forested hiking leads to Terminal Geyser, where clouds of steam rise out of a multicolored canyon and billow into the sky. Little Willow Lake lies just a mile southwest of the main trail for those seeking an additional destination.

DIRECTIONS TO TRAILHEAD: From Highway 36 in Chester, follow Feather River Road for just over a half mile to a junction and veer left on County Road 312, following signs for Drakesbad. Pass the turnoff to High Bridge Campground on the way to a junction, 6.1 miles from Highway 36, where County Road 311 veers left toward Domingo Springs Campground. Proceed on Road 312 past the entrance to Warner Valley Campground and through the residential community of Warner Valley. Cross a bridge over Warner Creek and travel 4.2 miles to a major fork, where Road 312 bends sharply to the left to cross Kings Creek and then continues toward Drakesbad. Enter national park land at 14 miles and continue another mile to the self-pay entrance station near the Warner Valley ranger station. Another mile leads to the entrance into Warner Valley Campground and the northbound Pacific Crest Trail trailhead. Continue ahead a short distance to the left-hand turn into the parking area for the Warner Valley Trailhead, 16.3 miles from Highway 36. The trailhead is equipped with a modern vault toilet, bear-proof trash cans, and picnic tables.

DESCRIPTION: Follow the Pacific Crest Trail southwest through open forest near the fringe of the extensive and lush meadows of the Drakesbad area, and continue along the north bank of spring-fed Hot Springs Creek. Along with such notable thermal features as Boiling Springs Lake and Devils Kitchen (as well as several unnamed hot springs), Hot Springs Creek is also fed by a number of cold springs trickling down the sides of Warner Valley, which keeps the summertime water temperature somewhere between 50 and 55 degrees. Watch for the dipper, a small, chunky, bobbing gray bird that feeds in the fast-flowing water. Mountain alder lines the creek and springs, with extensive patches growing in the meadows as well. Numerous species of water-loving wildflowers carpet the slopes before late July: white- or cream-colored flowers include Brewer's bittercress, white brodiaea, corn lily, Gray's lovage, long-stalked

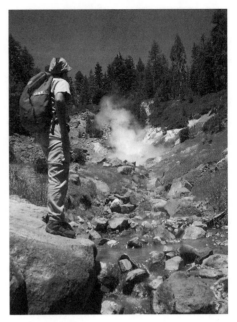

Terminal Geyser

starwort, Brewer's thistle, naked star tulip, and yarrow; yellow flowers include sticky cinquefoil, common dandelion, common large, and monkeyflower; pink flowers are most likely Oregon checker; red-violet flowers could be California blue-eyed grass or meadow penstemon; and blue-violet flowers might be alpine brookline or large-leaved lupine. Boardwalks span some of the boggy sections of meadow on the way to a wood-plank bridge across the creek.

Proceed across the hillside above the south bank, passing above the inviting-looking hot springs pool of the Drakesbad resort. At a Y-junction with a trail accessing Dream Lake, Devils Kitchen, and the horse trail from the resort's stables, follow signs for Boiling Springs Lake and veer left. Proceed on a steady climb along the PCT through a scattered to light forest of firs, incense cedars, ponderosa pines, and lodgepole pines, reaching another Y-junction at 0.9 mile.

To visit Boiling Springs Lake, which is definitely worth the short diversion, turn right at the junction and follow the Boiling Springs Lake circuit on a mild climb toward

THE BATTLE FOR TERMINAL GEYSER

In 1962, an oil company bulldozed a road to Terminal Geyser, which at the time was part of a 566-acre privately owned tract of land just outside the park boundary. Sixteen years later, without contacting the Park Service, Phillips Petroleum Corporation cleared a 1.5-acre site on their land and sunk a test well immediately below Terminal Geyser, within a stone's throw of the Pacific Crest Trail. Park officials were concerned about the negative side effects future drilling might have on Terminal Geyser and other nearby hydrothermal features such as Boiling Springs Lake and Devils Kitchen. After Phillips returned to the site a year later without notifying the Park Service, the Interior Department condemned the property and then issued a "declaration of taking" in 1980.

After years of litigation, Phillips Petroleum Corporation and its trustees were awarded more $11 million in damages. The Park Service had the well plugged in 1997 and began restoration of the site the next year. Nowadays, park visitors without previous knowledge are completely unaware of the travesty that once occurred at Terminal Geyser. The grassy slope on the far side of Willow Creek was the site that was cleared in 1978.

the lake. Soon come to the crossing of a seasonal stream that carries the geothermal outflow from the lake. A red warning sign nearby encourages visitors to stay on the trail and away from unstable ground for their own safety. After the crossing, you emerge from the forest and make a short uphill walk to where steamy Boiling Springs Lake is visible (see Trip 67 for information on the lake). The trail veers away at the south end of the lake, and climbs a bit into the trees in order to avoid steep and unstable slopes above the south shore. Just after crossing, the usually dry inlet the trail leads to a signed three-way junction southeast of the lake. Turn right, following signed directions toward Terminal Geyser and Little Willow Lake.

Head southeast on mild to moderately rising trail through mixed forest, which eventually gives way to a more open forest, where pinemat and greenleaf manzanita flourishes on the dry and sunny slopes. After gaining the top of a broad ridge, the trail begins a mild then moderate descent back into forest cover on the way to Terminal Geyser. At 2.5 miles from the trailhead, you rejoin the PCT at a signed junction.

Turn right (south) and walk about 25 feet to a second junction, where the PCT veers right toward Little Willow Lake, but you continue ahead toward Terminal Geyser.

Follow moderate then steeply descending tread past a red warning sign, then a sign with directions to the PCT. Where the grade eases, reach a third sign for Terminal Geyser ahead and Warner Valley behind. Near this last sign, the obscure tread of a seldom-used trail heads southeast to Willow Lake (see Trip 74). Now following the course of an old road, you curve around into the upper canyon of Willow Creek and head upstream toward the billowing cloud of steam above Terminal Geyser. Step across a pair of small, spring-fed rivulets and pass another warning sign on the approach to the geyser.

Continually churning out steam, Terminal Geyser is not really a geyser, which periodically erupts hot water, but a fumarole, which emits steam and gases. Back-dropped by colorful rocks, the fumarole spits out a continuous plume that rises above the surrounding treetops, while smaller openings in the crust scattered around the head of the canyon emit less dramatic wisps of steam. Without the typical guardrails that keep tourists a safe distance from more visited hydrothermal features in the park, you must observe this feature with caution. Even the water downstream from Terminal Geyser in nascent Willow Creek can be quite hot in places.

Once you've absorbed the full experience of Terminal Geyser, retrace your steps back up to the junction with the Pacific Crest Trail and turn left to follow the southbound PCT across a seasonal swale and then on a moderate, 230-foot climb through the forest to the top of a ridge. From there, the trail drops nearly an equal amount of elevation to the forest-rimmed shore of Little Willow Lake, 1 mile from the junction. Little Willow Lake can be considered a bona fide lake only during early season, as by midsummer it resembles a wet marsh, and by late summer it's a mudflat. Mosquitoes are problematic as well.

Once you've fully taken in the ambiance of Little Willow Lake, retrace your steps north-northeast to the junction of the PCT and the trail to Terminal Geyser. Continue north on the PCT, immediately passing the junction to Boiling Springs Lake and continuing northwest toward Warner Valley. A moderate ascent to the top of a broad ridge passes an open area carpeted with arrowleaf balsamroot's yellow flowers. Beyond this floral oasis, the conifers return and the grade eases before mildly descending trail leads away from the ridge.

Farther on, a brief stretch of trail through open forest and manzanita offers filtered views of Lassen Peak, Mt. Harkness, and Flatiron Ridge above Warner Valley. Head back into the trees and continue the gentle descent to a junction, where the PCT briefly merges with the Boiling Springs Lake circuit before veering away to soon reach a junction with the short lateral to the lake. From there, continue straight ahead (northwest) to retrace your steps 0.9 mile to the Warner Valley trailhead.

R Fires are prohibited, and camping is prohibited within a quarter mile of Boiling Springs Lake and Terminal Geyser, and at Little Willow Lake.

DRAKESBAD TRAILHEADS

Trip 69

Drake Lake

Ⓜ ╱ DH, BP

DISTANCE: 4.8 miles out and back

ELEVATIONS: 5640/6510, +875/-875

SEASON: June to mid-October

USE: Moderate

MAP: *Reading Peak*

INTRODUCTION: About 4 feet deep around the Fourth of July and half that by Labor Day, Drake Lake may not be the most desirable lake for swimmers and anglers, but this is a popular horseback ride for parties from the Drakesbad Guest Ranch, and a number of hikers and some backpackers visit the forest-rimmed lake with some regularity. For those who don't mind the steep climb, there are good views of Warner Valley and some of the surrounding peaks, and the lake itself can be a pleasant spot for a picnic lunch or an overnight camp.

DIRECTIONS TO TRAILHEAD: From Highway 36 in Chester, follow Feather River Road for just over a half mile to a junction and veer left on County Road 312, following signs for Drakesbad. Pass the turnoff to High Bridge Campground on the way to a junction, 6.1 miles from Highway 36, where County Road 311 veers left toward Domingo Springs Campground. Proceed on Road 312 past the entrance to Warner Valley Campground and through the residential community of Warner Valley. Cross a bridge over Warner Creek and travel 4.2 miles to a major fork, where Road 312 bends sharply to the left to cross Kings Creek and then continues toward Drakesbad. Enter national park land at 14 miles and continue another mile to the self-pay entrance station near the Warner Valley ranger station. Another mile leads to the entrance into Warner Valley Campground

Drake Lake

To Corral Meadow

Sifford Lake

Pacific Crest Trail

Warner Valley CG

Drakesbad

Self-Pay
Fee Station

Dream
Lake

Hot

Springs

Devils Kitchen

T

S

312

Creek

Warner Valley Trailhead

69

Pacific Crest Trail

Boiling Springs Lake

▲7139'

Lassen Volcanic National Park

Drake Lake

Panther

Creek

0   .25   .5 mile
0   .25   .5 kilometer

To North Arm Rice Creek   ▲ Sifford Mountain   To Little Willow Lake

and the northbound Pacific Crest Trail trailhead. Continue ahead a short distance to the left-hand turn into the parking area for the Warner Valley Trailhead, 16.3 miles from Highway 36. The trailhead is equipped with a modern vault toilet, bear-proof trash cans, and picnic tables.

DESCRIPTION: Follow the Pacific Crest Trail southwest through open forest near the fringe of the extensive and lush meadows of the Drakesbad area, and continue along the north bank of spring-fed Hot Springs Creek. Along with such notable thermal features as Boiling Springs Lake and Devils Kitchen (as well as several unnamed hot springs), Hot Springs Creek is also fed by a number of cold springs trickling down the sides of Warner Valley, which keeps the summertime water temperature somewhere between 50 and 55 degrees. Watch for the dipper, a small, chunky, bobbing gray bird that feeds in the fast-flowing water.

Mountain alder lines the creek and springs, with extensive patches growing in the meadows as well. Numerous species of water-loving wildflowers carpet the slopes before late July: white- or cream-colored flowers include Brewer's bittercress, white brodiaea, corn lily, Gray's lovage, long-stalked starwort, Brewer's thistle, naked star tulip, and yarrow; yellow flowers include sticky cinquefoil, common dandelion, common large, and monkeyflower; pink flowers are most likely Oregon checker; red-violet flowers could be California blue-eyed grass or meadow penstemon; and blue-violet flowers might be alpine brookline or large-leaved lupine. Boardwalks span some of the boggy sections of meadow on the way to a wood-plank bridge across the creek.

Proceed across the hillside above the south bank, passing above the inviting-looking hot springs pool of the Drakesbad resort. At a Y-junction with a trail accessing Dream Lake, Devils Kitchen, and the horse trail from the resort's stables, veer left and make a very short climb to a second junction, where the PCT continues ahead but you turn right on the fainter tread of the trail to Drake Lake. Immediately cross the usually dry channel of Boiling Springs Lake's outlet, and then briefly climb alongside it before the gradient eases, as the trail turns southwest. Soon cross the first of many spring-fed rivulets you'll see over the next half mile or so. Fortunately, most of the springs are below the trail, sparing you from having to plow through thick alder groves. At the first rivulet, look for Sierra corydalis, a spreading, water-loving plant that superficially resembles a large lupine. However, further inspection of the erect rows of pale-pink flowers reveals a closer resemblance to the larkspur, which makes the Sierra corydalis a member of the buttercup family. Pass a few giant aspens before crossing a smaller rivulet, and then follow the trail on a rolling traverse through a shady white fir forest, with occasional views of the spring-fed Drakesbad Meadow below. At 1.3 miles from the trailhead, you reach a junction with a connector to the Devils Kitchen Trail.

Heading west from the junction, a more moderate climb leads through a forest that now includes western white pines. Soon the forest opens, which creates habitat for a healthy understory of pinemat manzanita. An afternoon ascent of this essentially shadeless slope can be hot, so an early start is recommended when the weather forecast calls for high temperatures. The tread is rocky and has been churned up by horses along this section, which makes the steep climb seem even more tedious.

Midway up the slope, you can stop and rest at switchbacks, taking the opportunity to scan the countryside and enjoy the view  of Warner Valley and such notable peaks as Pilot Mountain, Saddle Mountain, Mt. Harkness, Reading Peak, and Lassen Peak. Fortunately, the steep climb slackens where the trail returns to forest cover. Reach lodgepole- and grass-rimmed Drake Lake, where a few small campsites will tempt overnighters.

O Adventurous souls can follow the disappearing tread of a trail that supposedly continues south from the lake and into the North Arm Rice Creek drainage—more of a cross-country route than a bona fide trail.

R Wilderness permits are required for overnight stays, and fires are prohibited.

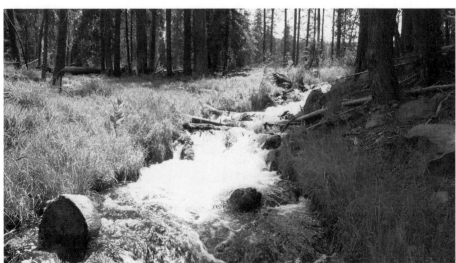

Hot Springs Creek tributary

Trip **70**

Dream Lake and Devils Kitchen

E ✎ DH

DISTANCE: 5.6 miles out and back

ELEVATIONS: 5640/6095, +800/-800

SEASON: June to mid-October

USE: Moderate

MAP: *Reading Peak*

INTRODUCTION: Hydrothermal wonders abound at the end of this short trail to the basin of Devils Kitchen, where visitors can enjoy close views of bubbling mud pots and venting fumaroles amid a rainbow of colored rock. You will encounter far fewer people here than at places like Sulphur Works and Bumpass Hell, which attract hordes of tourists. In addition to the hydrothermal area, the trail offers an easy hike to Dream Lake, where fishing and swimming are popular activities, as is beaver watching. Since part of the trail to Devils Kitchen passes through the rich Drakesbad Meadow, hikers can also enjoy some of the vibrant wildflower displays through midsummer.

DIRECTIONS TO TRAILHEAD: From Highway 36 in Chester, follow Feather River Road for just over a half mile to a junction and veer left on County Road 312, following signs for Drakesbad. Pass the turnoff to High Bridge Campground on the way to a junction, 6.1 miles from Highway 36, where County Road 311 veers left toward Domingo Springs Campground. Proceed on Road 312 past the entrance to Warner Valley Campground and through the residential community of Warner Valley. Cross a bridge over Warner Creek and travel 4.2 miles to a major fork, where Road 312 bends sharply to the left to cross Kings Creek and then continues toward Drakesbad.

Enter national park land at 14 miles and continue another mile to the self-pay entrance station near the Warner Valley ranger station. Another mile leads to the entrance into Warner Valley Campground and the northbound Pacific Crest Trail trailhead. Continue ahead a short distance to the left-hand turn into the parking area for the Warner Valley Trailhead, 16.3 miles from Highway 36. The trailhead is equipped with a modern vault toilet, bear-proof trash cans, and picnic tables.

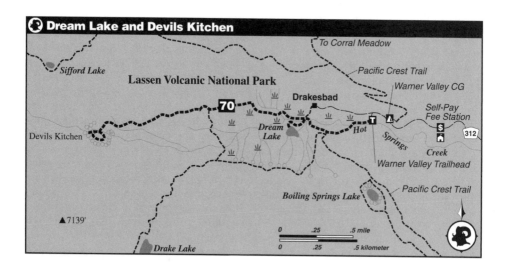

Dream Lake and Devils Kitchen

DESCRIPTION: Follow the Pacific Crest Trail southwest through open forest near the fringe of the extensive and lush meadows of the Drakesbad area, and continue along the north bank of spring-fed Hot Springs Creek. Along with such notable thermal features as Boiling Springs Lake and Devils Kitchen (as well as several unnamed hot springs), Hot Springs Creek is also fed by a number of cold springs trickling down the sides of Warner Valley, which keeps the summertime water temperature somewhere between 50 and 55 degrees. Watch for the dipper, a small, chunky, bobbing gray bird that feeds in the fast-flowing water. Mountain alder lines the creek and springs, with extensive patches growing in the meadows as well. Numerous species of water-loving wildflowers carpet the slopes before late July: white- or cream-colored flowers include Brewer's bittercress, white brodiaea, corn lily, Gray's lovage, long-stalked starwort, Brewer's thistle, naked star tulip, and yarrow; yellow flowers include sticky cinquefoil, common dandelion, common large, and monkeyflower; pink flowers are most likely Oregon checker; red-violet flowers could be California blue-eyed grass or meadow penstemon; and blue-violet flowers might be alpine brookline or large-leaved lupine. Boardwalks span some of the boggy sections of meadow on the way to a wood-plank bridge across the creek.

Proceed across the hillside above the south bank, passing above the inviting-looking hot springs pool of the Drakesbad resort. At a Y-junction, veer right, leaving the PCT and following directions for Devils Kitchen, whose trail crosses bridges and boardwalks to a three-way junction.

To visit Dream Lake, turn left, cross a bridge over Hot Springs Creek, and make a short, moderate climb through mixed forest to the grass-tinged and forest-rimmed shore of the lake. Although Dream Lake was originally artificially made, a family of beavers has taken over the duties of maintaining the lake, and a beaver lodge can be viewed near the lake's outlet and beaver dam (be careful not to disturb the animals). Your best chance of observing one of these furry

> **MARMOTS**
>
> Marmots may be seen in Drakesbad Meadow, but their burrows are a more common sight. The chubby rodents burrow into high spots in the meadow and occasionally under logs—very atypical marmot dwelling sites. Typically, marmots make their burrows in rock piles, such as talus slopes, but the meadow is lacking in such rocky areas.

rodents is during early-morning and evening periods. The small lake is stocked with trout, although it receives plenty of pressure from anglers from Drakesbad Guest Ranch. The spring-fed waters are not as warm as you might think, given the lake's size and relatively low elevation, but Dream Lake is nevertheless an acceptable swimming hole, particularly for nonguests of the resort who are barred from using the hot springs pool.

Return to the junction and head west toward Devils Kitchen through Drakesbad Meadow. After a lengthy traverse of the meadow, the trail bends and climbs a few vertical feet to higher ground. At 1.4 miles from the trailhead, you reach a three-way junction with a connector to the Drake Lake Trail.

Proceed ahead (west) from here on a mild to moderate climb through mixed forest, and hop over a thin, seasonal stream on the way toward Devils Kitchen. Nearing the hydrothermal area, you will no doubt smell the rotten egg odor of your destination well before arriving at the Devils Kitchen loop. Drop down to cross an alder-lined tributary of Hot Springs Creek, follow the creek briefly, and then make a very short climb to the top of a low ridge, where equestrians must dismount and tie up their horses. Cross the ridge to head into the main canyon of Hot Springs Creek, which you cross on a wood bridge. On the far side, warning signs advise you to remain on the trail at all times, as you could be severely burned upon breaking through the thin crust and plunging into the boiling water below. On the far side of the creek, a short climb leads up a hillside, where the sight of bubbling mud pots and wisps of steam emanating from vents downstream herald your approach to Devils Kitchen and the start of the loop trail.

On the loop through Devils Kitchen, you'll see numerous fumaroles and mud pots amid a riot of odd-colored rock. A substantial stream flows right through the middle of Devils Kitchen, carving a way through the soft, easily erodible, decayed rock. The icy stream cascades into the basin and then exits at the east end only a few degrees warmer. Another significant difference from other hydrothermal areas is the considerable amount of vegetation present in the Devils Kitchen basin, including the unusual pairing of incense cedars with Labrador teas (here, above 6000 feet, incense cedars are at the top of their range, while Labrador teas are at the bottom of their range). Labrador teas can be recognized by their small, shiny leaves, which, when rubbed between fingers emit a turpentine odor. After enjoying the marvels of Devils Kitchen, retrace your steps to the trailhead.

[O] The return route can be turned into a semiloop by hiking back 1.3 miles to the three-way junction with a trail toward Drake Lake and turning right. Head south through forested terrain to a boulder hop of an alder-lined creek about 130 yards before a bridged crossing of Hot Springs Creek, lined with alders and aspens. From the creek, a mild climb leads to a junction with the trail to Drake Lake, where you should turn left (east) and pass above and across several spring-fed creeks on the way to a junction with the Pacific Crest Trail. From there, turn left and follow the PCT a very short distance to a second junction with your original route to Devils Kitchen and then continue northeast through lush vegetation to a bridged crossing of Hot Springs Creek. From the crossing, the trail follows the north bank of the creek back to the trailhead.

[R] Fires are prohibited, and camping is prohibited within a quarter mile of Devils Kitchen.

DRAKESBAD TRAILHEADS

Trip 71

Sifford Lakes

(M)/ DH, BP

DISTANCE: 4.2 miles out and back

ELEVATIONS: 5685/7200, +1515/-1515

SEASON: Mid-June to mid-October

USE: Moderate

MAP: *Reading Peak*

INTRODUCTION: The Sifford Lakes are a group of nearly a dozen small lakes and ponds nestled into a bench above the lip of Hot Springs Creek canyon. Distinct trail leads to the first two lakes in the chain, and the remainder can easily be reached via short and straightforward cross-country routes. Most of the traffic seems to emanate from visitors staying at the Drakesbad Guest Ranch, but most people go no farther than the first lake, so it's reasonable to expect solitude at the others. Surrounded by open forest, Sifford Lakes usually shed their snow by mid-June and typically warm up for decent swimming by early July. However, anglers should look elsewhere to practice their craft, as the shallow lakes are devoid of fish. Backpackers will find fairly good campsites around the first two lakes, and nearby cliffs offer excellent views of the terrain both near and far.

DIRECTIONS TO TRAILHEAD: From Highway 36 in Chester, follow Feather River Road for just over a half mile to a junction and veer left on County Road 312, following signs for Drakesbad. Pass the turnoff to High Bridge Campground on the way to a junction, 6.1 miles from Highway 36, where County Road 311 veers left toward Domingo Springs Campground. Proceed on Road 312 past the entrance to Warner Valley Campground and through the residential community of Warner Valley. Cross a bridge over Warner Creek and travel 4.2

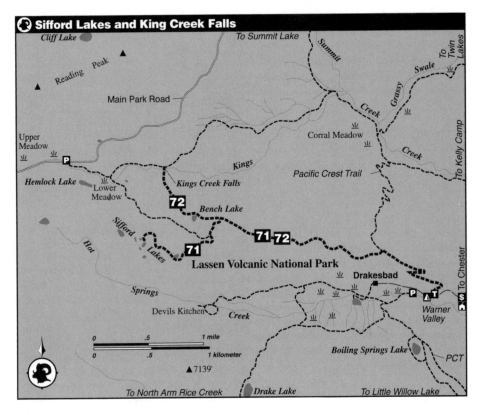

Sifford Lakes and King Creek Falls

miles to a major fork, where Road 312 bends sharply to the left to cross Kings Creek and then continues toward Drakesbad. Enter national park land at 14 miles and continue another mile to the self-pay entrance station near the Warner Valley ranger station. Another mile leads to the entrance into Warner Valley Campground—a handful of sites above Hot Springs Creek are to the left of the road, while the majority of the 18 sites and the northbound Pacific Crest Trail trailhead are up the road to the right. Turn right and follow the campground access road to the small parking area opposite the trailhead, which has vault toilets.

DESCRIPTION: Beneath the cover of Jeffrey pines, incense cedars, and white firs, the well-graded Pacific Crest Trail heads southwest, immediately crossing a tiny, spring-fed creek before climbing the north wall of Hot Springs Creek canyon to the first of three long switchbacks. The forest thins above the first switchback, allowing good views of Drakesbad and the canyon below. Above the last switchback, the trail surmounts the lip of the canyon wall, returns to forest, and reaches a junction at 1.2 miles from the trailhead.

Leaving the PCT, turn left (southwest), initially on gently graded tread, followed by a moderate climb along a lateral moraine. Although the westward climb closely follows the brink of Hot Springs Creek canyon, views are somewhat limited, thanks to a dense forest of white and red firs. Farther on, the firs yield to an open Jeffrey pine forest with plenty of shrubs, particularly greenleaf manzanita and tobacco brush. Western white pines and lodgepole pines join the forest as you climb to an open knoll, followed by a short drop to a Y-junction in a shallow bowl with a trail to Bench Lake, 2.7 miles from the trailhead.

Veer left and make a stiff, quarter-mile climb to gentler terrain and a three-way junction with your spur trail to Sifford Lakes. Proceed ahead (west) and follow undulating trail that weaves across open slopes carpeted with pinemat manzanita amid widely scattered pines and firs. After climbing the final rise, the first lake appears, 0.5 mile from the junction. The small and mostly shallow lake is just deep enough for decent swimming. Being surrounded by an open forest of lodgepole pines, western white pines, hemlocks, and firs, the lake usually sheds its snow by mid-June and warms up to a decent temperature by early July. From mid-July to late August, the water temperature hovers in the mid- or upper 60s, which ranks this as one of the park's warmest lakes. Use trails lead to campsites near the brink of the upper part of Hot Springs Creek canyon, with views straight down rock cliffs to the valley floor.

Well-defined tread leads away from the first lake to the next lake in the chain, a slightly larger body of water, rimmed with an open forest similar in composition to the first lake. Slightly better campsites with more solitude are scattered around the lakeshore. Nearby cliffs provide a stunning view that includes such notable landmarks as Lassen Peak and Lake Almanor.

While defined tread ends at the second Sifford Lake, the remaining lakes on the bench are just a straightforward cross-country jaunt away to the northwest.

Wilderness permits are required for overnight stays, and fires are prohibited.

DRAKESBAD TRAILHEADS

Trip 72

see map on p.210

Kings Creek Falls

M / DH

DISTANCE: 7.6 miles out and back

ELEVATIONS: 5685/6980/6820, +1460/-1460

SEASON: Late June to mid-October

USE: Moderate

MAP: *Reading Peak*

INTRODUCTION: This trip is the long way to picturesque Kings Creek Falls, but you won't have to contend with the crowds on this route, at least until you reach the falls. The other benefit to this route is that the steep climbing is done during the first half of the journey, which makes the return all downhill—exactly opposite of the more popular, 1.2-mile trail from the Kings Creek Trailhead. A 2.25-mile extension provides an opportunity to see Kings Creek Cascades and Lower Kings Creek Meadow, and to reach the Sifford Lakes trail junction, from which you could extend the trip even farther to visit the Sifford Lakes described in Trip 71.

DIRECTIONS TO TRAILHEAD: From Highway 36 in Chester, follow Feather River Road for just over a half mile to a junction and veer left on County Road 312, following signs for Drakesbad. Pass the turnoff to High Bridge Campground on the way to a junction, 6.1 miles from Highway 36, where County Road 311 veers left toward Domingo Springs Campground. Proceed on Road 312 past the entrance to Warner Valley Campground and through the residential community of Warner Valley. Cross a bridge over Warner Creek and travel 4.2 miles to a major fork, where Road 312 bends sharply to the left to cross Kings Creek and then continues toward Drakesbad. Enter national park land at 14 miles and continue another mile to the self-pay entrance station near the Warner Valley ranger station. Another mile leads to the entrance into Warner Valley Campground—a handful of sites above Hot Springs Creek are to the left of the road, while the majority of the 18 sites and the northbound Pacific Crest Trail trailhead are up the road to the right. Turn right and follow the campground access road to the small parking area opposite the trailhead, which has vault toilets.

DESCRIPTION: Beneath the cover of Jeffrey pines, incense cedars, and white firs, the well-graded Pacific Crest Trail heads southwest, immediately crossing a tiny, spring-fed creek before climbing the north wall of Hot Springs Creek canyon to the first of three long switchbacks. The forest thins above the first switchback, allowing good views of Drakesbad and the canyon below. Above the last switchback, the trail surmounts the lip of the canyon wall, returns to forest, and reaches a junction at 1.2 miles from the trailhead.

Leaving the PCT, turn left (southwest), initially on gently graded tread, followed by a moderate climb along a lateral moraine. Although the westward climb closely follows the brink of Hot Springs Creek canyon, views are somewhat limited, thanks to a dense forest of white and red firs. Farther on, the firs yield to an open Jeffrey pine forest with plenty of shrubs, particularly greenleaf manzanita and tobacco brush. Western white pines and lodgepole pines join the forest as you climb to an open knoll, followed by a short drop to a Y-junction in a shallow bowl with a trail to Bench Lake, 2.7 miles from the trailhead.

Continue northwest from the junction, initially on gently graded trail before a steep climb attacks the hillside ahead through an open forest of lodgepole pines, western white pines, and firs, with a groundcover primarily of pinemat manzanita. The stiff climb abruptly ends when you reach the basin holding forest-rimmed Bench Lake, a lackluster lake that becomes even more so after midseason, when the water level drops significantly. Just past the lake, the trail

resumes the steep climb before dropping into the Kings Creek drainage in dense forest that now includes mountain hemlocks. With the roar of the creek reverberating through the canyon, you follow a descending traverse to a bridge of twin, flat-topped logs spanning the churning stream and a junction on the far bank, 3.75 miles from the trailhead.

Turn right (east) and head downstream a short distance from the junction to a viewpoint of Kings Creek Falls. Situated on the very brink of the falls and guarded by a cable, the overlook provides a fine aerie from which to gaze at the 50-foot cascade. Some visitors scramble down the steep slope to the base of the falls, but this is not a maintained trail—exercise extreme caution if you choose to descend the potentially loose and slippery rocks. Because of the fall's aspect, photographers should plan on a visit from late morning to shortly after

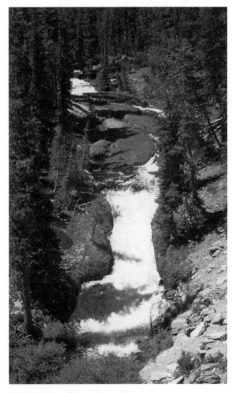

Cascade on Kings Creek

noon, as this is the only time when the falls are bathed in sunlight.

O It's possible to alter the return route to create a 2.25-mile semiloop. Return to the junction near the bridge over Kings Creek, and instead of heading back over the bridge, continue upstream on a moderate climb under forest cover. A short distance past a horse trail (a quarter mile from the junction), you break out of the trees at the base of a very steep section of trail that travels next to Kings Creek Cascades, a series of tumbling cataracts and rapidly swirling pools where the creek plummets through a narrow gash of rock. The dramatic scenery provides plenty of opportunities to catch your breath during the steep but short ascent. Just beyond the top of the cascades is a junction with the horse trail bypass of the cascades, a short lateral to a viewpoint, and the continuation of the trail to the Kings Creek Trailhead. Continue ahead toward the Kings Creek Trailhead on a mildly rising climb to a junction near the east end of Lower Kings Creek Meadow.

Leave the Kings Creek Trail and turn left (south) across the lower end of the meadow to a log crossing of Kings Creek (may be a wet ford in early season). From there, the trail heads southeast on a nearly level grade through open forest for a half mile or so before dropping more steeply toward the Sifford Lakes junction (if you wish to visit the lakes, see Trip 71). From the junction, continue the descent northeast and then east to the junction at the close of the loop. From there, turn right, and retrace your steps to the trailhead.

R Fires are prohibited, and camping is prohibited at Kings Creek Falls, as well as at the upper and lower meadows.

DRAKESBAD TRAILHEADS

Trip 73

Corral Meadow Loop

M **Q** DH, BP

Distance:	9.6 miles loop
Elevations:	5685/6980/5685, +1885/-1885
Season:	Late June to mid-October
Use:	Moderate
Map:	*Reading Peak*

INTRODUCTION: This loop follows less-traveled routes to a couple of the park's significant features, Corral Meadow, a popular camping area along the Pacific Crest Trail, and Kings Creek Falls, a dramatic 50-foot waterfall.

DIRECTIONS TO TRAILHEAD: From Highway 36 in Chester, follow Feather River Road for just over a half mile to a junction and veer left on County Road 312, following signs for Drakesbad. Pass the turnoff to High Bridge Campground on the way to a junction, 6.1 miles from Highway 36, where County Road 311 veers left toward Domingo SpringsCampground. Proceed on Road 312 past the entrance to Warner Valley Campground and through the residential community of Warner Valley. Cross a bridge over Warner Creek and travel 4.2 miles to a major fork, where Road 312 bends sharply to the left to cross Kings Creek and then continues toward Drakesbad. Enter national park land at 14 miles and continue another mile to the self-pay entrance station near the Warner Valley ranger station. Another mile leads to the entrance into Warner Valley Campground—a handful of sites above Hot Springs Creek are to the left of the road, while the majority of the 18 sites and the northbound Pacific Crest Trail trailhead are up the road to the right. Turn right and follow the campground access

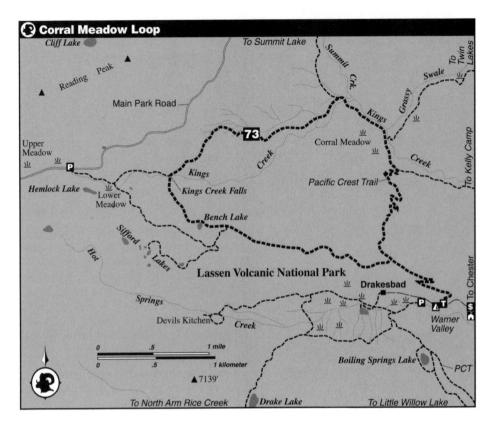

Corral Meadow Loop

Cliff Lake

To Summit Lake

Summit Crk.

To Twin Lakes

Swale

Reading Peak

Main Park Road

Grassy Swale

Kings

73

Corral Meadow

To Kelly Camp

Upper Meadow

P

Creek

Creek

Hemlock Lake

Lower Meadow

Kings

Kings Creek Falls

Pacific Crest Trail

Bench Lake

Sifford

Hot Lakes

Lassen Volcanic National Park

To Chester

Drakesbad

Springs

P T

Warner Valley

Devils Kitchen

Creek

S

0   .5   1 mile

0   .5   1 kilometer

Boiling Springs Lake

PCT

▲7139'

To North Arm Rice Creek

Drake Lake

To Little Willow Lake

road to the small parking area opposite the trailhead, which has vault toilets.

DESCRIPTION: Beneath the cover of Jeffrey pines, incense cedars, white firs, and a few sugar pines, the well-graded Pacific Crest Trail heads southwest, immediately crossing a tiny, spring-fed creek and climbing lava flows on the north wall of Hot Springs Creek canyon to the first of three long switchbacks. The forest thins above the first switchback, allowing good views of Drakesbad and the canyon. Drought-resistant vascular plants seen along the trail may include two penstemons: mountain pride, with crimson-colored flowers, and derived penstemon, with blue flowers. The tiny, very common Torrey's monkey flower makes a brief display with pink flowers, as does the fork-toothed ookow, with tight clusters of blue-violet flowers. All four of these species have tubular flowers.

Dry, rocky habitats also suit many ferns, although people tend to associate these plants with shady and moist environments. Along the dry part of the ascent, Sierra cliff-brake, Indian's dream, imbricate sword fern, and Eaton's shield fern may be present. Shrubs include snowbush, which is never common anywhere in its range, and huckleberry oak, which is the dominant shrub in mid-elevations of the Sierra. However, in Lassen Volcanic, this shrub is restricted to the sunny slopes of Hot Springs Creek canyon and Warner Valley. Above the last switchback, the trail surmounts the lip of the canyon wall, returns to forest (now minus the Jeffrey pines and sugar pines of below), and reaches a junction at 1.2 miles from the trailhead.

Head northwest to remain on the PCT, and follow gently rising tread, as the white firs give way to red firs and western white pines. Hike over the western part of Flatiron

Ridge, composed of relatively flat layers of lava flows topped with glacial sediments. From there, a well-graded, switchbacking descent leads down the north side of the ridge toward the floor of the Kings Creek canyon. Reach a junction near the outskirts of Corral Meadow, 2.7 miles from the trailhead, where the Kings Creek Trail heads downstream toward Kelly Camp (see Trip 66).

Head left (northwest) and continue on the PCT across a thin rivulet and a boardwalk over a marshy area filled with lush vegetation, including numerous corn lilies. Under forest canopy, the trail skirts the east edge of Corral Meadow, filled with grasses, plants, and willows, on the way to another junction, 3.1 miles from the trailhead, where the PCT fords Kings Creek and heads upstream through Grassy Swale. Nearby, on a low bench adjacent to Kings Creek, several campsites will lure overnighters with the opportunity to fall asleep to the soothing sound of the rushing creek.

From the junction, your route leaves the PCT, heading north to make a brief but steep climb above the level of the creek, where you'll find a good view across the canyon of Grassy Swale Creek cascading toward a union with Kings Creek. Drop down and follow the west bank of Kings Creek, hopping across some seasonal rivulets, to where the trail crosses to the far side of the stream. The crossing, which is made via a combination of rocks and logs, is not particularly easy, even in late season (you may want to pack along an extra pair of flip-flops or sandals). Safely across Kings Creek, hop over a side stream and reach a junction with a trail to Summit Lake, 3.75 miles from the trailhead.

Continue west-southwest upstream through thick and lush vegetation to an easy boulder hop of a spring-fed tributary. Past the stream crossing, the path moves farther away from Kings Creek and climbs through a mixed forest of lodgepole pines, white firs, and western white pines. About 0.75-mile from the junction, you reach a verdant meadow filled with lush, water-loving plants and flowers. From there, the trail crosses several spring-fed streams and then crests a minor ridge before a short descent leads to a viewpoint above Kings Creek Falls.

Situated on the very brink of the falls and guarded by a cable, the overlook provides a fine aerie from which to gaze at the 50-foot cascade. Some visitors scramble down the steep slope to the base of the falls, but it is not a maintained trail—exercise extreme caution if you choose to descend the potentially loose and slippery rocks. Because of the fall's aspect, photographers should plan on a visit from late morning to shortly after noon, as these are the only times when the falls are bathed in sunlight.

A short walk from the falls leads to a junction, where the trail ahead continues 1.1 miles to the Kings Creek Meadow Trailhead on the main park road. However, your loop continues by turning left and crossing Kings Creek on a wood bridge. From the bridge, the trail makes a brief climb to the base of a long cliff with an extensive talus slope, where a bit of exploration will reveal a couple of shallow caves near the base. Continue climbing to a low spot in a lateral moraine that dams chest-deep Bench Lake. The lake apparently loses a significant amount of water through glacial sediments, for by Labor Day it is barely more than a mud hole. (Slightly smaller but deeper, the first Sifford Lake nearby is a much more attractive destination). From Bench Lake, the trail descends a gully between a pair of moraines to a junction with a lateral to Sifford Lakes, 6.8 miles from the trailhead.

Continue southeast along the crest of a lateral moraine through mostly open forest with an understory of pinemat and greenleaf manzanita, and tobacco brush. After 1.5 miles from the Sifford Lakes junction, you close the loop at the junction with the PCT. From there, turn right to retrace your steps 1.2 miles to the trailhead at the Warner Valley Campground.

R Wilderness permits are required for overnight stays. Fires and camping are prohibited at Kings Creek Falls.

Introduction to the Southern Borderlands

The southern borderlands comprise a very loosely defined region south of Lassen Volcanic that encompass a wide range of trails, most of which see very little use—especially outside of hunting season usually beginning sometime in October. Slightly less scenic than the more noteworthy lands within the park, the surrounding area still has many subtle attractions, including picturesque lakes, wildflower-filled meadows, and serene forests, and is more than worthy of a visit.

Access

State highways 32, 36, and 172 provide the main access to the southern borderlands area.

Amenities

About 10 miles west of Chester, the St. Bernard Lodge offers a restaurant, tavern, stables, and seven guest rooms. Call (530) 258-3382 for reservations or for restaurant hours, as the restaurant is generally not open every day of the week. Farther west, past the junction of Highway 32 and just before the junction of Highway 172, is Childs Meadow Resort, equipped with motel, cabins, a small store, and a cafe (530-595-3383 or 888-595-3383). A short distance down Highway 172 is the Mill Creek Resort, with a rustic building housing a restaurant, small store, and post office. The all-year resort also offers housekeeping cabins and a campground with shower and laundry facilities (except during winter). Call (888) 595-4449 for reservations or more information. The small town of Mineral offers the most centralized services, with gas stations, a convenience store, and cabin rentals. The all-year Lassen Mineral Lodge (530-595-4422) offers a general store, restaurant, lodging, and an RV park.

Ranger Stations and Visitor Information

Lassen Volcanic National Park headquarters is located near the west end of Mineral.

Campgrounds						
Campground	Fee	Elevation	Season	Restrooms	Running Water	Bear Boxes
Domingo Springs (Plumas 312, 8.5 miles NW of 36)	$13	5200′	May to October	Vault	Yes	No
Willow Springs (Lost Creek Road, 29N19, 4 miles N of 36)	$11	5200′	May to October	Vault	No	No
Elam (Hwy. 32, 3.3 miles SW of 32/36 Jct.)	$15	4600′	May to October	Vault	Yes	No
Alder Creek (Hwy. 32, 7.5 miles SW of 32/36 Jct.)	$11	3900′	April to November	Vault	No	No
Potato Patch (Hwy. 32, 10.5 miles S of 32/35 Jct.)	$14	3400′	May to October	Vault	Yes	No
Gurnsey Creek (Hwy. 36, 2.5 miles N of 35/32 Jct.)	$13	5000′	May to October	Vault	Yes	No
Hole in the Ground (28N06A, 3.3 miles SW of Hwy. 172)	$12	4300′	May to October	Vault	Yes	No
Battle Creek (Hwy. 36, 6.5 miles W of 36/89 Jct.)	$18	4800′	May to October	Flush	Yes	No

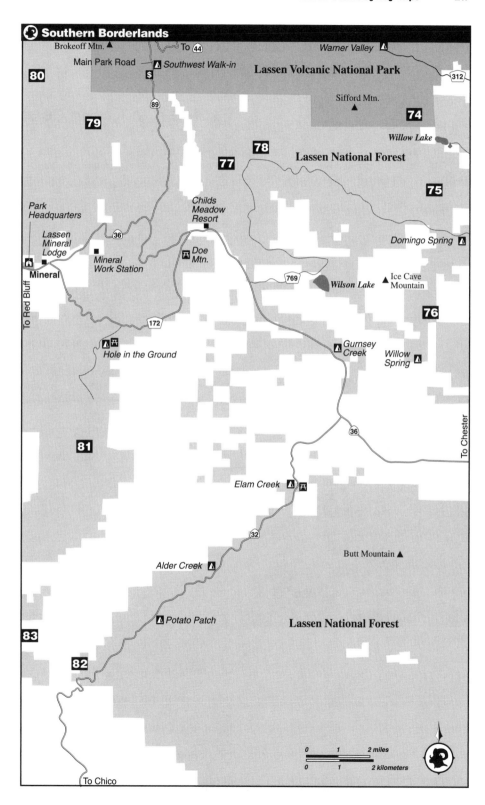

Southern Borderlands

Brokeoff Mtn. ▲

To (44)

Warner Valley △

Main Park Road

△ Southwest Walk-in

Lassen Volcanic National Park

80

$ S

(89)

Sifford Mtn.
▲

(312)

79

74

78

77

△ Willow Lake

Lassen National Forest

75

Park
Headquarters

Childs
Meadow
Resort

Lassen
Mineral
Lodge

(36)

Domingo Spring △

■ Doe
Mtn.

Ice Cave
Mountain ▲

△ Mineral

■ Mineral
Work Station

(769)

Mineral

Wilson Lake

To Red Bluff

76

(172)

△ Hole in the Ground

△ Gurnsey
Creek

Willow
Spring △

(36)

To Chester

81

Elam Creek △ △

△ Alder Creek

(32)

Butt Mountain ▲

83

△ Potato Patch

Lassen National Forest

82

0   1   2 miles

0   1   2 kilometers

To Chico

The nearest Forest Service ranger station is near the west end of Chester.

Good to Know Before You Go

Drives to the Ishi Wilderness are long and the roadbeds are marginal. The trails are also poorly maintained; only the most accessible trail in the Ishi Wilderness has been included in this guide. Adventurous souls interested in visiting other trails in the area should prepared for difficult driving conditions and very poor trails.

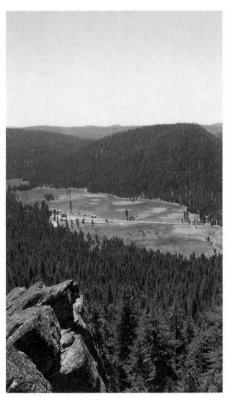

Canyon Overlook

Trip **74**

Willow Lake to Terminal Geyser

M ∕ DH

DISTANCE:	4.4 miles out and back
ELEVATIONS:	5445/5795, +500/-500
SEASON:	June to mid-October
USE:	Light
MAPS:	*Mount Harkness, Reading Peak*

INTRODUCTION: The 2.8-mile trail from Drakesbad to Terminal Geyser is a popular hike, especially for guests lodging at the resort—this slightly shorter trail from Willow Lake to the same destination is not. The first half of the route is an essentially flat hike around the shore of aptly named Willow Lake and the extensive meadow above the northwest shore. The second half is a moderate climb through forest cover to the geyser, which is actually not a geyser, which periodically erupts hot water, but a fumarole, which emits steam and gases. Whatever the correct designation, Terminal Geyser provides an interesting hydrothermal show, and the hike is a fine complement to an overnight stay at the primitive Willow Lake Campground.

DIRECTIONS TO TRAILHEAD: From Highway 36 in Chester, follow Feather River Road for just over a half mile to a junction and veer left on County Road 312, following signs for Drakesbad. Pass the turnoff to High Bridge Campground on the way to a junction, 6.1 miles from Highway 36, where County Road 312 continues toward Drakesbad, but you veer left on Highway 311 toward Mineral. Follow Highway 311 for 0.4 mile, then turn right onto Forest Road 29N14 (a dirt road signed for Willow Lake), and then proceed almost 4 miles to the end of the road at the primitive Willow Lake Campground.

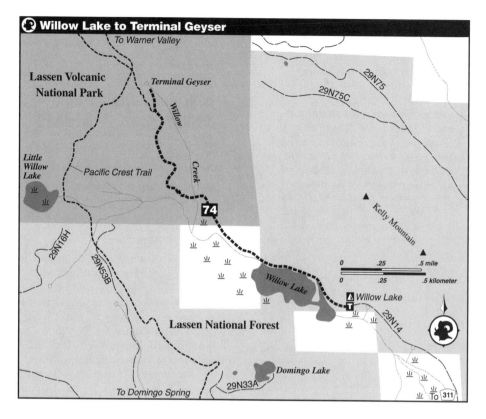

Willow Lake to Terminal Geyser

DESCRIPTION: The trail begins at the north end of the campground and heads toward the east shore of aptly named Willow Lake, through a forest of white firs, incense cedars, and ponderosa pines. Although the primitive campground is devoid of picnic tables, some are inexplicably scattered alongside the shoreline trail. A few tiny rivulets spill across the trail as you walk toward the end of the lake, where an extensive swath of meadow is covered with grasses, sedges, and cattails.

 Near the lake's northwest end, signs herald your entry into Lassen Volcanic National Park. Through tall grasses and wildflowers, the sometimes boggy path follows the right-hand edge of the meadows for a while before bending over to a crossing of thin Willow Creek, 1.25 miles from the trailhead.

From the creek, the trail continues across a slender section of meadow before heading into the trees. Shortly after entering the forest, you reach an informal junction, where barely discernible tread heads west to the bank of the creek draining Little Willow Lake (the trail shown on the USGS map that connects to an old road north-northeast to Terminal Geyser has been abandoned). The previously gently graded trail now attacks the hillside with a vengeance on a weaving ascent through dense forest. After a stiff 0.75-mile climb, the characteristic odor of sulfurous gases heralds your arrival at a junction with a trail from the Drakesbad area. Turn right and follow the course of an old road on an arcing approach to roaring Terminal Geyser. Continually churning out steam, Terminal Geyser is technically a fumarole, not a geyser, the result of a cold stream flowing over a steam vent.

DISASTER AVERTED

The area around Terminal Geyser appears pristine, but this was not always the case. In 1978, Phillips Petroleum Company, involved in geothermal exploration, drilled and capped the "Walker O" well on the broad area at the end of the road that now serves as the last 180 yards of trail. Tapping the underground steam for power would have led to the geyser's demise, but this disaster was averted beginning in 1980, when the National Park Service condemned the private inholding. Subsequently, the well was removed and the access road was abandoned in 1999, thereby restoring the area around Terminal Geyser to a more unspoiled state.

[O] With shuttle arrangements, you could continue north from the junction near Terminal Geyser to the Drakesbad area.

[R] Fires are prohibited, and camping is prohibited within a quarter mile of Terminal Geyser.

DOMINGO SPRINGS TRAILHEAD

Trip **75**

Pacific Crest Trail: Northbound to Drakesbad

(M) **/** DH

DISTANCE: 8.2 miles point to point

ELEVATIONS: 5110/6240/5640, +1725/-1200

SEASON: June to mid-October

USE: Light

MAPS: *Stover Mountain, Mount Harkness, Reading Peak*

INTRODUCTION: Hikers can certainly find shorter and easier routes to Little Willow Lake and Terminal Geyser, but this route along the famed Pacific Crest Trail offers a more solitary journey. In fact, solitude is nearly guaranteed between the Domingo Springs Trailhead and the Terminal Geyser junction. Campsites are few and far between, and the ones that do exist are marginal at best, making this 8.2-mile section of the PCT better suited for a dayhike, provided a car shuttle can be arranged. Be forewarned: After early season, Little Willow Lake is not a recommended destination for anyone except those who enjoy mosquitoes and mud holes.

DIRECTIONS TO TRAILHEAD: START: From Highway 36 in Chester, follow Feather River Road for just over a half mile to a junction and veer left on County Road 312, following signs for Drakesbad. Pass the turnoff to High Bridge Campground on the way to a junction, 6.1 miles from Highway 36, where County Road 312 continues toward Drakesbad, but you veer left on Highway 311 toward Mineral. Follow Highway 311 past Domingo Springs Campground, where, shortly, the pavement ends and gravel road begins, and continue to a wide pullout on the right, 0.4 mile from the campground and 8.8 miles from Highway 36.

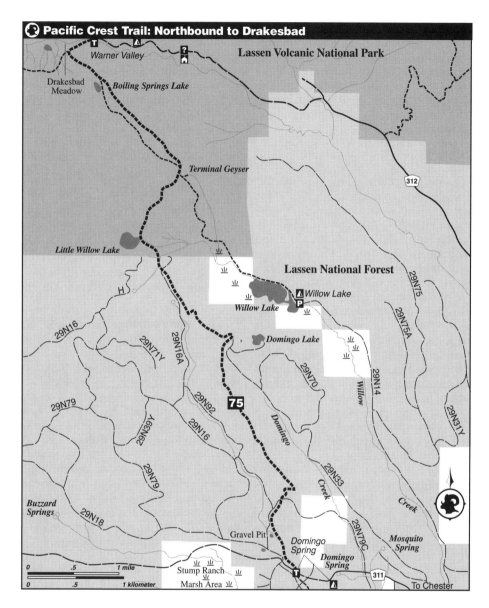

Pacific Crest Trail: Northbound to Drakesbad

Lassen Volcanic National Park

Warner Valley

Drakesbad Meadow · Boiling Springs Lake

Terminal Geyser

312

Little Willow Lake

Lassen National Forest

29N75

H

Willow Lake

Willow Lake

29N16

29N71Y

29N16A

Domingo Lake

29N75A

29N70

Willow

29N14

29N79

29N69Y

29N92

29N16

75

Domingo

29N33

Creek

29N31Y

29N79

Buzzard Springs

29N18

Creek

Gravel Pit

Domingo Spring

Domingo Spring

29N79C

Mosquito Spring

0   .5   1 mile

0   .5   1 kilometer

Stump Ranch

Marsh Area

311

To Chester

END: From Highway 36 in Chester, follow Feather River Road for just over a half mile to a junction and veer left on County Road 312, following signs for Drakesbad. Pass the turnoff to High Bridge Campground on the way to a junction, 6.1 miles from Highway 36, where County Road 311 veers left toward Domingo Springs Campground. Proceed on Road 312 past the entrance to Warner Valley Campground and through the residential community of Warner Valley. Cross a bridge over Warner Creek and travel another 4.2 miles to a major fork in the road, where Road 312 bends sharply to the left to cross Kings Creek and then continues toward Drakesbad. Enter national park land at 14 miles and continue another mile to the self-pay entrance station near the Warner Valley ranger station. Another mile leads to the entrance into Warner Valley

Campground and the northbound Pacific Crest Trail trailhead. Continue ahead a short distance to the left-hand turn into the parking area for the Warner Valley Trailhead, 16.3 miles from Highway 36. The trailhead is equipped with a modern vault toilet, bear-proof trash cans, and picnic tables.

DESCRIPTION: From the trailhead, the Pacific Crest Trail heads northwest, briefly following the course of an old road that soon dwindles to single-track trail through a shady forest of firs and pines. Traverse a volcanic rubble slope to the edge of a grass-filled meadow just to the left of the lodgepole-pine-lined trail. A shallow pond in the midst of the meadow is a remnant of an old gravel pit. Beyond the meadow, you leave the lodgepoles behind, as the trail climbs up a hillside through white firs, incense cedars, sugar pines, and ponderosa pines. Cross an old logging road a couple of times before the trail merges with the road for a while. Single-track resumes and bends northwest for a protracted traverse along a ridge. Along this nearly 3-mile traverse, you have occasional views northwest of Lassen Peak and east of Willow Lake, capped off by the view from a rock cliff about 3 miles from the trailhead.

From the viewpoint, the trail contours west, drops to a saddle, and traverses northwest across the west slope. Up the canyon to the west, a seemingly well-used dirt road can be seen climbing toward a broad saddle. The now descending trail closely parallels this road and then briefly merges with an abandoned section of it just south of the park boundary. As shown on the USGS map, this road used to go all the way to Terminal Geyser, but the Park Service wisely abandoned the road in 1999. Single-track trail leaves the old roadbed and follows a flower-lined course to the crossing of a seasonal stream before reaching the well-signed park boundary, 4.5 miles from the trailhead.

From the border, the trail climbs through the forest to the swale carrying the seasonal

outlet from Little Willow Lake. Then it climbs more steeply along the north bank of the creek to the lake, which, except in early season when the lake is knee deep, could be more accurately described as a wet marsh. By late season, a shrinking pond has retreated to the southwest corner of the basin, and the surrounding area is little more than a field of drying mud. Mosquitoes seem to be quite at home here through midsummer, and if your trip coincides with their season's zenith, you may want to hurry past this uninspiring spot.

Beyond Little Willow Lake, the trail climbs moderately through thick forest to the top of a ridge and then descends to a junction with a lateral to Terminal Geyser, offering a short side trip to one of the more interesting hydrothermal features in the park.

⑤ **SIDE TRIP TO TERMINAL GEYSER:** Turn right at the junction, and follow moderate then steeply descending tread past a red warning sign, then a sign with directions to the PCT, and, where the grade eases, a third sign for Terminal Geyser ahead and Warner Valley behind. Near this last sign, the very obscure tread of a seldom-used trail heads southeast to Willow Lake (see Trip 74). Now following the course of an old road, you curve around into the upper canyon of Willow Creek and head upstream toward the billowing cloud of steam above Terminal Geyser. Step across a pair of small, spring-fed rivulets and pass another warning sign on the approach to the geyser.

Continually churning out steam, Terminal Geyser is not really a geyser, which periodically erupts hot water, but a fumarole, which emits steam and gases. Back-dropped by colorful rocks, the fumarole spits out a continuous plume that rises above the surrounding treetops, while smaller openings in the crust scattered around the head of the canyon emit less dramatic wisps of steam. Without the guardrails that typically keep tourists a safe distance from popular hydrothermal features, you must observe this feature with caution. Even the water downstream from Terminal Geyser in Willow Creek can be quite hot in places.

END SIDE TRIP

From the Terminal Geyser junction, the PCT makes a steady climb on well-graded tread through an increasingly light forest. Near the top of the climb, the forest is open enough to allow pinemat manzanita to flourish on the sunlit slopes. From the trip's high point, you began a protracted descent toward the Warner Valley Trailhead. Back in the trees, you reach a junction with the loop around Boiling Springs Lake, which, similar to Terminal Geyser, is well worth the minor diversion. Away from the circuit around Boiling Springs Lake, the PCT continues past a couple more junctions before bending northeast above flower-bedecked Drakesbad Meadow to a bridge across Hot Springs Creek and a short walk through lush foliage to the trailhead.

R Fires are prohibited within Lassen Volcanic, and camping is prohibited within a quarter mile of Terminal Geyser and Boiling Springs Lake.

HIGHWAY 36 TRAILHEAD

Trip **76**

Pacific Crest Trail: Highway 36 to Domingo Springs

Ⓜ / DH

DISTANCE:	9.9 miles point to point
ELEVATIONS:	5110/6240/5640, +1725/-1200
SEASON:	June to mid-October
USE:	Light
MAP:	*Stover Mountain*

INTRODUCTION: Solitude is the chief attraction along this section of the Pacific Crest Trail, as the route between Highway 36 and County Road 311 receives little use. For the most part, the path travels through featureless sections of private and public land that have been logged. However, the trip has a few worthwhile attributes, including Stover Spring, periodic views of Lassen Peak, and a bridged crossing of North Fork Feather River.

DIRECTIONS TO TRAILHEAD: START: The Pacific Crest Trail crosses Highway 36 about 6 miles west of the junction with Highway 89, on the western edge of Chester. Parking is available in a wide dirt area on the north side of the highway. PCT signs mark the highway crossing.

END: From Highway 36 in Chester, follow Feather River Road for just over a half mile to a junction and veer left on County Road 312, following signs for Drakesbad. Pass the turnoff to High Bridge Campground on the way to a junction, 6.1 miles from Highway 36, where County Road 312 continues toward Drakesbad, but you veer left on Highway 311 toward Mineral. Follow Highway 311 past Domingo Springs Campground, where, shortly, the pavement ends and gravel road begins, and continue

Pacific Crest Trail: Highway 36 to Domingo Springs

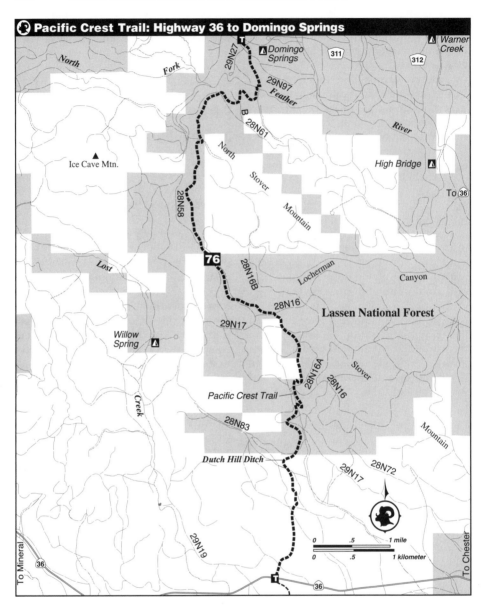

to a wide pullout on the right, 0.4 mile from the campground and 8.8 miles from Highway 36.

DESCRIPTION: Head north from the parking area on gently graded trail beneath a mixed forest of Jeffrey pines, sugar pines, incense cedars, and white firs. Very soon, you pass a junction with an interpretive trail to the right and proceed past several trail signs through a logged forest owned by the Collins Pine Company. Reach the crossing of the first of several dirt roads on the way to Marian Creek, which, throughout most of the hiking season, is little more than a string of dry boulders. Beyond the creek, the grade increases to a moderate ascent that leads across a remnant of the Dutch Hill Ditch.

DUTCH HILL DITCH

The construction of the Dutch Hill Ditch was begun in 1874, to carry water from Rice Creek 33 miles to the Dutch Hill Mine near Seneca. Utilizing stretches of open ditch, short sections of flume, two tunnels, and 8 miles of iron pipe, the project was abandoned in 1884, following the California legislature's ban on hydraulic mining.

Continue a moderate climb away from the ditch onto Forest Service land to the crossing of yet another logging road. Shortly thereafter, the trail merges with the gently graded course of an abandoned road before the moderate climb resumes. After more road crossings, single-track trail eventually draws near to a lushly lined swale below Stover Spring. A primitive camping area lies next to the swale, 3.2 miles from Highway 36, which sees very little use outside of hunting season, despite the easy access via a dirt road. Farther on, water gushes from a pipe below Stover Spring into a small, artificial pond; however, after midsummer, water from the pipe diminishes to a trickle.

Beyond Stover Spring, the PCT follows a mostly uninteresting course for several miles through previously logged forest on an arcing, mostly upward traverse along the south and west slopes of North Stover Mountain, paralleling and crossing numerous logging roads along the way to the top of a viewless ridge cloaked in sugar pines and white firs. Eventually, the trail begins a descent toward North Fork Feather River, with occasional views of Lassen Peak to the north. A seemingly unnecessary climb interrupts the descent for a bit, before the trail bends down into the river canyon. Cross a stout bridge over the river, 9 miles from Highway 36, and proceed to a switchback on the far side. Just upstream from the switchback are passable campsites for backpackers interested in an overnight stay.

A steep but short climb leads out of the narrow gorge, and then gently graded trail travels through previously logged forest of Jeffrey pines, lodgepole pines, white firs, and a few incense cedars. Walk across a couple of logging roads on the way to the Domingo Springs Trailhead along County Road 311.

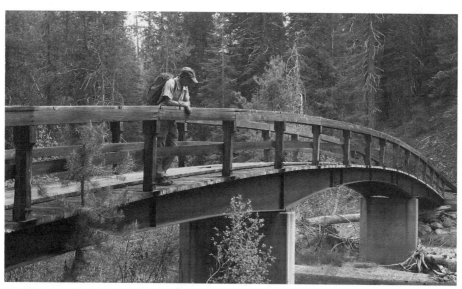

A bridge over North Fork Feather River

SPENCER MEADOW TRAILHEAD

Trip **77**

Spencer Meadow Loop

🆖 ⋔ DH, BP

DISTANCE: 13.2 miles semiloop

ELEVATIONS: 4930/6675/4930, +2230/-2230

SEASON: June to mid-October

USE: Light

MAPS: *Childs Meadow, Reading Peak, Lassen Peak*

INTRODUCTION: The Spencer Meadow Loop has all the necessary elements for a great hike: cool forests, flower-dotted meadows, a tumbling stream with a waterfall, and far-ranging views. The only element lacking from this trip is people, as most hikers in the area opt for hikes in the more popular, neighboring Lassen Volcanic National Park. The relatively low elevation means that the Spencer Meadow Loop sheds the winter snow earlier than trails in the park, making this a fine early-season opportunity hike. The description follows the Meadow Route (cool forests, flower-dotted meadows) and then returns via the Canyon Route (tumbling stream, waterfall, far-ranging views).

DIRECTIONS TO TRAILHEAD: Take Highway 36 to the Spencer Meadow Trailhead, 5 miles east of the junction with Highway 89 and 0.3 mile east of Childs Meadow Resort. Park on the broad shoulder on the north side of the highway, near the trailhead signboard.

DESCRIPTION: Well-maintained tread climbs east from the highway, through a mixed forest of incense cedars, ponderosa pines, white firs, and a few sugar pines and black oaks to the crossing of a tiny stream coursing down a narrow, V-shaped swale. The moderate climb continues across the forested hillside

until the trees part just enough to allow a brief view of Childs Meadow below. Back under forest cover, ascending trail leads near a thin, spring-fed rivulet that drains into the meadow. Above a set of switchbacks, the trail draws closer to and then crosses over the stream on the way to a junction with the Canyon Route at the start of the loop, 2 miles from the trailhead.

Proceed ahead (north) from the junction on the Meadow Route, as the grade eases to a pleasant, mildly ascending stroll across the gentle slopes of broad and lengthy Wild Cattle Mountain. You now enter a lighter forest of Jeffrey pines, lodgepole pines, and red and white firs, and the additional sunlight aids a scattered understory of greenleaf and pinemat manzanita. Eventually, the trail drops slightly to a Y-junction with the lateral to Blue Lake at 3.4 miles (see Trip 78).

Continue ahead (north) on a mild ascent, passing well to the right of a spring-fed stream. Farther on, Mt. Conard makes a brief appearance through a gap in the forest, and farther still, Brokeoff Mountain temporarily pops into view. The views are soon left behind, as the trees close in again, and you stroll across a forest floor carpeted with lush plants and seasonal wildflowers. ❀ Beyond this forested vale, the trail makes a short, moderate ascent to a meadow, where the grade mellows once again. After an extended walk, the grade increases on the way to a junction, where the Canyon Route and the Meadow Route reunite, 5.2 miles from the trailhead.

Pressing north toward Spencer Meadow, you resume a moderate climb through a forest of lodgepole pines, western white pines, and firs. Soon, the grade eases and the forest parts near the edge of the large, grassy meadow, where you walk through a dilapidated fence and pass the remnants of a wood structure and a couple of primitive campsites. From the south end of Spencer Meadow, Mt. Conard and the tip of Lassen Peak rise above the verdant grasses and ❀ scattered wildflowers. The route of the sometimes indistinct trail comes to a fairly easy boulder hop of Canyon Creek, and then passes along the western fringe of the

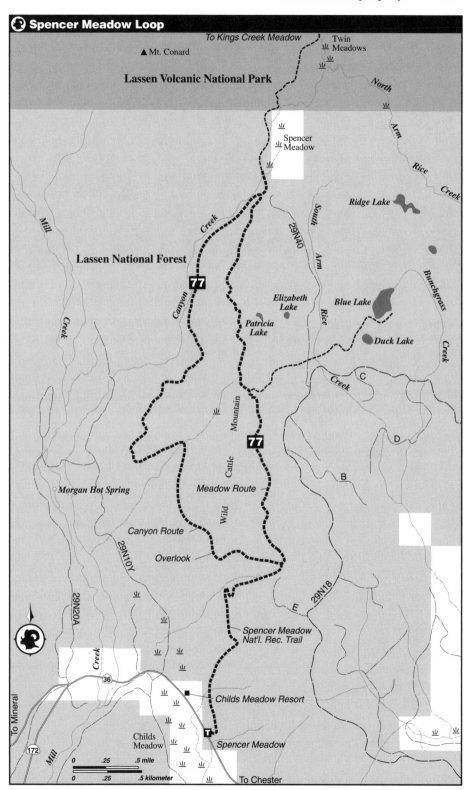

Spencer Meadow Loop

To Kings Creek Meadow

Twin Meadows

▲ Mt. Conard

Lassen Volcanic National Park

Spencer Meadow

North

Arm

Rice

Creek

Ridge Lake

Mill

Creek

Canyon

Lassen National Forest

77

29N40

South

Arm

Rice

Bunchgrass

Elizabeth Lake

Blue Lake

Patricia Lake

Duck Lake

Creek

Creek

C

D

Mountain

77

B

Morgan Hot Spring

Cattle

Meadow Route

Wild

Canyon Route

29N10Y

Overlook

29N18

E

29N20A

Spencer Meadow
Nat'l. Rec. Trail

Creek

36

Childs Meadow Resort

To Mineral

Childs Meadow

T

Spencer Meadow

172

Mill

0   .25   .5 mile

0   .25   .5 kilometer

To Chester

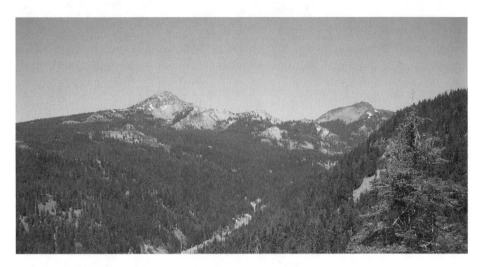

Brokeoff Mountain and Mill Creek Canyon from Canyon Route

meadow through a lodgepole pine forest. At the far end of the meadow, the trail climbs up the hillside to avoid an extensive patch of willows and crosses a flower-lined stream flowing into the meadow. Shortly afterward, you reach a fence at the boundary of Lassen Volcanic (Trip 11 describes the route north from Spencer Meadow to the Kings Creek Trailhead in reverse).

After enjoying the delightful scenery of Spencer Meadow, retrace your steps to the junction with the Canyon Route and turn right (west) to follow the Canyon Route through a forest of western white pines, lodgepole pines, and firs into the drainage of Canyon Creek. Within earshot but seldom within sight of the creek, the trail heads downstream through the trees, which occasionally allow for fleeting glimpses of Brokeoff Mountain. After about a mile from the junction, keep alert for an indistinct use trail that heads a short distance toward the creek for a view of a 50-foot waterfall. Eventually, the trail begins to move away from the creek and ends up high on the canyon wall, following a descending traverse across the west slope of Wild Cattle Mountain. Around 2.5 miles from the junction, you reach a shrub-covered slope with a grand view up Mill Creek canyon of

Brokeoff Mountain, Mt. Diller, and Pilot Pinnacle, and a downstream view of Childs Meadow.

Away from the edge of the canyon, gently graded trail veers northeast into the forested drainage of a tributary and then crosses the lushly lined stream before resuming the traverse of the canyon rim. Pass a small meadow on an elevated section of trail and continue through the trees until an open forest of Jeffrey pines, incense cedars, and black oaks heralds your arrival at Canyon Overlook, 4 miles from the junction. A sweeping view unfolds of Mill Creek canyon and Childs Meadow more than 1000 feet below. From the overlook, the trail mildly ascends through the forest to the lower junction of the Canyon and Meadow routes at the close of the loop. From there, turn right to retrace your steps 2 miles to the trailhead.

[O] By continuing north from Spencer Meadow through Lassen Volcanic, trails lead to trailheads along the main park road at the Southwest Campground, Bumpass Hell, and Upper Kings Creek Meadow.

[R] Wilderness permits are required for overnight stays in Lassen Volcanic, and fires are prohibited.

SPENCER MEADOW TRAILHEAD

Trip **78**

Blue Lake

see map on p.230

Ⓜ ✓ DH, BP

DISTANCE: 9.4 miles out and back

ELEVATIONS: 4930/6315, +1965/-1965

SEASON: June to mid-October

USE: Light

MAPS: *Childs Meadow, Reading Peak*

INTRODUCTION: This trip is for those who consider the journey as important as the destination. Blue Lake won't knock anyone's socks off for beauty; it has a fairly standard look for a Lassen lake, with a shoreline rimmed by generic trees. To further discourage hikers, the first 2 miles of trail requires a continuous, moderate climb from the Spencer Meadow Trailhead. From there, the grade is fairly gentle and the trail lightly used. Solitude should be expected along the trail and at the lake, which offers a couple of primitive campsites for interested backpackers.

DIRECTIONS TO TRAILHEAD: Take Highway 36 to the Spencer Meadow Trailhead, 5 miles east of the junction with Highway 89 and 0.3 mile east of Childs Meadow Resort. Park on the broad shoulder on the north side of the highway, near the trailhead signboard.

DESCRIPTION: Well-maintained tread climbs west from the highway, through a mixed forest of incense cedars, ponderosa pines, white firs, and a few sugar pines and black oaks to the crossing of a tiny stream coursing down a narrow, V-shaped swale. The moderate climb continues across the forested hillside until the trees part just enough to allow a brief view of Childs Meadow below. Back under forest cover, ascending trail leads near a thin, spring-fed rivulet

that drains into the meadow. Above a set of switchbacks, the trail draws closer to and then crosses over the stream on the way to a junction with the Canyon Route at the start of the loop, 2 miles from the trailhead.

Proceed ahead (north) from the junction on the Meadow Route, as the grade eases to a pleasant, mildly ascending stroll across the gentle slopes of broad and lengthy Wild Cattle Mountain. You now enter a lighter forest of Jeffrey pines, lodgepole pines, and red and white firs, and the additional sunlight aids a scattered understory of greenleaf and pinemat manzanita. Eventually, the trail drops slightly to a Y-junction with the lateral to Blue Lake at 3.4 miles.

Head northeast, away from the Spencer Meadow Trail, and proceed on less-used tread for a short climb over a forested hill. Descend the far side of the hill through open forest and shrubby patches with the aid of a couple switchbacks to a crossing of Forest Road 29N40 at the bottom of the slope. A short distance from the road, make an easy boulder hop of South Arm Rice Creek and then start a climb up the next hill. Near the crest, Lassen Peak and Mt. Conard appear through the trees, shortly followed by Duck Lake just below the trail. Follow the crest through open forest to a clearing on the southwest side of Blue Lake, where an informal junction leads to shady but primitive campsites above the south and west shores.

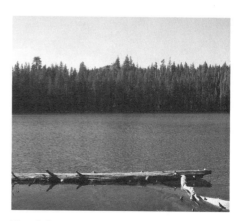

Blue Lake

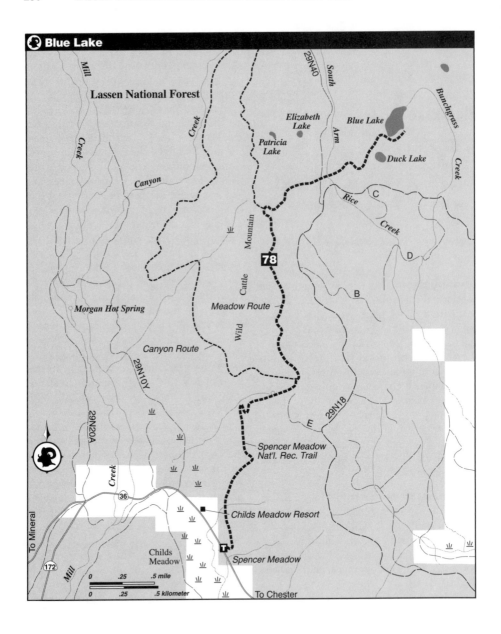

Trip **79**

Heart Lake via Glassburner Meadow

Ⓜ ╱ DH, BP

DISTANCE: 12.6 miles out and back

ELEVATIONS: 5925/7485/6590, +2250/-2250

SEASON: June to mid-October

USE: Light

MAP: *Lassen Peak*

INTRODUCTION: Considerably longer than the Digger Creek Trail to Heart Lake (Trip 80), this is for hikers and backpackers who don't mind the extra distance in return for a bit more solitude (although Heart Lake doesn't receive that much use from either of these trails). Heart Lake is surrounded by trees but unlike at many of Lassen Volcanic lakes, Brokeoff Mountain can be seen towering above the treetops from the west shore.

DIRECTIONS TO TRAILHEAD: Leave Highway 36 at 2.25 miles west of the Highway 89 junction and turn northwest onto Forest Road 30N16. Proceed for 2.1 miles, turn left on Forest Road 29N22, and continue almost 2 miles to a rocky road on the right, signed HEART LAKE TRAILHEAD that travels up Plantation Gulch. Most sedans should park near the junction, but high-clearance vehicles may be able to go up the road 0.4 mile to the start of the actual trail.

DESCRIPTION: Walk northeast up the initially steep road, which soon mellows to more of a moderate climb through open forest and shrub-covered slopes, with intermittent views north to Brokeoff Mountain. Reach the wide turnaround at the trailhead, and then follow single-track into a thicker forest of lodgepole pines, western white pines, and

firs. Very soon, the trail leads across a thin rivulet draining Plantation Gulch, followed by a more open forest of firs and Jeffrey pines on a climb of a moraine with good views of the Martin Creek drainage below. Cross the head of the moraine, and then follow undulating trail toward a creek draining lower Glassburner Meadow, a boggy clearing carpeted with grasses, lined with willows, and edged with lodgepole pines. Wildflowers, including asters and buttercups, add color to the meadow through midsummer.

Head upstream on a moderate climb to where the trail makes a log crossing of the creek, bordered by alders, wildflowers, plants, and grasses. Continue up the left bank, past a pair of springs bubbling out of the hillside where the creek originates. Beyond the springs, a section of gently graded trail leads past some low rock cliffs, where you may start to notice mountain hemlocks joining the forest, before a moderate climb resumes on sometimes rocky trail to the Lassen Volcanic boundary, 3.7 miles from the trailhead.

From the park boundary, follow a lupine-lined path across a rocky ridge with a brief view of Brokeoff Mountain's summit. (On the USGS map, the trail that connects the Spencer Meadow Trail to the Brokeoff Mountain Trail has been abandoned and no longer exists.) Once past the ridge, a descending traverse leads out of the park and back onto Forest Service land across the southwest base of Brokeoff Mountain and above Twin Meadows through a forest of mountain hemlocks, western white pines, and firs.

At 4.8 miles, you cross over a flower-lined creek, past which the trail becomes hard to discern through a tangle of deadfalls and associated debris. The alignment of the trail basically follows a level traverse across the forest floor for 0.3 mile to a sloping, open swath of vegetation bordering the next creek, a tributary of Digger Creek like the previous one. Cross the verdant swath of flowers, which include knee-high corn lilies, and pick up a faint path on the far side near an old, wood trail marker. Proceed a short

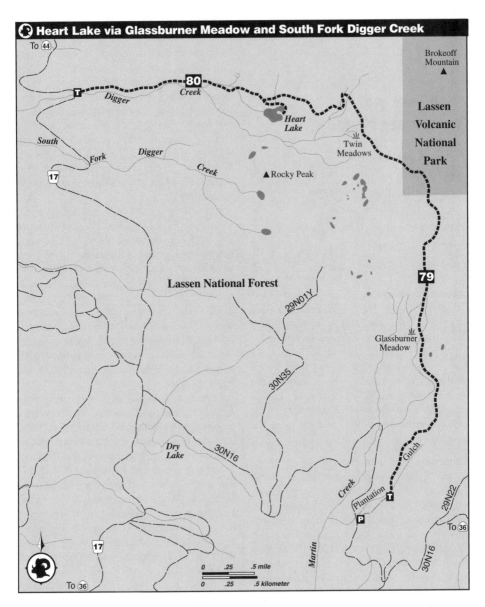

Heart Lake via Glassburner Meadow and South Fork Digger Creek

To 44

Brokeoff
Mountain
▲

Digger Creek

80

Heart
Lake

Lassen
Volcanic
National
Park

Twin
Meadows

South

Fork   Digger

Creek

17

▲Rocky Peak

Lassen National Forest

29N01Y

79

Glassburner
Meadow

30N35

Dry
Lake

30N16

Creek   Gulch

Plantation   T

P

29N22

To 36

17

Martin

30N16

0   .25   .5 mile

0   .25   .5 kilometer

To 36

distance to a third creek coursing through a similarly verdant but narrower swath of flowers. Immediately after this crossing, the trail turns downstream and soon crosses back over the creek, following the sprightly watercourse for a while before bending away through scattered to light forest.

On a moderate to moderately steep descent, follow a rocky crest down open slopes covered with pinemat manzanita and a sprinkling of lupine. Farther down the slope, you continue dropping through thicker stands of forest and pockets of meadow to a junction between the trail from the Digger Creek Trailhead and the lateral to Heart Lake, 6 miles from the trailhead.

Turn left and proceed through cool forest to a patch of meadow bordering the northeast shore of Heart Lake. Good campsites can be found on the east-shore peninsula, although horse packers seem to use the area with some regularity. Although you can easily negotiate your way around the lake to meet the South Fork Digger Creek Trail above the west shore, discernible tread disappears on the south side of the lake. Another batch of good campsites will tempt overnighters near the west shoreline, where lakeside views include Brokeoff Mountain. Though mostly shallow, this trout-stocked lake is fairly deep in the middle, offering the opportunity for a refreshing swim.

R Fires are prohibited in Lassen Volcanic National Park.

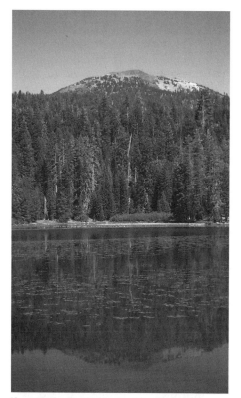

Heart Lake back-dropped by Brokeoff Mountain

SOUTH FORK DIGGER CREEK TRAILHEAD

Trip **80**

see map on p.232

Heart Lake via South Fork Digger Creek

M ✗ DH, BP

DISTANCE: 4.2 miles out and back

ELEVATIONS: 5755/6585, +970/-970

SEASON: June to mid-October

USE: Light

MAP: *Lassen Peak*

INTRODUCTION: Those in search of a short and easy hike to a lakeshore lunch spot, campsite with a view, or a fine swimming hole will be pleased with the 2-plus-mile journey to Heart Lake via the trail along South Fork Digger Creek. One-third the distance to the lake of the southern part of the Heart Lake Recreation Trail, the northern part is the more popular route, although such popularity is relative, as visitation to the lake is minimal. As with most Lassen lakes, mosquitoes may be problematic until midsummer.

DIRECTIONS TO TRAILHEAD: Forest Road 17 runs almost 22 miles across Lassen Volcanic's western borderlands, connecting Highway 36 and Highway 44. This major road leaves Highway 36 at the east end of the Battle Creek Bridge, about 0.1 mile east of Battle Creek Campground, and 1.1 miles west of Lassen Volcanic headquarters in Mineral. Forest Road 17 leaves Highway 44 at 1.1 miles west of the junction with Highway 89. The South Fork Digger Creek Trailhead is on Forest Road 17, 9.7 miles north of Highway 36 and 12 miles south of Highway 44. Limited parking is available on the east shoulder near the trailhead. (The Digger Creek Trail, shown on USGS maps and described in earlier editions of this guide, no longer exists.)

DESCRIPTION: Follow the well-shaded north bank of South Fork Digger Creek east for 0.4 mile to where the trail veers away from the creek and climbs through the trees for another 0.8 mile to a wet meadow hemmed in between two glacial moraines. With the meadow marking the midpoint of the route, climb gently a quarter mile east, then more steeply up to a small saddle near Rocky Peak. From there, the trail turns northwest and soon crosses a second, small saddle before a brief descent leads to a creek that drains Twin Meadows. After a quarter-mile traverse over a low, broad surface, you spy Heart Lake through the trees and soon reach the west shore.

Good campsites will tempt overnighters near the west shoreline, where lakeside views include Brokeoff Mountain. Additional campsites may be found on the lake's east shore peninsula, albeit without the views. Though mostly shallow, this trout-stocked lake is fairly deep in the middle, offering the opportunity for a refreshing swim. Continuing on the trail around the north shore leads to a junction a good distance north of the lake, with the trail from Glassburner Meadows and a lateral to the east shore. Although you can easily negotiate your way around the lake from the east side back to the South Fork Digger Creek Trail, discernible tread disappears on the south side of the lake.

Trip **81**

Mill Creek Trail

Ⓜ ⟋ DH, BP

DISTANCE: 12.2 miles out and back

ELEVATIONS: 4545/3365, +2170/-2170

SEASON: May to November

USE: Light

MAP: *Lassen Peak*

INTRODUCTION: From its origin on the remnant slopes of ancient Mt. Tehama, Mill Creek tumbles through the southwest corner of Lassen Volcanic and across Forest Service land toward the Sacramento Valley. River runners and anglers regard sections of this creek as special places to ply their crafts. This section of the fabled stream has a 14-mile stretch of little-used trail that heads downstream through varied zones of vegetation that include montane forest, chaparral, and oak woodland. Despite what Mill Creek Trail's name implies, the creek stays out of sight for most of the journey, which is generally high above the water across the steep slopes of the canyon; indeed, the first unobstructed, bona fide view of the creek doesn't come for 7.5 miles. However, dayhikers will find a walk along the first 6 miles to be a pleasant, forested stroll, and backpackers will find some little-used campsites near 4.25 and 6 miles.

DIRECTIONS TO TRAILHEAD: From Highway 36, either 9 miles east of Mineral or 9 miles west of the 36/32 junction, follow the Highway 172 loop to Forest Service Road 28N06 and turn south. Proceed on FS 28N06 past the turnoff for Hole in the Ground Campground to the trailhead at the end of the road, 4.5 miles from 172.

DESCRIPTION: Before the trailhead was relocated, the Forest Road 28N06 used to cross Rocky Gulch and then continue

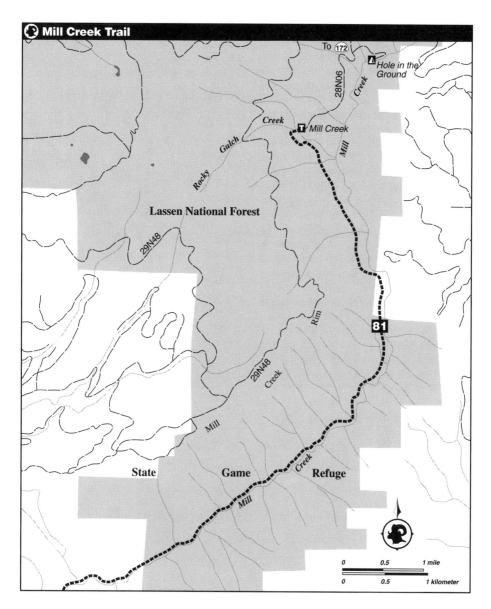

Mill Creek Trail

To (172)

Hole in the Ground

28N06

Creek

Creek

Mill Creek

Creek

Gulch

Mill

Rocky

Lassen National Forest

29N48

Rim

81

29N48

Creek

Mill

State   **Game**   Creek   **Refuge**

Mill

| 0 | 0.5 | 1 mile |
| 0 | 0.5 | 1 kilometer |

downstream about a mile to the old trail-head. Nowadays, you head away from the gravel turnaround at the new trailhead by following a rough section of single-track trail across a hillside and down a bank to a boulder hop of Rocky Gulch Creek. After the creek, the trail switchbacks twice and climbs up the slope before winding down to meet the alignment of the old road, well above the course of unseen Mill Creek to the left. Follow the realigned trail downstream through the road cut between a forest of primarily Douglas firs with a smattering of incense cedars and sugar pines. On the way to the old trailhead, cross a year-round stream and a number of seasonal swales.

Beyond the old trailhead, the path continues through a narrower swath of vegetation along the course of an old jeep road well above the level of Mill Creek, which remains out of sight at the bottom of a steep-sided, V-shaped canyon. As you continue downstream on mildly descending tread, a few oaks start to intermix with the Douglas firs, ponderosa pines, incense cedars, and sugar pines. Pass through a dilapidated gate and cattle guard in an old fence line just short of the 3-mile mark. Around 4 miles, near Big Bend, a sharp bend in the creek, the creek can finally be seen for the first time through gaps in the forest. About a quarter mile farther, hop across a side stream and proceed another quarter mile to a little-used campsite, the first developed site on the journey so far. Just down the trail, a tributary stream spills between moss-covered rocks into a picturesque pool, providing an excellent water source for dayhikers needing to replenish their supplies, or overnighters who elect to use the campsite.

Continue downstream, hopping over a few more rivulets, as the trail begins a series of undulations, still through thick forest. Just after the 6-mile mark, a barely noticeable use trail plunges down the hillside to primitive campsites on a small flat near the edge of the creek. Mill Creek slows down just enough at this spot to offer a pool suitable for an afternoon swim.

O Although most hikers generally go no farther than this pool, the Mill Creek Trail continues downstream another 8 miles to primitive Black Rock Campground on the edge of Ishi Wilderness, dropping another 2400 feet in the process. Accessing the campground and wilderness trailhead requires a very long drive, partially on rough dirt roads, which makes a shuttle trip highly impractical (see Trip 83). About 1.5 miles from the camping area, the trail enters a zone of chaparral, offering the first open views of the canyon and the tumbling creek. Seldom-used campsites should be available for backpackers around 9, 11, and 13 miles from the Rocky Gulch Trailhead. Watch for poison oak, rattlesnakes, and ticks in the lower canyon.

R Fishing in Mill Creek is catch-and-release only from the last Saturday in April through November 15. Anglers must use artificial lures with barbless hooks.

DEER CREEK TRAILHEAD

Trip 82

Deer Creek Trail

Ⓜ ⚲ DH, BP

DISTANCE: 4.8 miles out and back

ELEVATIONS: 3220/2970, +650/-650

SEASON: March to late November

USE: Light

MAP: Onion Butte

INTRODUCTION: When the Lassen high country is buried in snow, the Deer Creek Trail offers a wonderful opportunity to get out on the trail, especially in spring, when the stream is strong and Lower Deer Creek Falls is in full glory. Summers can be hot at

this elevation—hike early or late in the day to avoid the heat. Most parties go no farther than the falls, which are definitely the high point of the journey, but the trail continues to a decent camping area before merging with a dirt road. Deer Creek offers anglers some challenging catch-and-release fishing between late April and mid-November.

DIRECTIONS TO TRAILHEAD: From its junction at Highway 36, follow Highway 32 southwest toward Chico for 11.2 miles to a parking area on the east shoulder, just before a red bridge across Deer Creek. The bridge is approximately 40 miles from Chico.

DESCRIPTION: The trail begins on the opposite shoulder from the parking area, near a trail sign somewhat obscured by the surrounding vegetation. Follow single-track trail southwest through mixed forest of Douglas firs, incense cedars, ponderosa

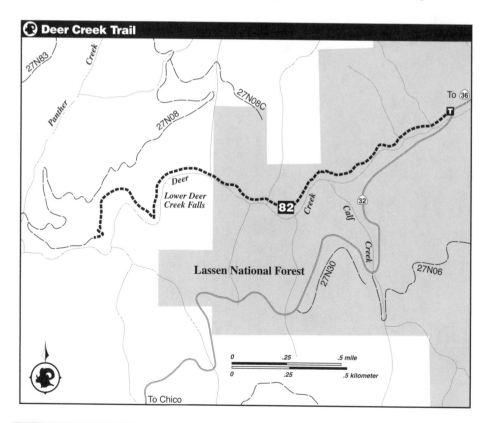

Deer Creek Trail

pines, and canyon live oaks down to the north bank of tumbling Deer Creek. Along with a healthy understory of shrubs and plants, poison oak—common in the foothills—is prevalent along the trail. The highway parallels the trail on the opposite bank for the first half mile, but the roar of the creek drowns out most of the road noise. During that stretch, the trail briefly dips into side gullies to cross over a couple thin rivulets running down the slope toward the main creek. About 0.4 mile from the trailhead, the trail passes just below a shallow cave.

The surroundings seem a bit wilder where the highway veers south to cross Calf Creek, and you follow the undulating trail downstream, enjoying periodic views of the creek through openings in the primarily oak woodland. Pass a couple campsites (better ones can be found farther along the trail)

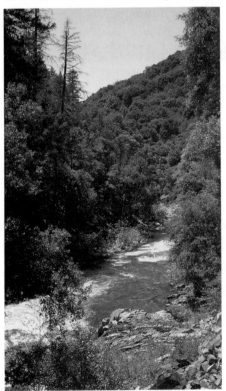

Deer Creek

and continue to an unmarked path that veers away from the main trail toward a view of Lower Deer Creek Falls, 1.7 miles from the trailhead. Here, the falls plunge 15 feet over the lip of a rocky chute and tumble downstream through a series of dramatic cataracts. Use trails lead both to a view from above the falls, on top of a rock rib that juts into the canyon, and from below the falls at a streamside vantage point. Nearby, the remains of an old fish ladder appear above the north bank of the creek.

Away from the dramatic climax of the trip, the trail continues downstream, passing a camping area on a gently sloping, oak-shaded bench above a placid stretch of the creek that is suitable for a dip. A stiff climb leads back into mostly coniferous forest, which now includes some California nutmeg. High above the creek, seemingly in the middle of nowhere, a blank signboard appears that offers no information that might explain such a curious placement. Beyond the sign, the trail begins a stiff descent to a flat above the creek, where the trail ends and a spur road to Forest Road 27N08 begins. Crude markings on tree trunks indicate that camping and fires are banned in this area.

O Legal camping can be reached by following the spur road west a half mile from the end of the trail to Road 27N08, and then turning left and walking 0.3 mile to a primitive campground on the right just before a bridge over Deer Creek. From the primitive campground, Forest Road 27N08 continues another 6 miles to a junction with Highway 32, for those who may be interested in arranging a shuttle.

R Fishing in Deer Creek is catch-and-release only from the last Saturday in April through November 15. Anglers must use artificial lures with barbless hooks.

Trip **83**

Mill Creek Trail-Ishi Wilderness

M / DH, BP

DISTANCE: 13.2 miles out and back

ELEVATIONS: 2100/1500, +1400/-1400

SEASON: March to late November

USE: Light

MAPS: *Barkley Mountain, Panther Spring*

INTRODUCTION: Named for the last survivor of the Yahi Yani tribe, the Ishi Wilderness is a remote foothills community of deep canyons and dark volcanic rock. Hiking the Mill Creek Trail through Ishi Wilderness requires a high level of commitment, as just getting to the trailhead requires a multihour drive, a good portion of which is on a rough dirt road built as a fire break by the Civilian Conservation Corps in the 1930s. The low elevation ensures snow-free hiking throughout most of the year, and a springtime trip offers the added bonus of a fine wildflower display. Kayakers and anglers are drawn to this section of creek for river running and excellent catch-and-release fishing. A few cautions are worth noting: At this elevation, poison oak is prevalent, rattlesnakes inhabit the canyon, and ticks can be bothersome, especially in spring.

DIRECTIONS TO TRAILHEAD: Leave Highway 36 about 23 miles east of Red Bluff and 84 miles westbound of Susanville, and turn southeast on Paynes Creek Road at a sign for Tehama Wildlife Refuge. Proceed for 0.3 mile to a right turn onto Plum Creek Road, immediately past a store, and cross a bridge

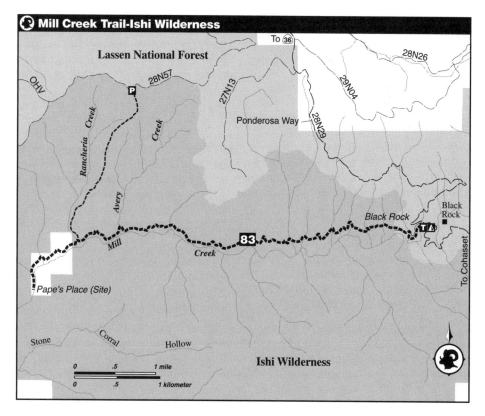

over Paynes Creek, passing through a tiny community with the same name. Pass the entrance to the Tehama Wildlife Refuge and Ishi Conservation Camp on the way to Plum Creek Ridge, and then proceed along the ridge to a junction with Ponderosa Way.

Turn right on the gravel Ponderosa Way, following signed directions for Black Rock. Cross Antelope Creek at 12.4 miles and enter Lassen National Forest at 14 miles, where a sign indicates the road ahead is not maintained between November and May. Proceed on dirt road, crossing over the middle and south forks of Antelope Creek on the way to a junction at 21.1 miles, with a road accessing the Peligreen Jeep Trail on the right. Remain on Ponderosa Way, which climbs nearly to the top of Round Mountain and passes a junction with the road to Long Point before beginning a lengthy descent into Mill Creek canyon. Just before the creek crossing, a road angles sharply right that you follow shortly to the primitive Black Rock Campground and the Mill Creek Trailhead.

DESCRIPTION: The trail begins near the west end of the campground and makes a brief climb west before leveling off and merging with a dirt road that provides access to the private ranch ahead. Cross a small stream spilling across the road; single-track trail resumes just before a gate at the ranch's property line. The trail climbs up the hillside and just above a fence line across sloping meadowlands and oak woodland, passing through a gate on the way to a small, spring-fed stream that provides water for the ranch house below. Beyond the creek, open views across the ranch emit

a pastoral feel, especially in spring when the green meadowlands are sprinkled with flowers, creating a fine backdrop for the dark, volcanic hulk of Black Rock. After hopping across a couple more spring-fed creeks, you leave the ranch behind to enter true wilderness.

The trail follows an undulating course down the canyon, bending in and out of small side canyons carrying tiny rivulets. The open forest is composed of canyon live oaks, blue oaks, and California black oaks, with a smattering of gray pines, California juniper, and stands of ponderosa pines. A diverse understory includes such shrubs as honeysuckle, currant, mountain mahogany, manzanita, wild lilac, and redbud. Shortly after passing through another gate, a grass-covered bench below the trail offers the first passable campsites near the 2-mile mark. Just beyond the camp area, the trail draws close to Mill Creek and divides into two paths; take the upper route, which soon climbs into a side canyon and then travels across grassy slopes high above the creek.

Continue the downstream journey across grassy hillsides and pockets of woodland, dipping occasionally into side canyons along the way. Just before the crossing of Rancheria Creek, you meet the faint tread of a trail climbing the north canyon wall to the Peligreen Jeep Trail. Another mile leads to the end of the trail at the site of Pape's Place along the bank of the creek.

R Fishing in Mill Creek is catch-and-release only from the last Saturday in April through November 15. Anglers must use artificial lures with barbless hooks.

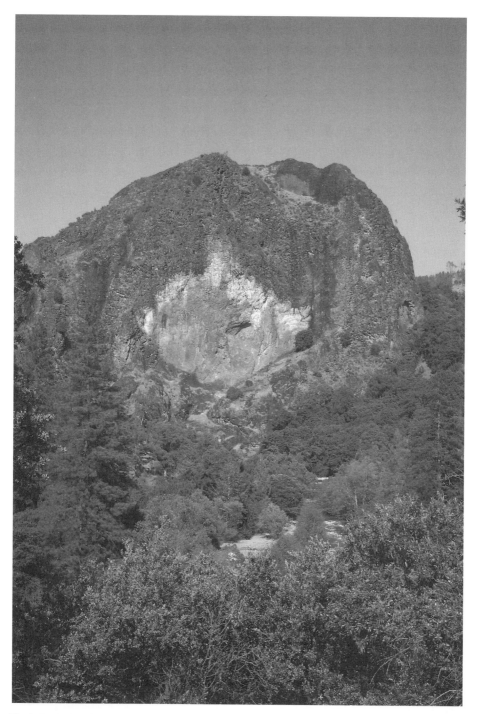

Black Rock, Ishi Wilderness

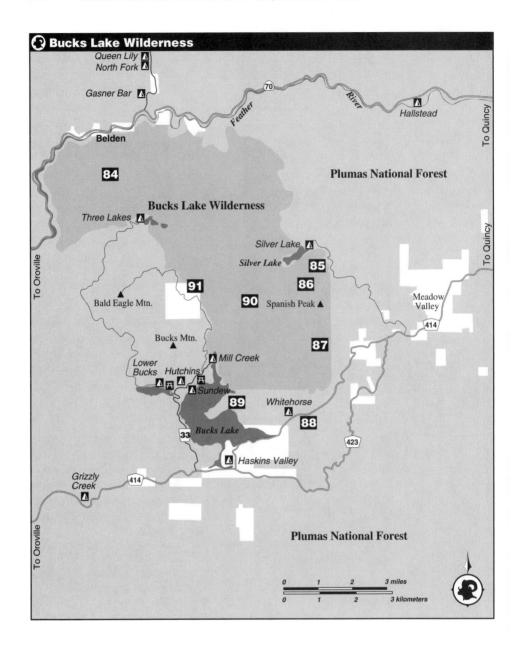

Chapter 6

Bucks Lake Wilderness Trips

Introduction to Bucks Lake Wilderness

Approximately 21,000 acres of backcountry north and east of Bucks Lake was set aside as Bucks Lake Wilderness in 1984. While Bucks Lake has long been a popular summer resort area, and the lake today is abuzz with motorboats, water skiers, and jet skis, the 45 miles of trails nearby are generally lightly used, offering hikers and backpackers some of the most serene experiences in northern California. The wilderness is characterized by an escarpment that runs north-south near the east edge, offering stunning views of Northern California. Below this escarpment, a glaciated granite cirque holds several stunning lakes, fine destinations for either a dayhike or an overnight stay. Most of the rest of the wilderness is sheltered by a serene mixed forest, broken by a smattering of wildflower-carpeted meadows or refreshing brooks. To the north, the wilderness plunges steeply toward the bottom of the North Fork Feather River canyon through open pockets of chaparral and a mixed forest of conifers and oaks.

The first trip described in this section begins at a low elevation near the banks of North Fork Feather River and climbs steeply through a forest of black oaks, Douglas firs, ponderosa pines, and incense cedars along with open sections of chaparral to the Three Lakes area. Next are hikes from Silver Lake, on the east side of the wilderness, to Gold Lake and Spanish Peak, and trails in the Bucks Creek and Bucks Summit area on the south side. Rounding out the chapter is a backpacking loop trip through the wilderness and an out-and-back trip to Three Lakes from the Mill Creek Trailhead on the west side of the wilderness.

Access

Primary access to the Bucks Lake area is via the Bucks Lake Road (Plumas County Road 414), heading west from the town of Quincy. The road splits just west of Meadow Valley, with a steep climb along Bucks Creek Road (Road 414) over Bucks Summit, and a longer, less steep route along Big Creek Road (Road 423), built primarily for recreational vehicles. The two roads reunite in Haskins Valley, just south of Bucks Lake, and then continue as the Quincy-Oroville Highway toward Oroville. Forest Service roads provide access to trailheads and campgrounds around the lake. State Highway 70 provides access to the Pacific Crest trailhead for entry into the north end of Bucks Lake Wilderness.

Amenities

Quincy is a full-service community offering numerous gas stations, stores, and lodging. General stores near the south end of Bucks Lake provide limited supplies.

Campgrounds

Campground	Fee	Elevation	Season	Restrooms	Running Water	Bear Boxes
Whitehorse (SE of Bucks Lake)	$14	5200′	May to October	Vault	Yes	No
Haskins Valley (PG&E; S of Bucks Lake)	$15	5180′	May to October	Vault	Yes	No
Grizzly Creek (SW of Bucks Lake)	$18	5400′	May to October	Vault	Yes	No
Sundew (NE shore of Bucks Lake)	$18-20	5100′	May to October	Vault	Yes	No
Hutchins Group (NE shore of Bucks Lake)	$60	5100′	May to October	Vault	Yes	No
Lower Bucks (Lower Bucks Lake)	$14	5000′	May to October	Vault	Yes	No
Mill Creek (N arm of Bucks Lake)	$18-20	5100′	May to October	Vault	Yes	No
Gansner Bar (FS 27N26, North Fork Feather River)	$18	2300′	April to October	Flush	Yes	No
North Fork (FS 27N26, North Fork Feather River)	$18	2600′	May to October	Flush	Yes	No
Queen Lilly (FS 27N26, North Fork Feather River)	$18	2600′	May to October	Flush	Yes	No
Hallstead (W of FS27N26 on I-70)	$18	2800′	May to October	Flush	Yes	No

Ranger Stations and Visitor Information

The Quincy Ranger District office is located at 159 Lawrence Street in the town of Quincy.

Good to Know Before You Go

Wilderness permits are not required for overnight stays in Bucks Lake Wilderness, although the Forest Service requests that all overnight visitors self-register at the trailhead.

Trip **84**

Pacific Crest Trail to Three Lakes

S / DH, BP

DISTANCE: 15.8 miles out and back

ELEVATION: 2340/6130, +5090/-5090

SEASON: June to November

USE: Light

MAPS: *Belden, Storrie, Bucks Lake*

INTRODUCTION: Only mildly masochistic hikers and backpackers will find this trip appealing, as the trail starts low near the North Fork Feather River and follows a brutally steep climb for the first few miles

before adopting a more humane grade for the remainder of the nearly 8-mile trip. During the hot summer months, beginning at such a low elevation will ensure nearly unbearable temperatures for the entire ascent out of the canyon. Survivors of the canyon climb still face many more miles of hiking in order to reach Three Lakes. If getting to the lakes is your goal, the route from the Mill Creek trailhead is much more appealing (see Trip 91). If all of these warnings haven't deterred you from taking this hike, I'd be happy to pass on the name of a well-respected therapist. (That said, and while the climb out of the North Fork Feather River is characterized as a grunt, the periodic views from the trail are certainly worth the effort for those up to the task.)

DIRECTIONS TO TRAILHEAD: Follow Hwy. 70 to the signed turnoff for Belden, approximately 50 miles east of Oroville, and leave the highway to drive across a bridge over North Fork Feather River. Proceed through

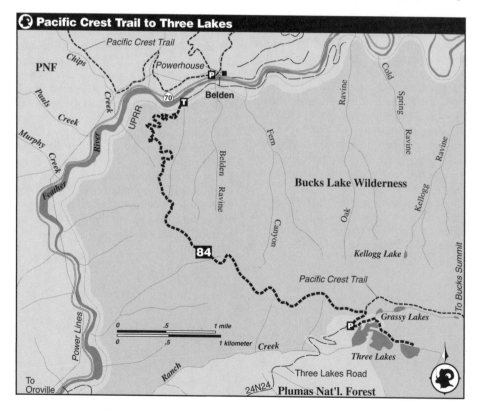

the tiny community of Belden. Continue past the equestrian trailhead, where the pavement gives way to a dirt-and-gravel surface, to the end of the road near the railroad tracks. Park on the narrow shoulder.

DESCRIPTION: Carefully cross to the far side the railroad tracks to the start of the trail. Proceed past a Pacific Crest Trail sign through plentiful trailside foliage across a rocky gully and into Douglas fir forest on the way to the first of many switchbacks to come. California laurels, black and live oaks, incense cedars, and ponderosa pines accompany the Douglas firs in this plant community. Lining the path are such shrubs as dogwood, broadleaf maple, thimbleberry, and bracken fern. Keep your eyes alert for poison oak, which is a common plant on the lower part of the trail. Soon, the trail leads into Bucks Lake Wilderness near some trail signs and a registration box.

Switchbacks zigzag across the steep slope, with the trail passing over a seasonal stream a few times on the way to the edge of a deep ravine. Turning upstream, the path proceeds well above the ravine on an unrelenting, winding march up the south wall of North Fork Feather River canyon. Above the head of the ravine, after nearly 40 switchbacks, the trail breaks out of the forest onto a slope carpeted with dry shrubs, including chinquapin, tobacco brush, and manzanita. Here you have a sweeping view of the river canyon below, which provides a vivid picture of the upward extent of your progress.

Having conquered the canyon wall, the grade eases to a mild to moderate climb. Although the hardest part of the journey is now behind you, the Three Lakes area is still a significant distance away. Head across open slopes carpeted with manzanita, chinquapin, tobacco brush, and lesser amounts of wild cherry, where the single-track trail eventually merges with the track of an old fire road. Follow the old road through a couple minor saddles, where you can see Lassen Peak to the north. From the last saddle, the route continues to a shady bend, beyond which you make a gentle, half-mile traverse to the Three Lakes area and resume single-track trail just before a three-way junction.

Leaving the PCT, turn right on the lateral and descend moderately through open forest, past a Bucks Lake Wilderness sign to another junction. The way ahead leads to the Three Lakes Road, but you turn left and soon catch a glimpse of the lower lake and the dam at the far end. After crossing an old, wood bridge over a narrow creek, the path continues through a dense forest of white firs, western white pines, lodgepole pines, and a few sugar pines. Arrive at the middle lake, a natural body of water rimmed by gray cliffs that is much more scenic than the artificial lower lake. Beyond a couple of passable campsites, the encroach- ing water at the far end of the middle lake inundates the trail, where thick brush makes circumventing the obstacle quite difficult—at least not without getting your feet wet. Once past this minor inconvenience, the trail makes a short climb to the upper lake, clearly the most attractive of the Three Lakes. Unfortunately, this lake offers only small, marginal campsites above the north- west shore. Deteriorating tread continues above the lakeshore but disappears entirely in thick brush before reaching the far end of the lake.

Trip **85**

Gold Lake

Ⓜ ↗ DH, BP

DISTANCE: 3.4 miles out and back

ELEVATION: 5785/5960, +425/-425

SEASON: June to November

USE: Light

MAP: *Bucks Lake*

INTRODUCTION: A short hike to a glacier-carved lake is the highlight of this trip on the east side of Bucks Lake Wilderness. The trail begins near the primitive Silver Lake Campground, which may be attractive to backpackers, since the small campsites and

narrow access road are unsuitable for motor homes and large trailers. Gold Lake offers a few tiny campsites for those seeking more of a backcountry experience.

DIRECTIONS TO TRAILHEAD: From Quincy, follow Bucks Lake Road west for 8 miles to the Silver Lake Road (Forest Road 24N29X), and turn right (northwest). Make a 6-mile climb on this dirt-and-gravel road to Silver Lake. Just past the primitive campground, the road narrows to one lane on the approach to the trailhead near the end of the road. Park in the small parking area near the north shore of Silver Lake. The trailhead is equipped with modern vault toilets. The water from Silver Lake is used as a domestic water supply for residents of Meadow Valley, so swimming is not allowed at the inviting lake. (However, the lake loses its allure by late summer, when the water level drops significantly, and the

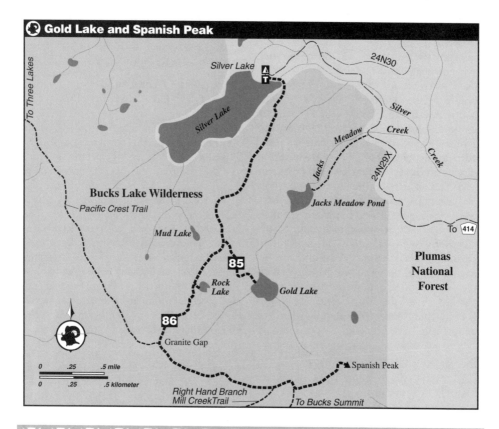

lake becomes a shallow, unattractive, rock-studded, oversized puddle.)

DESCRIPTION: Find the start of the trail near a signboard, and follow a broad path east and then south across the top of the earthen dam on the northeast shore of Silver Lake. Here, the trail leaves the lakeshore path and ascends terrain carpeted with manzanita, tobacco brush, and huckleberry oak, and dotted with Jeffrey pines and white firs. As the steady climb continues, you soon cross into Bucks Lake Wilderness and gain the crest of a moraine, offering fine over-the-shoulder views of Silver Lake, which sparkles in the customary sunshine.

Drop off the moraine and then resume an undulating climb while enjoying good views of swampy Jacks Meadow Pond to the east and Spanish Peak to the south. As you continue, Gold Lake springs into sight, nestled on a bench below the northwest face of the flat-topped peak. A short stretch of moderately steep climbing on sandy tread leads to a junction marked by a 4-by-6-foot post with the trail to Gold Lake.

Follow the left-hand trail on an easy traverse through shrubs, grasses, and boulders over glacier-polished terrain, interrupted briefly by the crossing of a seasonal swale and a tiny stream shooting down a rocky gorge. A short climb from the gorge leads to a rocky perch in the notch of a prominent cleft on the edge of the lake's basin. From this notch, make a short but steep descent and clamber through boulders to an informal junction above the Gold Lake shoreline, where the left-hand path heads to the outlet, and the other path plunges steeply to the lakeshore. Because the lake is hemmed in on all sides by the steep rock walls of a cirque, campsites are few and far between, with the only passable options on spartan sandy patches above the west shore. The water is quite chilly until early August, when the temperature rises enough for refreshing swimming. Rocks near the northeast shore offer good diving opportunities.

Trip **86**

see map on p.247

Silver Lake to Spanish Peak

Ⓜ ╱ DH

DISTANCE:	7.2 miles out and back
ELEVATION:	5785/7017, +1965/-1965
SEASON:	Mid-June to November
USE:	Light
MAP:	*Bucks Lake*

INTRODUCTION: A good, stiff climb brings ample rewards in the form of stunning views from the summit of 7017-foot Spanish Peak, which lies just inside the eastern border of Bucks Lake Wilderness. After the climb, visitors have the option of taking a refreshing dip in Rock or Gold lakes, but not in Silver Lake, which is the domestic water supply for Meadow Valley.

DIRECTIONS TO TRAILHEAD: From Quincy, follow Bucks Lake Road west for 8 miles to the Silver Lake Road (Forest Road 24N29X), and turn right (northwest). Make a 6-mile climb on this dirt-and-gravel road to Silver Lake. Just past the primitive campground, the road narrows to one lane on the approach to the trailhead near the end of the road. Park in the small parking area near the north shore of Silver Lake. The trailhead is equipped with modern vault toilets. The water from Silver Lake is used as a domestic water supply for residents of Meadow Valley, so swimming is not allowed at the inviting lake. (However, the lake loses its allure by late summer, when the water level drops significantly, and the lake becomes a shallow, unattractive, rock-studded, oversized puddle.)

DESCRIPTION: Find the start of the trail near a signboard, and follow a broad path east and then south across the top of the earthen dam on the northeast shore of Silver Lake. Here, the trail leaves the lakeshore path and ascends terrain carpeted with manzanita, tobacco brush, and huckleberry oak, and dotted with Jeffrey pines and white firs. As the steady climb continues, you soon cross into Bucks Lake Wilderness and gain the crest of a moraine, offering fine over-the-shoulder views of Silver Lake, which sparkles in the customary sunshine.

Drop off the moraine and then resume an undulating climb while enjoying good views of swampy Jacks Meadow Pond to the east and Spanish Peak to the south. As you continue, Gold Lake springs into sight, nestled on a bench below the northwest face of the flat-topped peak. A short stretch of moderately steep climbing on sandy tread leads to a junction with the Gold Lake Trail, 1.3 miles from the trailhead.

Continue heading southwest, past the junction, where level trail passes through the vicinity of Mud Lake. As its name implies, Mud Lake isn't exactly the beauty queen of the area's lakes, and, unfortunately, its poor aesthetic quality was exacerbated after a recent fire, which left the shallow body of water with a charred forest of dead snags. It is now vaguely reminiscent of Tolkien's description of Mordor in the Lord of the Rings trilogy.

Leaving the burned area behind, your ascent eventually resumes, with western white pines briefly joining the forest before you return to open, brushy terrain. Early-summer hikers may be treated to a fine display of wildflowers on the way to a junction with a lateral on the left to Rock Lake, 1.5 miles from the trailhead.

S **SIDE TRIP TO ROCK LAKE:** Head southwest from the trail, and climb through brush and boulders to the lip of the lake's basin. Drop down from the lip through a forest of pines and firs to the east side of the aptly named lake, where large rocks line a shoreline back-dropped by rocky bluffs and outcrops. Pockets of conifers shade a few campsites. **END OF SIDE TRIP**

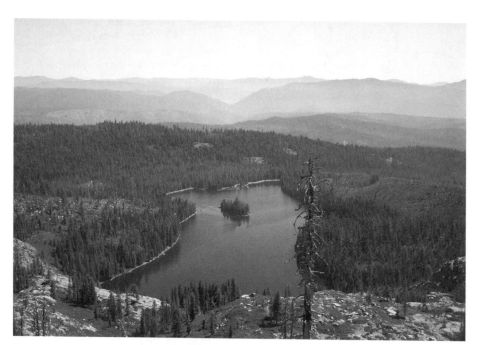

Silver Lake from Pacific Crest Trail ridge

Climb more steeply from the Rock Lake junction with improving views of Silver, Rock, and Mud lakes below. Switchbacks lead up a rocky gully toward Granite Gap and a junction with the Pacific Crest Trail in a grove of pines and firs, 2.2 miles from the trailhead.

Turn left (southeast) and follow the well-defined tread of the PCT on a traverse along the rim of Gold Lake's cirque (the lake is usually out of sight along this traverse). After a half mile, you crest a low ridge and drop into a flat, broad saddle to a junction with the Right Hand Branch Mill Creek Trail, marked by a post. Remain on the PCT and head west, back into the forest briefly before you enter open terrain carpeted with pinemat manzanita on the way to a junction with the lateral to Spanish Peak, 3.1 mile from the trailhead.

Leaving the PCT, you proceed ahead (west) toward Spanish Peak on mildly rising tread through pinemat manzanita and red firs. Break out of the trees near the top, passing by the dilapidated shack that once served as the outhouse for the seasonal ranger for the lookout that once stood atop the peak. A short climb leads to the summit, and a sweeping view across northern California includes Lassen Peak and Lake Almanor to the north and Sierra Buttes to the southeast. Scattered around the summit, a few remnants from the old lookout remain, including the concrete foundation.

A faint use trail leads away from the lookout site, heading northwest toward the edge of the escarpment. Enter into forest cover and pass a dry campsite before the path dies out near the edge of the cirque holding Gold Lake below. The view straight down into the cirque is quite impressive, and includes Rock Lake, Mud Lake, and a piece of Silver Lake, as well as Gold Lake. For a refreshing swim on your return, take the lateral southeast to Gold Lake (see Trip 85).

BUCKS SUMMIT TRAILHEAD

Trip **87**

Bucks Summit to Spanish Peak

M / DH

DISTANCE: 9.4 miles out-and-back
ELEVATION: 5785/7017, +1632/-1632
SEASON: Mid-June to November
USE: Light
MAP: *Bucks Lake*

INTRODUCTION: Great views from the site of a former fire lookout are the chief rewards of this trip along a section of the storied Pacific Crest Trail. The journey is a contrast in environments, as the first half climbs through mostly open and dry, shrub-covered terrain, while the second half ascends slopes of shady forest and verdant meadows. The final 0.4 mile follows the route of the abandoned road that once served the fire lookout atop Spanish Peak, where you'll have unobstructed views to the north, east, and south.

DIRECTIONS TO TRAILHEAD: From Quincy, take the Bucks Lake Road west to Bucks Summit, and park in the large parking area near the northbound Pacific Crest Trail.

DESCRIPTION: Head northbound from the well-signed start of this section of the Pacific Crest Trail through a stand of Jeffrey pines that soon give way to open slopes of head-high shrubs, including tobacco brush, chinquapin, and manzanita. The dry vegetation is replaced momentarily by lush foliage near seeps and piped stream crossings, as you continue the steady climb aided by an occasional switchback. Fine views of the surrounding countryside may ease the strain of the ascent, especially when the temperatures are high.

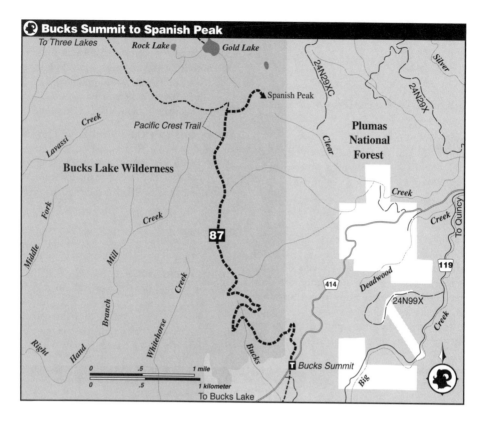

Bucks Summit to Spanish Peak

To Three Lakes   Rock Lake   Gold Lake

Silver

24N29XC   Spanish Peak   24N29X

Lavassi Creek   Pacific Crest Trail

Plumas
National
Forest

Clear

Bucks Lake Wilderness

Creek

Middle Fork   Mill   Creek

Creek   87   Creek

To Quincy

Branch   Whitehorse Creek   414   Deadwood   119

Right   Hand   24N99X

Creek

Bucks   Bucks Summit

0   .5   1 mile

0   .5   1 kilometer

To Bucks Lake   Big

Eventually, you leave the bushy, open slopes for alternating stands of shady forest and pockets of verdant meadow. During peak season, a fine assemblage of ferns and flowers, including corn lily, lupine, paintbrush, and larkspur, borders sections of the trail. Just after a patch of pinemat manzanita is a junction with the lateral to the top of Spanish Peak.

Leaving the PCT, you proceed right toward Spanish Peak on mildly rising tread through pinemat manzanita and red firs. Break out of the trees near the top, passing the dilapidated shack that once served as the outhouse for the seasonal ranger who staffed the lookout that once stood atop the peak. A short climb leads to the summit, and a sweeping view across northern California includes Lassen Peak and Lake Almanor to the north and Sierra Buttes to the southeast. Scattered around the summit, a few remnants from the old lookout remain, including the concrete foundation.

A faint use trail leads away from the lookout site, heading northwest toward the edge of the escarpment. Enter into forest cover and pass a dry campsite before the path dies out near the edge of the cirque holding Gold Lake below. The view straight down into the cirque is quite impressive, and includes Rock Lake, Mud Lake, and a piece of Silver Lake, as well as Gold Lake.

Trip 88

Bucks Creek Loop

E ↻ DH

DISTANCE:	4.3 miles loop
ELEVATION:	5180/5485, +315/-315
SEASON:	June to November
USE:	Light
MAP:	*Bucks Lake*

INTRODUCTION: Although it was designed primarily as a route for mountain bikers, hikers will also enjoy this short loop around a headwaters section of tumbling Bucks Creek. The gently graded trail passes through stands of thick forest and pockets of flower-filled meadows on a 4.3-mile circuit between the southeast arm of Bucks Lake and Bucks Summit. Although most of the route follows single-track or closed dirt road, to complete the loop, hikers will have to walk a 0.4-mile stretch of Bucks Lake Road immediately below Bucks Summit.

DIRECTIONS TO TRAILHEAD: From Quincy, take Bucks Lake Road west to the Bucks Creek Trailhead, near the southeast arm of Bucks Lake, 2 miles west of Bucks Summit. Park along the shoulder of the road as space allows.

DESCRIPTION: Find the start of the trail on the northeast side of the short bridge over Bucks Creek, marked by a small sign reading BUCKS CREEK LOOP TRAIL, 4.3 MILES. Follow the path along the creek's north side and through mixed forest for 0.3 mile to White Horse Campground, and then stroll along the paved access road past campsites to the far side of the campground, where a

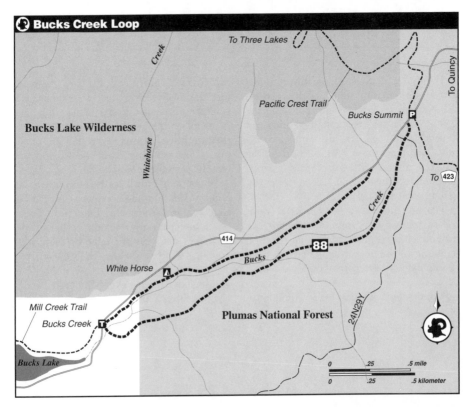

stout wood bridge spans Whitehorse Creek. Beyond the bridge, the trail veers away from the highway, crosses a rivulet, and then comes alongside Bucks Creek for a while. Eventually, the trail bends northeast and makes a mild climb along the course of an abandoned road toward Bucks Summit. The road meets Bucks Lake Road at 1.75 miles, requiring hikers to carefully walk the pavement for the next 0.4 mile to the resumption of single-track trail. Pass a dirt road on the right before reaching signed trail angling sharply to the right (south).

Follow the trail 0.1 mile to the crossing of the dirt road you previously passed, and follow the track of an old road through mixed forest to the south of an alder-and-willow-lined stretch of Bucks Creek. Farther on, pass pockets of flower-filled meadow, parts of which can be quite boggy in early season. Just beyond the 4-mile mark, hop across a seasonal stream and continue along the trail as it bends west and proceeds through the forest toward Bucks Lake Road and the conclusion of the loop at the south end of the bridge over Bucks Creek.

BUCKS CREEK TRAILHEAD

Trip **89**

Bucks Creek to Mill Creek Campground

M / DH

DISTANCE: 5 miles point to point

ELEVATION: 5180/5165, +200/-215

SEASON: June to November

USE: Light

MAP: *Bucks Lake*

INTRODUCTION: Generally, this is an easy, 5-mile, lakeside stroll through shady forest. However, when snowmelt swells the feeder streams emptying into Bucks Lake, a couple of fords can be quite treacherous—check with the Forest Service for current stream conditions in early season. Even later in the summer, you may want to pack a pair of sandals or old tennis shoes for the fords of Mill Creek and Right Hand Branch Mill Creek. Aside from these two potential difficulties, the trail is a pleasant walk along the quiet, east side of Bucks Lake, near the boundary of Bucks Lake Wilderness, with plenty of fine views of the lake backdropped by forested hillsides.

DIRECTIONS TO TRAILHEAD: START: From Quincy, take Bucks Lake Road west to the Bucks Creek Trailhead, near the southeast arm of Bucks Lake, 2 miles west of Bucks Summit. Park along the shoulder of the road as space allows.

END: Follow Bucks Lake Road to a junction with the Oroville-Quincy Highway in Haskins Valley, turn right, and proceed to a junction with Forest Road 33, just west of Haskins Bay and Bucklin Dam. Head north for 4.4 miles to a Y-junction and veer right onto Forest Road 24N69X, as Road 33 on the left turns to dirt, and follow paved road 0.5 mile to Mill Creek Campground.

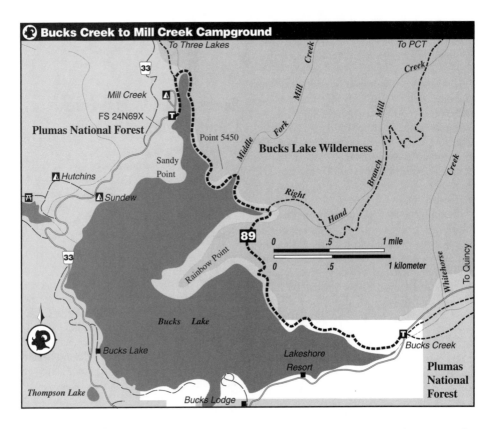

Park in the day-use area. The campground is equipped with running water and vault toilets.

DESCRIPTION: Head southwest on gently graded trail alongside a short stretch of Bucks Creek through a mixed forest of white firs, incense cedars, ponderosa pines, lodgepole pines, and western white pines until the trail reaches the southeast arm of Bucks Lake. Proceed along the shoreline trail, where you have good views across the lake's surface to the south shore until the trees obscure the view. Soon pass through a boggy area, where alders and aspens intermix with the conifers, and early-season wildflowers line the path. Continue the mellow stroll, stepping over a number of small, seasonal streams on the way toward Rainbow Point. The trail leaves the shoreline to climb directly over Rainbow Point, pass-

ing through Bucks Lake Wilderness on the way to a small cove. Head down to a ford of Right Hand Branch Mill Creek, which may be difficult during high water—search upstream for a downed log. Safely across the creek, you reach a junction at 2.6 miles from the trailhead, where the right-hand trail heads up the creek for nearly 5 miles to a connection with the Pacific Crest Trail.

Continue along the forested lakeshore trail, crossing a rock outcrop with a good view across the lake, before veering into the next side canyon and a usually ankle-deep ford of Middle Fork Mill Creek. The trail wraps around Point 5450 and then crosses a seasonal, alder-lined stream. Reach a stretch of open forest, where the white beach of Sandy Point glistens in the sun across the north arm of the lake. Back into the forest, the trail follows the shore across more seasonal streams toward the top of the north arm, where a moderate ascent leads across an open slope covered with tobacco brush. Briefly enter the wilderness on the way to the top of the climb, head back into forest, and then drop steeply toward a ford of Mill Creek, which may be very difficult in early season.

From the west bank of Mill Creek, climb up the hillside to a junction with the Mill Creek Trail. Turn left (south) and walk 0.4 mile to the end of the trail. Proceed to the day-use parking area of Mill Creek Campground.

MILL CREEK CAMPGROUND TRAILHEAD

Trip **90**

Bucks Lake Wilderness Loop

M **Q** DH, BP

DISTANCE: 18 miles loop

ELEVATION: 5170/6960/5170, +3800/-3800

SEASON: June to November

USE: Light

MAP: *Bucks Lake*

INTRODUCTION: Hermits will love this trail, as few other than Pacific Crest Trail thru-hikers favor this route. Generally, you will only see other humans on boats when you're hiking the 3-mile stretch of trail along the northeast shore of Bucks Lake. In spite of this loop's lack of popularity, it has much to offer, including scenic lakes, cascading streams, wildflower-filled meadows, shady forests, wide-ranging views, and side trips to Three Lakes and Spanish Peak. Established campsites are few and far between, requiring a bit of logistical planning as to where to camp.

DIRECTIONS TO TRAILHEAD: Follow Bucks Lake Road west from Quincy to a junction with the Oroville-Quincy Highway in Haskins Valley, turn right, and proceed to a junction with Forest Road 33, just west of Haskins Bay and Bucklin Dam. Head north for 4.4 miles to a Y-junction and veer right onto Forest Road 24N69X, as Road 33 on the left turns to dirt, and follow paved road 0.5 mile to Mill Creek Campground. Park in the day-use area. The campground is equipped with running water and vault toilets.

DESCRIPTION: The first leg of the loop is the least enjoyable stretch of trail, which climbs steeply and follows close to or directly on a dirt road before better conditions prevail

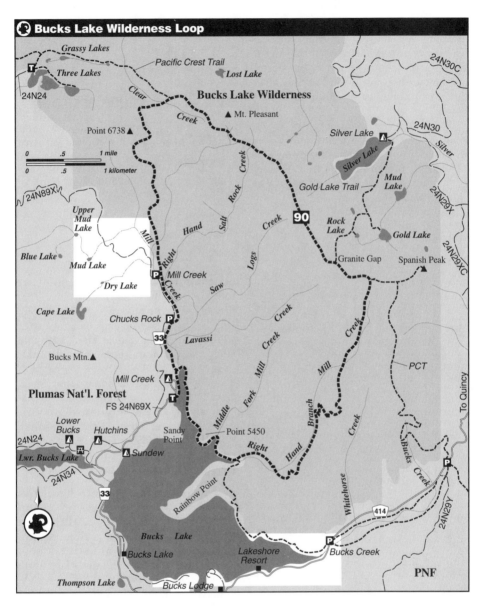

beyond the Mill Creek Trailhead. From Mill Creek Campground, follow single-track trail north for a quarter mile to a junction with the Mill Creek Trail, above the ford of Mill Creek just before it pours into the northern arm of Bucks Lake. Beyond the junction, the grade increases substantially on a climb toward Chucks Rock. Fortunately, a mixed forest of conifers shades most of the brutally

steep route. Just below Chucks Rock, the trail crosses Forest Road 33 and continues a short distance to cross the road again higher up the slope. According to *A Guide to Bucks Lake Wilderness* (Plumas National Forest, 1991), a trail continues from here to the Mill Creek Trailhead, although I was unable to find any discernible trail in 2007. Unless you prefer a quest for the holy grail of trails, the most efficient route follows the road to the trailhead. Fortunately again, the road is much more pleasantly graded than the section of trail below.

Single-track trail resumes beyond the Mill Creek Trailhead, and immediately crosses Mill Creek to follow gently graded trail through a light forest of white firs and lodgepole pines to a boulder hop over the creek. The tread briefly disappears in a small, grassy meadow on the far side but is easily found again just past a snow survey marker, where the trail reenters forest cover. Leaving Mill Creek, the lupine-lined trail begins a moderate climb through shady forest with occasional pockets of meadow carpeted with grasses, sedges, shrubs, and wildflowers in early to midseason. Progressing up the trail, you may notice cow pies scattered across the area. Unfortunately, part of the wilderness is still used for cattle grazing, a practice that dates back to the early 1900s. For a bovine-free experience, visit the area prior to August 1 or after September 30. Around the 1.5-mile mark, the trail draws alongside an alder-lined tributary of Mill Creek and then continues climbing to a high point, south-southeast of Point 6738. Nearby, an unmarked junction with a use trail on the right drops down to a horse camp, where a faint path continues to a water source at a nascent stream.

From the high point, the trail descends toward the Three Lakes area and passes through a pair of meadows, the tread temporarily disappearing in the verdant vegetation of the second one. Continue the descent, hopping across a trio of thin, lushly lined rivulets and passing a shallow pond bordered by tall grasses and covered with lily pads. Just past the pond, you reach a three-way junction with the Pacific Crest Trail, 3.3 miles from the trailhead.

[S] **SIDE TRIP TO THREE LAKES:** To visit Three Lakes, turn left (west) and follow the gently graded PCT past the pond and alongside an alder-lined seasonal stream that drains into the pond from Grassy Lakes. A fern-lined section of trail leads through open forest with evidence of a fire on the right-hand

hillside. Continue past Grassy Lake, which, except in early season, will appear to be more like a grassy meadow with a small pond at the far end. Reach a junction with the unmaintained trail to Kellogg Lake on the right, a second-rate body of water made more unappealing after the fire. Proceed ahead a short distance to a junction with a lateral heading south-southwest to Three Lakes.

Leaving the PCT, the lateral descends moderately through open forest, past a Bucks Lake Wilderness sign to another junction. The way ahead leads to the Three Lakes Road, but you turn left and soon catch a glimpse of the lower lake and the dam at the southwest end. After crossing an old, wood bridge over a narrow creek, the path continues through a dense forest of white firs, western white pines, lodgepole pines, and a few sugar pines to the middle lake, a natural body of water rimmed by gray cliffs that is much more scenic than the artificial lower lake. Beyond a couple passable campsites, the encroaching water at the northeast end of the middle lake inundates the trail, where thick brush makes circumventing the obstacle quite difficult, at least not without getting your feet wet. Once past this minor inconvenience, you make a short climb to the upper lake, clearly the most attractive of the Three Lakes. Unfortunately, this lake offers only small, marginal campsites above the northwest shore. Deteriorating tread continues above the lakeshore but disappears entirely in thick brush before you reach the far end of the lake. **END OF SIDE TRIP**

From the PCT junction, you head southeast on a flower-lined path through open to light forest, crossing a seasonal swale and passing a small, flower-filled meadow on the way to a crossing of Clear Creek, where a small campsite is just above the stream. After a while, the trail draws alongside the creek near some cascades and a small pool before quickly moving away again. Climbing moderately through light forest, the path approaches and crosses a number of lushly lined rivulets below the southwest slope of Mt. Pleasant, reaching a high point marked by a sign simply reading MT. PLEASANT, directly south of the broad-topped peak, 1.8 miles from the junction.

A short, mild descent leads to the start of a gently undulating traverse along the northeastern escarpment between Mt. Pleasant and Spanish Peak. Beginning in thick forest, the traverse eventually leads out of the trees to impressive views of the lakes below in their granite basins, and the terrain beyond, including the deep gash of North Fork Feather River, a slice of Sierra Valley, nearby Meadow Valley, and the more distant Quincy area. The traverse lasts for 2.5 miles, with stands of forest occasionally interrupting the stunning views. At Granite Gap, in one such stand of forest, you reach a junction with the trail to Silver Lake, 4.4 miles from the PCT/Three Lakes junction. Continuing ahead, a section of open forest allows more views before thicker forest returns on the way to a saddle and a junction with the Right Hand Branch Mill Creek Trail, 0.6 mile farther.

[S] **SIDE TRIP TO SPANISH PEAK:** Before continuing the loop on the Right Hand Branch Mill Creek Trail, consider a 0.8-mile extension to the marvelous view from the old lookout site on top of Spanish Peak. Remain on the southbound PCT, and travel through forest briefly before entering open terrain carpeted with pinemat manzanita on the way to a junction with the lateral to Spanish Peak.

Turn left and proceed toward Spanish Peak on mildly rising tread through pinemat manzanita and red firs. Break out of the trees near the top, passing by the dilapidated shack that served as the outhouse for the seasonal ranger who staffed the lookout that once stood atop the peak. A short climb leads to the summit and a sweeping view across northern California that includes Lassen Peak and Lake Almanor to the north and Sierra Buttes to the southeast. Scattered around the summit, a few remnants from the old lookout remain, including the concrete foundation.

A faint use trail leads away from the lookout site, heading northwest toward the edge of the escarpment. Enter into forest cover and pass a dry campsite before the path dies out near the edge of the cirque holding Gold Lake below. The impressive view straight down into the cirque includes Rock Lake, Mud Lake, and a piece of Silver Lake, as well as Gold Lake. **END OF SIDE TRIP**

Leave the PCT and follow the Right Hand Branch Mill Creek Trail south over a low rise before embarking on a nearly continuous, nearly 5-mile descent to the east shore of Bucks Lake. Beyond the low rise, the trail enters a small meadow, where the tread is momentarily lost in the lush vegetation—cairns should help keep you on course. Step across the usually dry streambed in the uppermost part of the canyon and continue to a second, larger meadow, where, once again, the trail disappears for a while in the thick grasses (again, cairns should be an aid). Follow the creek, which by now should be flowing with water, to an easy crossing, 1.1 miles from the PCT junction.

Beyond the crossing, the trail moves away from the creek for a spell, more or less traversing across the east side of the canyon for the next mile. The traverse ends at the beginning of an extended, switchbacking descent that leads steeply down the forested hillside. After a couple of miles and numerous switchbacks, the trail drops to a boulder hop of the main branch of the creek. A level spot just above the creek is the closest thing to a campsite along the Right Hand Branch Mill Creek Trail so far.

Beyond the crossing, a couple more short switchbacks lead to a tiny rivulet that is easily negotiated, and soon afterward you get your first glimpse through the trees of Bucks Lake's blue waters. Hop across a second rivulet just before a junction with the Mill Creek Trail, 4.9 miles from the PCT junction.

Turn right (west-northwest) and proceed along the forested lakeshore path. A sandy beach near the junction offers a possible campsite, albeit with the noise from passing pleasure craft slicing across the surface. Veer into the next side canyon and a usually ankle-deep ford of Middle Fork Mill Creek. The trail wraps around Point 5450, where overnighters may find better campsites on the bluff overlooking the lake. Cross a seasonal, alder-lined stream and reach a stretch of open forest, where the white beach of Sandy Point glistens in the sun across the north arm of the lake. Back into the forest, the trail follows the shore across more seasonal streams, surrounded by lush vegetation. Toward the end of the north arm, a moderate ascent leads across an open slope covered with tobacco brush. Briefly enter the wilderness on the way to the top of the climb, head back into forest, and then drop steeply toward a ford of Mill Creek, which may be very difficult in early season.

From the west bank of Mill Creek, climb up the hillside to a junction with the Mill Creek Trail. Turn left (south), and retrace your steps 0.4 mile to the end of the trail and proceed to Mill Creek Campground.

MILL CREEK TRAILHEAD

Trip **91**

Three Lakes

M ✗ DH, BP

DISTANCE:	10.6 miles out and back
ELEVATION:	5870/6580/6125 +1350/-1350
SEASON:	June to November
USE:	Light
MAP:	*Bucks Lake*

INTRODUCTION: Three Lakes lie at the northwest tip of Bucks Lake Wilderness, with one uninspiring, artificial lake outside the wilderness boundary and two more natural, picturesque lakes within the wilderness. Motorized access is available to the lower lake via the four-wheel-drive Three Lakes Road, but the number of users appears to be quite light. Few hikers take the 5.3-mile route to the uppermost lakes, which offers solitude and serenity to those up to the task. Overnighters will find campsites to be few and far between, but they seem to be more than adequate for the small amount of campers.

DIRECTIONS TO TRAILHEAD: Follow Bucks Lake Road west from Quincy to a junction with the Oroville-Quincy Highway in Haskins Valley, turn right, and proceed to a junction with Forest Road 33, just west of Haskins Bay and Bucklin Dam. Head north for 4.4 miles to a Y-junction with Forest Road 24N69X to Mill Creek Campground. Veer left to remain on Road 33, which narrows and turns to dirt. Proceed past Chucks Rock, near where the Mill Creek Trail crosses the road, and reach the Mill Creek Trailhead at 6.6 miles from Bucks Lake Road. Park as space allows.

DESCRIPTION: Head west from the trailhead and immediately hop over Mill Creek before turning north to follow gently graded trail

Three Lakes

Kellogg Lake

Kellogg Lake Trail

To 70

Clear Creek

Bucks Lake Wilderness

Lost Lake

25N81

25N80

Plumas National Forest

24N30C

24N30

Grassy Lakes

P

Three Lakes

24N24

Point 6738 ▲

Pacific Crest Trail

Mill Creek Trail

Mt. Pleasant ▲

Silver Lake

24N89X

91

Mill

Creek

Jacks Meadow Pond

Gold Lake

▲ Bald Eagle Mtn.

Plumas National Forest

24N89XA

Dry Lake

Mill Creek

Saw

Logs

Creek

Spanish Peak

Cape Lake

Bucks Mountain ▲

Mill Creek

33

T Mill Creek

Chucks Rock

P

Creek

Bucks Lake

0   .5   1 mile

0   .5   1 kilometer

To Bucks Summit

through a light forest of white firs and lodge-pole pines to a boulder hop over the creek. The tread briefly disappears in a small, grassy meadow on the far side but is easily found again just past a snow survey marker, where the trail reenters forest cover. Leaving Mill Creek, the lupine-lined trail begins a moderate climb through shady forest with occasional pockets of meadow carpeted with grasses, sedges, shrubs, and wildflowers in early to midseason. Progressing up the trail, you may notice cow pies scattered across the area. Unfortunately, part of the wilderness is still used for cattle grazing, a practice that dates back to the early 1900s. For a bovine-free experience, visit the area prior to August 1 or after September 30. Around the 1.5-mile mark, the trail draws alongside an alder-lined tributary of Mill Creek and then continues climbing to the high point of the trip, south-southeast of Point 6738. Nearby, an unmarked junction

with a use trail on the right drops down to a horse camp, where a faint path continues to a water source at a nascent stream.

From the high point, the trail descends toward the Three Lakes, passing through a pair of meadows; the tread temporarily disappears in the verdant vegetation of the second one. Continue the descent, hopping across a trio of thin, lushly lined rivulets, and pass a shallow pond bordered by tall grasses and covered with lily pads. Just past the pond, you reach a three-way junction with the Pacific Crest Trail, 3.3 miles from the trailhead.

Turn left (west) and follow the gently graded PCT past the pond and alongside an alder-lined seasonal stream that drains into the pond from Grassy Lakes. A fern-lined section of trail leads through open forest with evidence of a fire on the right-hand hillside. Continue past Grassy Lake, which, except in early season, will appear to be more like a grassy meadow with a small pond at the far end. Reach a junction with the unmaintained trail to Kellogg Lake, a second-rate body of water made more unappealing after the fire. Proceed a short distance to a junction with a lateral to Three Lakes.

Leaving the PCT, turn south-southwest on the lateral and descend moderately through open forest, past a Bucks Lake Wilderness sign to another junction. The way ahead leads to the Three Lakes Road, but you turn left and soon catch a glimpse of the lower lake and the dam at the far end. After crossing an old, wood bridge over a narrow creek, the path continues through a dense forest of white firs, western white pines, lodgepole pines, and a few

sugar pines. Arrive at the middle lake, a natural body of water rimmed by gray cliffs that is much more scenic than the artificial lower lake. Beyond a couple of passable campsites, the encroaching water at the far end of the middle lake inundates the trail, where thick brush makes circumventing the obstacle quite difficult, at least not without getting your feet wet. Once past this minor inconvenience, the trail makes a short climb to the upper lake, clearly the most attractive of the Three Lakes. Unfortunately, this lake offers only small, marginal campsites above the northwest shore. Deteriorating tread continues above the lakeshore but disappears entirely in thick brush before reaching the far end of the lake.

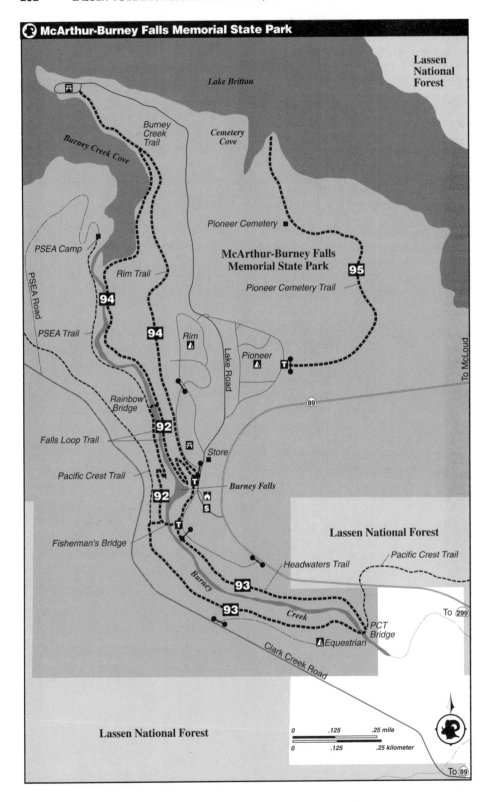

Chapter 7

McArthur-Burney Falls Trips

Introduction to McArthur-Burney Falls Memorial State Park

McArthur-Burney Falls Memorial State Park is a gem of natural beauty situated between Lassen Peak and Mt. Shasta, just off Highway 89. With an elevation just below 3000 feet, the park is open all year, although the highest visitation occurs between late spring and early fall. The namesake falls are spectacular, higher in height—reaching 129 feet—and greater in volume—pumping more than 100 million gallons of water a day—than any of the waterfalls within Lassen Volcanic.

This state park is blessed with a fine network of trails, including short loops around the falls, the headwaters of Burney Creek, and to Lake Britton. An out-and-back journey to a pioneer cemetery and the shore of Lake Britton completes the quartet of trails within the park.

Many visitors come simply to camp, fish, and relax, as the park boasts a couple of campgrounds, fair fishing in the waters of both Burney Creek and Lake Britton, and a boat ramp on the south shore of the lake. Although swimming and fishing are better at other locations in the greater Lassen area, Lake Britton attracts a fair number of both swimmers and anglers during the summer months.

Access

The park is just off Highway 89, about 6 miles north of the junction with Highway 299.

Amenities

The state park has a general store onsite. Wireless Internet service is available near the store. In 2007, 24 new cabins were constructed near the campground. Cabins have no electricity or plumbing, but they do have propane heat. Single-room cabins with two single bunk beds rent for $65 per night, and two-room cabins with four single bunk beds rent for $85 per night. The nearest full-service communities are Fall River Mills (on Highway 299, 11.5 miles northeast of the junction with Highway 89) and Burney (on Highway 299, 5 miles southwest of the junction of Highway 89).

Ranger Stations and Visitor Information

The park headquarters is located just inside the park entrance.

Good to Know Before You Go

There is a day-use fee for entry into McArthur-Burney Falls Memorial State Park.

Campgrounds

Campground	Fee	Elevation	Season	Restrooms	Running Water	Bear Boxes
Pioneer	$15-20	2925'	May to October	Flush	Yes	Yes
Rim	$15-20	2925'	Open all year	Flush	Yes	Yes

BURNEY FALLS TRAILHEAD

Trip **92**

Falls Loop

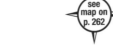

see map on p. 262

E ↻ DH

DISTANCE: 1 mile loop

ELEVATION: 2925/2765/2925, +170/-170

SEASON: March to November (open all year)

USE: Moderate

MAP: *Burney Falls*

INTRODUCTION: From the native Illmawi to the modern-day tourist, the watery splendor of Burney Falls has delighted passersby for thousands of years. The falls are created by the ice-cold waters of Burney Creek spilling over a lip of black basalt in twin cataracts and plunging 129 feet into an indigo-colored pool at the base. In addition, water from five underground aquifers above the falls passes through the porous basalt of the cliff face in countless white ribbons streaming down the dark rock. While the best view of the falls is from an overlook near the start of the trail, the short Falls Loop provides hikers an opportunity to experience Burney Falls and Burney Creek in a more intimate setting that incorporates two bridge crossings of Burney Creek. Interpretive signs along the way offer insights into the natural history of the area.

DIRECTIONS TO TRAILHEAD: Follow State Highway 89 to the entrance of McArthur-

Burney Falls Memorial State Park, 6 miles north of the State Highway 299 junction. Drive a short distance past the entrance station ($6 day-use fee) to the parking area on the right.

DESCRIPTION: Before embarking on the well-signed Falls Loop, take in the exceptional view of the falls from the overlook near the trailhead (don't forget your camera). Follow the paved trail, bordered by a rock wall and metal railing, on a switch-backing descent toward the base of the falls. About halfway down, a cool, fine mist rising from the thunderous falls offers a welcome respite from the typically hot summer temperatures. Reaching the bottom of the canyon, follow a short path away from the main trail, closer to the edge of a 22-foot-deep pool at the base of the falls. Buffeted and refreshed by the wind-driven spray, sightseers lining the broad pool gaze at the falls, which carries more than 100 million gallons of water each day.

Since most visitors never travel past the overlook, and few go no farther than the base of the falls, the rest of the Falls Loop offers hikers the possibility of serenity and seclusion. Head downstream on paved trail past more interpretive signs across a slope of blocky, black basalt alternating with cool stretches of Douglas fir forest interspersed with white and black oaks. Soon, you reach a junction with the Burney Creek Trail continuing ahead to Lake Britton (see Trip 94). Turn left at the junction, and cross a stout bridge arcing over the chilly waters of Burney Creek to a dirt trail that heads very briefly downstream to a junction. The PSEA Trail ahead continues downstream through Douglas firs, alders, and dogwoods to a

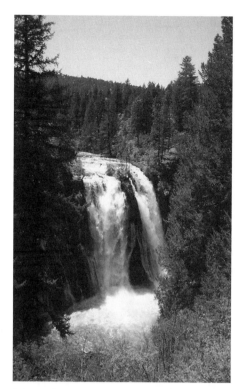

Burney Falls

Trip **93**

see map on p. 262

Headwaters Pool-Pacific Crest Trail Loop

E ↻ DH

DISTANCE:	1.7 miles loop
ELEVATION:	2925/2975/2925, +80/-80
SEASON:	March to November (open all year)
USE:	Moderate
MAP:	*Burney Falls*

INTRODUCTION: This short, easy stroll along Burney Creek to Headwaters Pool offers a fine diversion from the hubbub one normally encounters near Burney Falls overlook. The route combines the Headwaters Trail with a section of the famed Pacific Crest Trail to create a loop along Burney Creek above the falls to Headwaters Pool and back. Depending on the previous winter's snowpack and the extent of irrigation diversions, and despite the abundant volume of water pouring over the falls, Burney Creek may be dry above the spring-fed pool by midsummer.

DIRECTIONS TO TRAILHEAD: Follow State Highway 89 to the entrance of McArthur-Burney Falls Memorial State Park, 6 miles north of the State Highway 299 junction. Drive a short distance past the entrance station ($6 day-use fee), turn left, and follow paved road a short distance to the day-use parking area on the right. The trail begins on the south side of the parking area.

DESCRIPTION: Follow gently graded trail southeast below a set of power lines and into light mixed forest of Douglas firs, black and white oaks, ponderosa pines, and incense cedars, with tumbling Burney Creek just a stone's throw to the right. After a quarter mile, a long set of stairs from the

private camp on the west bank of Burney Creek Cove; the trail is open to the public as far as a gate at the camp's boundary, for those who don't mind the 1.5-mile, round-trip diversion.

Heading upstream from the junction, a brief, moderate climb leads to a switchback, from which you have a tree-filtered view of Burney Falls. Climb to the lip of the canyon and then follow pleasantly graded trail past more interpretive signs and a junction with a 0.1-mile connecter to the nearby Pacific Crest Trail. Continue upstream, above the falls, to Fisherman's Bridge. Cross to the east bank of Burney Creek, where a dirt path on the left leads down to the stream bank, while the main trail follows pavement on a short climb to the Fisherman's parking area, near the trailhead for the Headwaters Trail (see Trip 93). Following a sign marked FALLS OVERLOOK, RESTROOMS, stroll past the entrance station and shortly return to the trailhead area.

service road above leads across the trail and down to an abandoned, stone restroom building just above the creek. Farther on, a short, moderate climb leads to the bank of spring-fed Headwaters Pool, where the creek slows enough to tempt hikers into the water for a cool dip. A short distance above the pool, you reach a junction with the Pacific Crest Trail, 0.7 mile from the trailhead.

Turn right and follow the PCT over a footbridge spanning the creek and head into shadier forest on the south side of the stream. Pass around a burned area and by the edge of a large equestrian camp equipped with modern vault toilets, picnic tables, barbecues, and a small corral. Away from the camp, gently graded trail continues below a set of power lines to a four-way junction with a wide path from Clark Creek Road on the left. Turn right, following signed directions for Burney Falls, and almost immediately drop to a Y-junction with the Falls Loop. Head upstream (south) briefly, cross Fisherman's Bridge, and then follow a short section of paved trail back to the parking lot.

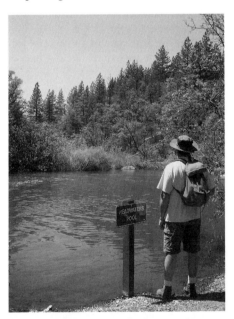

Headwaters Pool

BURNEY FALLS TRAILHEAD

Trip **94**

Burney Creek-Rim Trail Loop

see map on p. 262

E ↻ DH

DISTANCE: 2.8 miles loop

ELEVATION: 2925/2740/2925, +250/-250

SEASON: March to November (open all year)

USE: Moderate

MAP: *Burney Falls*

INTRODUCTION: This fine loop hits most of the highlights of McArthur-Burney Falls Memorial State Park: the watery drama of Burney Falls, the beauty of Lake Britton, the shady riparian habitat along Burney Creek, and the more arid environment along the rim of the creek's canyon.

DIRECTIONS TO TRAILHEAD: Follow State Highway 89 to the entrance of McArthur-Burney Falls Memorial State Park, 6 miles north of the State Highway 299 junction. Drive a short distance past the entrance station ($6 day-use fee) to the parking area on the right.

DESCRIPTION: Before embarking on the well-signed Falls Loop, take in the exceptional view of the falls from the overlook near the trailhead (don't forget your camera). Follow the paved trail, bordered by a rock wall and metal railing, on a switchbacking descent toward the base of the falls. About halfway down, a cool, fine mist rising from the thunderous falls offers a welcome respite from the typically hot summer temperatures. Reaching the bottom of the canyon, follow a short path leads away from the main trail, closer to the edge of a 22-foot-deep pool at the base of the falls. Buffeted and refreshed by the wind-driven spray, sightseers lining the broad pool gaze at the falls, which carries more than 100 million gallons of water each day.

Since most visitors never travel past the overlook, and few go no farther than the base of the falls, the rest of the trip to Lake Britton and back offers hikers some opportunity for serenity and seclusion. Head downstream on paved trail, past more interpretive signs, across a slope of blocky, black basalt alternating with cool stretches of Douglas fir forest sprinkled with white and black oaks. Soon, you reach a junction with the Falls Loop, which turns left and immediately crosses a bridge over Burney Creek.

Continuing ahead from the junction, follow the dirt path adjacent to the creek through a shady forest of Douglas firs, ponderosa pines, and incense cedars toward Lake Britton. Eventually, the trail moves away from the creek on the approach to the sluggish waters of Burney Creek Cove, where the PSEA camp appears on the opposite shore. Follow the shoreline to a junction with the Rim Trail, at 1.3 miles from the trailhead. This will be your return route.

Proceed ahead along the forested shoreline for another quarter mile to the end of the trail at the picnic parking area. Unless you are visiting during spring or fall, expect to see a flurry of activity from picnickers, swimmers, waders, boaters, and anglers who flock to the lake on hot summer days, especially weekends. After taking in the sights and sounds of Lake Britton, retrace your steps a quarter mile to the junction between the Burney Creek and Rim trails.

Turn left and make a moderate climb on the Rim Trail through thick forest for about a quarter mile until you gain gentler terrain on the rim of Burney Creek canyon. Mildly rising tread leads through a drier, more open forest on the canyon rim, eventually taking you along the west edge of Rim Campground. The trail ends at the edge of the closed Old Rim Camp Road. Take this road north and then northeast for 0.2 mile back to the trailhead.

PIONEER TRAILHEAD

Trip **95**

see map on p. 262

Pioneer Cemetery Trail

E ✔ DH

DISTANCE:	2.4 miles out and back
ELEVATION:	2905/2735, +175/-175
SEASON:	March to November (open all year)
USE:	Light
MAP:	*Burney Falls*

INTRODUCTION: This route follows the course of an old wagon road through a quiet forest to a pioneer cemetery and then continues to a secluded section of Lake Britton's shoreline. The cemetery has several historical headstones bearing the names of early pioneers who helped settle the region in the 1800s. Those who continue down the road to Cemetery Cove on Lake Britton may be fortunate to witness a bald eagle soaring above the tops of the Douglas firs.

DIRECTIONS TO TRAILHEAD: Follow State Highway 89 to the entrance of McArthur-Burney Falls Memorial State Park, 6 miles north of the junction of State Highway 299. Drive a short distance past the entrance station ($6 day-use fee), visitor center, and store and turn right into Pioneer Campground. Follow signs toward Campsites 75 and 76; the trailhead is located between them.

DESCRIPTION: The wide track of the old wagon road heads east on a gentle grade through a forest of incense cedars, pines, and oaks. After 0.3 mile, the road veers north and continues for another 0.3 mile before turning west and descending moderately through thickening forest. Reach the fenced cemetery, where a number of headstones occupy the site and clumps of lilac grace the air with their pleasant fragrance in spring.

Away from the cemetery, the wagon road appears to be infrequently used as it descends toward Cemetery Cove and the shore of Lake Britton. On the approach to the cove, the lake's waters can be seen through the forest, which now includes Douglas firs. Reach the cove and continue northeast along a use trail to the edge of a peninsula that offers good views of the hills beyond the water. Swimmers will have to hunt around for good access points, as the banks of the peninsula are severely undercut. When the mood strikes, retrace your steps to the trailhead.

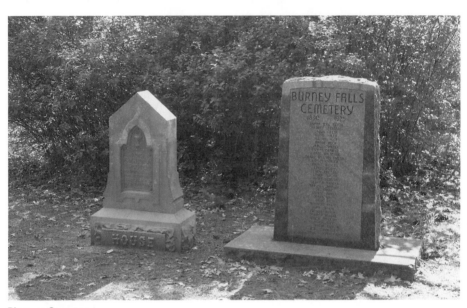

Pioneer Cemetery

Backpacks and Dayhikes Features Chart

Trip	Route	Solitude (Ratings: 1–10; 1 = crowded)	Difficulty	Length in Miles	Elevation Gain/Loss	Dayhike or Backpack	Season
1	↗	5	MS	7.0	+2700/-2700	DH	Mid-July to October
2	↗	5	M	3.2	+935/-935	DH	Mid-June to mid-October
3	↗	5	S	2.0	+1025/-1025	DH, BP	July to mid-October
4	↻	1	E	0.2	Negligible	DH	June to mid-October
5	↗	3	M	4.0	+400/-1200	DH	July to mid-October
6	↗	3	S	5.0	+1957/-1957	DH	Mid-July to early October
7	↗	8	M	3.4	+1075/-1075	DH	July to early October
8	↗	5	M	3.4	+705/-705	DH	Mid-July to early October
9	↗	7	E	2.4	+305/-305	DH	July to mid-October
10	↗	7	M	4.8	+700/-1360	DH	July to mid-October
11	↗	8	M	4.6	+750/-750	DH, BP	July to mid-October
12	↗	3	E	0.6	Negligible	DH	July to mid-October
13	↗	5	E	5.4	+750/-750	DH, BP	July to mid-October
14	↗	2	M	2.2	+475/-475	DH	July to mid-October
15	↺	4	M	8.4	+770/-770	DH	July to mid-October
16	↺	1	E	1.5	Negligible	DH	July to mid-October
17	↗	8	M	5.0	+650/-650	DH, BP	July to mid-October
18	↻	5	M	11.9	+1520/-1520	DH, BP	July to mid-October
19	↗	5	M	7.4	+1225/-1225	DH, BP	July to mid-October
20	↻	5	M	10.8	+1385/-1385	DH, BP	July to mid-October
22	↗	9	M	12.2	+665/-665	DH, BP	June to mid-October
23	↗	8	M	2.8	+625/-625	DH,	July to mid-October

Trip	Route	Solitude (Ratings: 1–10; 1 = crowded)	Difficulty	Length in Miles	Elevation Gain/Loss	Dayhike or Backpack	Season
24	↻	3	E	0.4	Negligible	DH	June to mid-October
25	↗	6	M	4.0	+990/-990	DH	Mid-June to mid-October
26	↗	6	M	6.6	+1250/-1250	DH	July to late October
27	↻	1	E	1.5	Negligible	DH	May to late October
28	↻	2	E	0.75	Negligible	DH	May to late October
29	↗	9	M	12.6	+850/-700	DH	June to mid-October
30	↗	7	M	9.5	+1075/-1075	DH, BP	Mid-June to late October
31	↻	4	E	1.6	+215/-215	DH	April to mid-November
32	↻	3	E	0.6	Negligible	DH	Late May through October
33	↗	8	M	3.0	+570/-40	DH	Late March to December
34	↗	5	E	4.0	+450	DH	March to mid-November
35	↗	8	M	5.8	+460/-460	DH	April to late November
36	↗	8	M	13.5	+675/-900	DH	April to mid-November
37	⟳	6	E	7.0	+750/-750	DH, BP	Mid-June to November
38	↗	7	MS	16.0	+1715/-1715	DH, BP	Mid-June to November
39	↗	7	S	6.0	+2399/-2399	DH	Mid-June to November
40	↻	4	E	2.3	+300/-300	DH	Early June to October
41	↗	9	MS	7.0	+2263/-2263	DH	Early July to October
42	⟳	5	MS	7.0	+1015/-1015	DH	Late May to October
43	↻	6	M	18.1	+1825/-1825	DH, BP	Late June to October
44	↻	8	M	19.3	+2450/-2450	DH, BP	Late June to October
45	↗	8	M	10.0	+600/-600	DH, BP	Mid-June to late October
46	↗	6	E	7.4	+430/-430	DH, BP	Mid-June to late October
47	↻	6	E	7.2	+570/-570	DH, BP	Mid-June to late October
48	↗	6	M	7.0	+585/-585	DH, BP	Mid-June to late October

Trip	Route	Solitude (Ratings: 1–10; 1 = crowded)	Difficulty	Length in Miles	Elevation Gain/Loss	Dayhike or Backpack	Season
49	↗	8	E	1.8	Negligible	DH	Late May to late October
50	↗	8	E	7.4	+810/-810	DH	Late May to late October
51	↻	7	M	7.2	+700/-700	DH, BP	Mid-June to late October
52	↗	4	E	4.5	Negligible	DH	May to late October
53	↗	6	E	1.2	+255/-255	DH	May to late October
54	↗	3	E	6.5	+450	DH	March to late December
55	↗	1	E	9.5	Negligible	DH	March to late October
56	↗	7	MS	3.8	+1846/-1846	DH	Early July to October
57	↻	7	E	6.3	+350/-350	DH	Mid-June to October
58	↗	7	E	0.8	+380/-380	DH	Mid-June to October
59	↗	7	E	1.4	+430/-430	DH	Mid-June to October
60	↻	8	E	6.5	+850/-850	DH, BP	Mid-June to October
61	↻	8	M	13.0	+1725/-1725	DH, BP	Mid-June to October
62	↻	8	M	7.2	+1160/-1160	DH, BP	Mid-June to October
63	↗	9	E	5.8	+1200/-1200	DH. BP	Mid-June to October
64	↻	9	M	18.7	+2700/-2700	DH, BP	Mid-June to October
65	↗	10	S	7.6	+2781/2781	DH	Mid-June to October
66	↗	10	M	8.0	+780/-780	DH	Mid-May to November
67	↻	7	M	2.4	+385/-385	DH, BP	Late May to mid-October
68	↻	7	M	5.8	+1185/-1185	DH	Late May to mid-October
69	↗	6	M	4.8	+875/-875	DH, BP	June to mid-October
70	↗	6	E	5.6	+800/-800	DH	June to mid-October
71	↗	3	M	4.2	+1515/-1515	DH, BP	Mid-June to mid-October
72	↗	8	M	7.6	+1460/-1460	DH	Late June to mid-October
73	↻	9	M	9.6	+1885/-1885	DH, BP	Late June to mid-October
74	↗	9	M	4.4	+500/-500	DH	June to mid-October
75	↗	9	M	8.2	+1725/-1200	DH	June to mid-October

Trip	Route	Solitude (Ratings: 1–10; 1 = crowded)	Difficulty	Length in Miles	Elevation Gain/Loss	Dayhike or Backpack	Season
76	↗	9	M	9.9	+1725/-1200	DH	June to mid-October
77	↻	9	MS	13.2	+2230/-2230	DH. BP	June to mid-October
78	↗	9	M	9.4	+1965/-1965	DH, BP	June to mid-October
79	↗	9	M	12.6	+2250/-2250	DH, BP	June to mid-October
80	↗	9	M	4.2	+970/-970	DH, BP	June to mid-October
81	↗	9	M	12.2	+2170/-2170	DH, BP	May to November
82	↗	8	M	4.8	+650/-650	DH, BP	March to late November
83	↗	9	M	13.2	+1400/-1400	DH, BP	March to late November
84	↗	9	S	15.8	+5090/-5090	DH, BP	June to November
85	↗	6	M	3.4	+425/-425	DH, BP	June to November
86	↗	6	M	7.2	+1965/-1965	DH	Mid-June to November
87	↗	7	M	9.4	+1632/-1632	DH	Mid-June to November
88	↻	6	E	4.3	+315/-315	DH	June to November
89	↗	8	M	5.0	+200/-215	DH	June to November
90	↻	9	M	18.0	+3800/-3800	DH, BP	June to November
91	↗	8	M	10.6	+1350/-1350	DH, BP	June to November
92	↻	3	E	1.0	+170/-170	DH	March to November
93	↻	5	E	1.7	+80/-80	DH	March to November
94	↻	5	E	2.8	+250/-250	DH	March to November
95	↗	8	E	2.4	+175/-175	DH	March to November

The Bear Facts and Other Animal Concerns

Bears

The last grizzly bear in California was shot and killed near Horse Corral Meadow in the southern Sierra Nevada during the early 1900s. Since then, the common American black bear has been the only bear species in the state, and it is therefore the only bear you may encounter in the Lassen Volcanic area.

Despite their name, black bears can range in color from black to cinnamon, and these quick, agile mammals often grow to be quite large—an adult male can weigh as much as 300 pounds. Active both day and night, these omnivores have a highly developed sense of smell. However, black bears subsist mainly on vegetation and are usually not aggressive animals, particularly toward humans. Bears that have not become accustomed to humans tend to be shy and retiring, avoiding contact at almost all costs.

The exception to this rule is black bears that have become familiar with human food and garbage through our carelessness—these bears can be destructive and potentially dangerous animals. Once bears discover human food sources from coolers, cars, backpacks, or garbage cans, reconditioning them to subsist on natural food sources is extremely difficult. Bears that frequent developed campgrounds in their quest for food tend to be the boldest and potentially most dangerous animals. Relocating these bears to backcountry areas has proven to be less than successful, as the bears generally find their way back to civilized areas, or become highly aggressive toward backcountry visitors. "Problem bears" eventually have to be destroyed.

Contrary to what some believe, bears are actually clever animals. Those accustomed to humans have figured out ways to thwart the standard practice of protecting food in the backcountry by hanging it from a tree using the counterbalance method. Nowadays, if you attempt to hang your food, a bear may climb a tree to snap the cord, break the branch holding the food bag, or simply dive bomb the sack in order to get at your food; or a mother bear may send a cub up the tree to the same end. Several years ago, park managers for Yosemite and Sequoia-Kings Canyon national parks, along with surrounding national forest managers, embarked on a plan to minimize encounters between bears and backcountry users. Popular backcountry campsites in these parks were equipped with bear-proof lockers, and bear-proof canisters were required in the most heavily visited areas and strongly suggested elsewhere. With a high degree of compliance, the plan has considerably reduced the bears' association of humans with food, resulting in a decline in human-bear encounters.

All human visitors to the park must take care to minimize the exposure of bears to our food and garbage. While bear canisters are not required in Lassen Volcanic, their use is strongly encouraged in the backcountry. The canisters may add a couple of pounds to a backpack, but that burden is offset by the sense of security the canisters provide. Campers at developed campsites should store food so that it is inaccessible to the bears and should dispose of all garbage in the appropriate bear-proof receptacles.

Following some simple guidelines should enhance your visit to Lassen Volcanic National Park:

Campgrounds

- Leave extra or unnecessary food and scented items at home.
- Store all food, food containers, and scented items in bear-proof lockers and latch them securely.
- Dispose of all trash in bear-proof trash receptacles.
- Do not leave food out at an unattended campsite.

Backcountry

- Don't leave your pack unattended while on the trail.
- Once in camp, empty your pack and open all flaps and pockets.
- Keep all food, trash, and scented items in a bear-proof canister.
- Pack out all trash.

Elsewhere

- Don't allow bears to approach your food—make noise, wave your arms, and throw rocks. Be bold but keep a safe distance and use good judgment.
- If a bear does get into your food, you are responsible to clean up and pack out the mess.
- Never attempt to retrieve food from a bear.
- Never approach a bear, particularly a cub.
- Report any incidents or injuries to the appropriate agency.

Other Animal Concerns

COUGARS: The chance of actually seeing a cougar (or mountain lion) in the backcountry is extremely small, as cougars are typically shy and wish to avoid human contact at nearly all costs. I have never seen a cougar in several decades of hiking in the backcountry and saw my first bobcat in 2006. Unlike black bears, cougars are strictly carnivorous, with mule deer as the preferred staple of their diet. When hunting for venison is poor, cougars will supplement their diet with smaller animals. A typical cougar kills an average of 36 deer per year, and the health of a particular deer population is often linked to the predatory success of these cats, as they thin the herd of the weakest members. Although cat-human encounters are rare, always hike with others in cougar country, especially at lower elevations. In the unlikely event of an encounter with one of these big cats, keep in mind the following guidelines:

- If you encounter a cougar, don't run, as they will mistake you for prey.
- Make yourself appear as large as possible—raise your arms and don't crouch or try to hide.
- Hold your ground or back away slowly while facing the cat.
- Never leave small children unattended; pick them up if the cat approaches.
- If the cougar seems aggressive, make noise, wave your arms, and throw rocks.
- If the animal attacks, fight back—don't play dead.
- Report any encounters to a ranger as soon as possible.

RATTLESNAKES: Although rattlesnakes inhabit the lower elevations of the Lassen backcountry, human encounters are relatively rare. Actual bites are even more unusual and almost never fatal in adults. While rattlesnakes live in a wide range of environments, pay special attention when hiking along streams below 5500 feet. These reptiles seek sun when the air temperature is cold and shade when the air temperature is hot; they are typically nocturnal during the hottest part of the summer. Rattlers are not aggressive and will seek an escape route unless cornered. If you happen upon a rattlesnake, quickly back away and give it some room. If you get bitten, seek immediate medical attention.

TICKS: Ticks are most common in the lower elevations, particularly in the foothills zone. Their numbers are higher in spring, especially following wet winters. Ticks are generally not a problem in the higher elevations during summer.

These blood-sucking pests would be just a simple nuisance if not for the fact that they can carry such maladies as Lyme disease and Rocky Mountain spotted fever. Although rare in the southern Cascades, these tick-borne conditions can be serious if not treated. If a tick has bitten you, consult a physician if you experience flulike symptoms, headache, rash, fever, or joint pain.

Myths, old wives tales, and urban legends abound about the best trick for removing a tick. The medically accepted method advises using a pair of tweezers to get a good hold on the body of the tick and then pull, using gentle traction to detach the pest from your flesh. Upon removal, check the wound to make sure the head was not left behind. Thoroughly wash the affected area with soap and water and then apply an antibiotic ointment to the wound. Monitor your health for the next several days to detect any symptoms of serious illness.

Prevention is the best medicine, so observe the following measures when traveling in tick country:

- Use an effective insect repellent on skin and clothing, and apply liberally.
- Wear light-colored, long-sleeved shirts and long pants with the pant legs tucked into socks.

- Inspect your entire body for bites at least once a day while in the backcountry.
- Check light-colored clothing thoroughly for any loose ticks.

MOSQUITOES: While not a major health concern, pesky mosquitoes can ruin an otherwise peaceful day in the mountains. Fortunately, the mosquito cycle in the Lassen area is waning by midsummer. The peak of the season varies from year to year, but usually coincides with the peak of wildflower season.

Unfortunately for the selected targets, mosquitoes seem to prefer some humans over others. For the afflicted, supposed deterrents can be the modern era's snake oil, from sleeping under a pyramid, ingesting a boatload of vitamin B, bathing in a vat of hand lotion, lighting aromatherapy candles, or using a device that emits a high-pierced shriek heard only by bugs and aliens. Although the only surefire protection against the ubiquitous mosquito is to stay at home, which isn't much of a solution, the following suggestions may enhance your enjoyment of the backcountry during the perpetual buzz of mosquito season:

- Use an insect repellent with deet as the active ingredient, and reapply often.
- Wear long-sleeved shirts and long pants. Articles of clothing infused with repellent, while expensive, will help keep the pests at bay.
- Select a mildly wind-prone campsite away from wet and marshy areas.
- Don't forget your tent.

Minimum-Impact Stock Regulations

- Horses and pack animals are allowed on designated trails except for the following: Manzanita Lake Trail, Lassen Peak Trail, Cinder Cone Trail, Reflection Lake Trail, Bumpass Hell Trail, Devils Kitchen, and Sulphur Works.

- Picketing and/or grazing of stock animals in the park are prohibited.

- Horses and pack animals are not permitted to travel cross-country while in the park.

- Stock parties camping in the park overnight are limited to one of the following designated sites and limitations:
  - Summit Lake and Butte Lake corrals: maximum of 8 animals and 10 people with parking limited to six-wheeled vehicles
  - Juniper Lake corral: maximum of 8 animals and 10 people with parking limited to four-wheeled vehicles

- Riding or tying stock animals in campgrounds, picnic areas, or within the immediate vicinity of eating or sleeping establishments or other areas of public gatherings is prohibited, except where trails and facilities are designated for such use.

Nonprofit Organizations

Lassen Association
PO Box 220
Mineral, CA 96063
(530) 595-3399
www.lassenloomis.info

Lassen Park Foundation
PO Box 3155
Chico, CA 95927
(530) 898-9309
www.lassenparkfoundation.org

The National Park Foundation
1201 Eye Street, NW
Suite 550B
Washington, DC 20005
(202) 354-6460
www.nationalparks.org

Sierra Club
Yahi Group
PO Box 2012
Chico, CA 95927
(530) 345-2696
http://motherlode.sierraclub.org/yahi

Snowlands Network
PO Box 2570
Nevada City, CA 95959
(530) 265-6424
www.snowlands.org

Quick Guide to Frequently Used Numbers and Websites

General

Caltrans (road conditions)	(800) 427-7623
Campground Reservations (NPS)	(877) 444-6777
Campground Reservations (USFS)	(877) 444-6777
Wilderness Press	(800) 443-7227

Lassen National Forest

Headquarters	(530) 257-2151
Almanor Ranger District	(530) 258-2141
Eagle Lake Ranger District	(530) 257-4188
Hat Creek Ranger District	(530) 336-5521

Lassen Volcanic National Park

Headquarters/Information	(530) 595-4444
Lassen Loomis Museum Association	(530) 595-3399
Lassen Park Foundation	(530) 898-9309
Loomis Museum	(530) 595-4444 ext. 5180
Manzanita Lake Camper Store	(530) 335-7557

Lodging

Childs Meadow Resort	(888) 595-3383 or (530) 595-3383
Drakesbad Guest Ranch	(530) 529-1512
Hat Creek Resort	(800) 568-0109
Lassen Mineral Lodge	(530) 595-4422
Mill Creek Resort	(888) 595-4449
Rancheria RV Park	(530) 335-7418
Rim Rock Ranch	(530) 335-7114
St. Bernard Lodge	(530) 258-3382

Plumas National Forest

Headquarters	(530) 283-2050
Feather River Ranger District	(530) 534-6500
Mt. Hough Ranger District	(530) 283-0555

Websites

Campground Reservations (NPS and USFS)	www.recreation.gov
Childs Meadow Resort	www.childsmeadowresort.com
Drakesbad Guest Ranch	www.drakesbad.com
Hat Creek Resort	www.hatcreekresortrv.com
Lassen Association	www.lassenloomis.info
Lassen Mineral Lodge	www.minerallodge.com
Lassen National Forest	www.r5.fs.fed.us/lassen
Lassen Park Foundation	www.lassenparkfoundation.org
Lassen Volcanic National Park	www.nps.gov/lavo
Mill Creek Resort	www.millcreekresort.net
Plumas National Forest	www.r5.fs.fed.us/plumas
Rancheria RV Park	www.rancheriarv.com
Rim Rock Ranch	www.rimrockcabins.com
St. Bernard Lodge	www.stbernardlodge.com
U. S. Geological Survey	www.store.usgs.gov
Wilderness Press	www.wildernesspress.com

Suggested Reading

Schaffer, Jeffrey P. *Pacific Crest Trail: Northern California from Tuolumne Meadows to the Oregon Border*. Berkeley, CA: Wilderness Press, 2003.

Schulz, Paul E. *Lassen Place Names*. Red Bluff, CA: Lassen Association, 1949.

Showers, David, and Mary Ann Showers. *A Field Guide to the Flowers of Lassen Volcanic National Park*. Mineral, CA: Lassen Association, 1996.

Strong, Douglas H. *Footprints in Time: A History of Lassen Volcanic National Park*. Red Bluff, CA: Lassen Association, 1998.

White, Mike. *Best Snowshoe Trails of California: 100 of the Finest Routes in the Cascades & the Sierra*. Berkeley, CA: Wilderness Press, 2005.

INDEX

A

alpine zone 13, 14
Atsugewi 3, 45

B

Badger Flat 94, 95
Barrett Lake 109, 110, 123, 124, 125
Barrett, Louis A. 5
Bathtub Lake 132, 133
bears 273–274
Beauty Lake 159
Bench Lake 81, 82, 212, 215
Big Bear Lake 89, 90
Big Meadow 5
Black Lake 153
Blue Lake 229
Boiling Springs Lake 199, 201, 202–203
Box Lake 124
Brewer, William H. 4, 40, 68
Brodt, Helen 4, 39, 68
Brokeoff Mountain 36–37, 56, 57, 58
Bucks Creek 252, 253, 254
Bucks Lake 253, 254, 255, 258
Bucks Lake Wilderness 243
Bumpass Creek 58, 59, 64, 74, 76
Bumpass Hell 62, 63, 64
Bumpass, Kendally Vanhook 64
Burney Creek 264, 265, 266, 267
Burney Creek Cove 267
Burney Falls 264, 265, 266
Butte Creek 133, 145
Butte Lake 130, 133, 143, 145

C

California State Geological Survey 4
Cameron Meadow 143, 185, 186
campgrounds 24–25
Canyon Creek 226, 228
Canyon Overlook 228
Caribou Lake 152, 154
Caribou Wilderness 130–131
Cemetery Cove 267, 268

Chaos Crags 44, 46, 98, 99, 103
Chaos Crater 98, 99
Chaos Jumbles 46, 103
Chester 160, 170, 194
Childs Meadow Resort 50, 216
Chucks Rock 256
Cinder Cone 4, 136, 137–138, 140
Cinder Cone National Monument 5
Civilian Conservation Corps 6
Clear Creek 257
Cliff Lake 72, 92, 93
Cluster Lakes 89, 90–91
Cold Boiling Lake 63, 65, 73, 74, 75
Collins, Walker 6
Conard Lake 76
Conard Meadows 74, 76
Conard, Arthur L. 6, 37
Cone Lake 148
Corral Meadow 84, 85, 86, 197, 198, 213, 215
cougars 274
Cowboy Lake 152
Crags Lake 98, 99
Crater Butte 142, 183
Crater Peak 127, 129
Crumbaugh Lake 63, 65, 73, 74, 75
Crystal Lake 176, 177
Cypress Lake 154, 155

D

Deer Creek 237, 238
Dersch family 42
Devastated Area 17, 42, 43–44, 97
Devils Half Acre 115
Devils Kitchen 207, 208–209
Diamond Peak 37, 38
Diamond Point 37
Diller, Joseph Silas 4
Dittmar, Michael E. 6
Drake Lake 204, 206
Drakesbad Guest Ranch 23, 170, 193
Dream Lake 207, 208
Duck Lake 229

Durbin Lake 109, 110
Dutch Hill Ditch 224–225

E

Eagle Lake 162–164
East Fork Hat Creek 92
East Sulphur Creek 58, 59, 74, 76
Echo Lake 85, 87, 88, 89, 91
Eiler Gulch 126, 127
Eleanor Lake 152–153
Emerald Lake (LVNP) 38–39
Emerald Lake (Caribou Wilderness) 154, 155
Englebright, Harry 6
eruptions 5, 6, 17, 43, 44, 69
Evelyn Lake 159
Everett Lake 125, 127

F

Fairfield Peak 141, 183
Fantastic Lava Beds 134, 137, 143
Feather Lake 91
Fernley Lassen Railroad 166
fishing 2
Forest Lake 56, 57

G

Gallatin Beach 163–164
Gem Lake 153
glaciers 16
Glassburner Meadow 231
Godfrey, Grover K. 4, 68
Gold Lake 247, 248
Granite Gap 249, 258
Grassy Creek 142, 184, 185, 186, 187, 192
Grassy Lake (Bucks Lake) 257, 260
Grassy Lake (Hat Creek Rim) 122
Grassy Swale 86
Grassy Swale Creek 86
grazing 4, 5
Great Western Power Company 5

H

Harkness, Harvey W. 4, 40
Harkness, Mt. 171, 172, 173, 194, 195–196
Hat Creek 94, 95, 116, 117–118
Hat Creek Hereford Ranch RV Park & Campground 51
Hat Creek Radio Astronomy Observatory 51
Hat Creek Resort 48
Hat Creek Rim Lookout 119, 122
Hat Creek Rim Overlook 114, 116
Hat Creek Valley 15, 17
Hat Lake 43, 96
Hat Mountain 42, 90
Hay Meadow 159
Headwaters Pool 265, 266
Heart Lake 231, 233, 234
Hemlock Lake 79
Hidden Lakes 160

Horseshoe Lake 138, 142, 179, 180, 182, 185, 187, 192
Hot Springs Creek 200, 202, 205, 208

I

Indian Lake 179, 180
Indian Meadow 159
Inspiration Point 177, 178
Ishi 3
Ishi Wilderness 218, 239

J

Jakey Lake 143, 146, 187, 188, 189
Jakey Lake Creek 186, 188, 189
Jewel Lake 152
Johnson, Harold T. "Bizz" 166
Juniper Lake 168, 173, 174–175, 179, 180

K

King, Clarence 4, 40
Kings Creek 78, 80, 81, 82, 84, 85, 86, 197, 198, 212, 215
Kings Creek Cascades 80, 81, 82, 211
Kings Creek Falls 80, 81, 82, 211, 212–213, 215
Kings Creek Meadows 74
Kohm Yah-mah-nee Visitor Center 8, 36

L

Lake Almanor 5, 167
Lake Britton 266, 267, 268
Lake Eiler 123, 124, 125
Lake Helen 38–39
Lassen Chalet 7
Lassen Mineral Lodge 50, 54, 218
Lassen Peak 1, 4, 5, 14, 16, 40, 43, 65–69, 97
Lassen Peak National Monument 5
Lassen Peak Trail 6, 65–69
Lassen Trail 3
Lassen, Peter 3, 4, 40, 68
Lily Pond 104
Little Bear Lake 89, 90
Little Willow Lake 201, 204, 220, 222
lodging 23–24
Long Lake 160
Loomis Museum 6, 7, 46
Loomis, Benjamin E. 5, 6, 44, 46, 101
Lost Creek 122
Lower Deer Creek Falls 237, 238
Lower Twin Lake 85, 86, 88, 89, 91, 138, 141, 183

M

Magee Lake 125, 127
Magee Peak 125, 127,128, 129
Maidu 3
Maidu, Mt. 14, 15
Main Park Road 1
Manzanita Creek 98, 100–101
Manzanita Creek Road 101, 102

Manzanita Lake 7, 46–47, 102–103
maps 26, 27
Marian Creek 224
McArthur–Burney Falls Memorial State Park 263
Middle Fork Mill Creek 254, 258
Mill Creek 234, 235–236, 239, 240
Mill Creek (Bucks Lake) 255, 257, 259
Mill Creek Falls 58, 59, 74, 76
Mill Creek Resort 50, 216
Mineral 6, 36, 50, 54, 216
Mineral Springs 5
mixed conifer forest 10, 11
mosquitoes 275
mountain chaparral 10, 11
mountain meadows 13
Mud Lake 249
Muir, John 38

N

Native Americans 2, 3
Nobles Emigrant Trail 3, 4, 45, 95, 136
Nobles Pass 45
Nobles Trail 42–43, 94–95, 105–106
Nobles, William H. 3, 4, 42, 46, 95
North Caribou Peak 155
North Divide Lake 153
North Fork Feather River 225
Northern California Power Company 47
nuees ardentes 44

O

Old Station 109
Old Station Visitor Center 48

P

Painted Dunes 137
Paradise Meadow 70, 96
Peak 8446 127, 129
Phillips Petroleum Corporation 7, 203, 220
Plantation Gulch 231
Point 5450 258–259
Posey Lake 159
Prospect Peak 134, 135

Q

Quincy 243

R

Rainbow Lake 138, 141, 183
Rainbow Point 254
Raker Memorial 36
Raker, John H. 5
rattlesnakes 274–275
Reading Peak 41
Reading, Pierson B. 41
Red Cinder 143, 146, 191
Red Cinder Cone 143, 146, 191
Red Cliff 127, 129

Reflection Lake 46
Ridge Lakes 60, 61
Right Hand Branch Mill Creek 254, 258
Rim Lake 154, 155
Rim Rock Ranch 48
Rock Lake 249
Rocky Gulch Creek 235
Roosevelt, Theodore 5

S

sagebrush-juniper woodland 10
Shadow Lake 72, 92, 93
Sierra pocket gophers 41
Sifford family 7, 23
Sifford Lakes 78, 79, 209, 210
Silver Lake (Bucks Lake) 248, 249
Silver Lake (Caribou Wilderness) 130
Silver Lake (LVNP) 89, 91
ski area 7, 8
Snag Lake 138, 142–143, 145, 147, 184, 185, 186, 192
Snell family 7
Sorahan, Elmer 43
South Arm Rice Creek 229
South Divide Lake 153
South Fork Digger Creek 233, 234
Spanish Peak 248, 250, 251, 258
Spattercone Nature Trail 106, 111–112
spattercones 111
Spencer Meadow 226 ,228
Spencer Meadow Trail 77, 226–228
St. Bernard Lodge 50, 170, 216
Stover Spring 225
subalpine zone 13
Subway Cave 106, 112–114
Sulphur Works 36, 61–62
Summertown 105
Summit Lake 83, 87
Summit Lake Ranger Station 42
Supan family 6, 36
Susan River 167
Susanville 160
Swan Lake 85, 86, 138, 141, 183

T

Tehama County Wagon Road 5
Tehama, Mt. 15, 37, 58, 68
Terminal Geyser 7, 201, 203, 218, 219, 220, 222
Terrace Lake 72, 92, 93
Thousand Lakes Volcano 15
Thousand Lakes Wilderness 107–108
Three Lakes 244, 246, 257, 259, 261
ticks 275
Tilman, Samuel E. 4
Trail Lake 155, 156, 157
Triangle Lake 148, 149, 150
Turnaround Lake 150–151
Twin Lakes (Caribou Wilderness) 150

Twin Lakes (LVNP) 87, 88, 89, 91
Twin Lakes (Thousand Lakes Wilderness) 125, 127
Twin Meadows 76, 77

U

Upper Kings Creek 77
upper montane forest 11, 12
Upper Twin Lake 85, 86–87, 88, 89, 91

W

Warner Valley 193
West Fork Hat Creek 94, 96
Wheeler Survey 4

Whitehorse Creek 253
Whitney, Josiah Dwight 4
Widow Lake 143, 145–146, 147, 148–149, 191
wilderness 7
wilderness permit 27–28, 30
Williams, Howel 37, 62
Willow Creek 203, 219, 222
Willow Lake 218, 219
Wilson, Woodrow 6

Y

Yahi 3
Yani 3

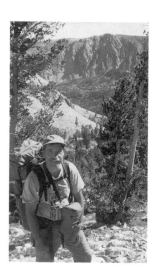

About the Author

Mike White was raised in the suburbs of Portland, Oregon, in the shadow of Mt. Hood (whenever the Pacific Northwest skies cleared enough to allow such things as shadows). His mother didn't drive, so walking was a way of life for her, as it became for her young son in tow. When Mike reached driving age, he began to explore further afield, hiking, backpacking, and climbing in the Cascades of Oregon and Washington. He further honed his outdoor skills while attending Seattle Pacific University.

After acquiring a B.A. in political science, Mike and his wife, Robin, relocated to the high desert of Reno, Nevada, where he was drawn to the beautiful and sunny Sierra. In the early 1990s, Mike left his last "real" job (with an engineering firm), and began writing full time. His first project for Wilderness Press was an update and expansion of Luther Linkhart's classic guide, *The Trinity Alps*. His first solo project was *Nevada Wilderness Areas and Great Basin National Park*. He is the author of the popular Snowshoe series, whose books include *Snowshoe Trails Tahoe*, *Best Snowshoe Trails of California*, and *Snowshoe Trails of Yosemite*. Mike's other titles include *Kings Canyon National Park*, *Sequoia National Park*, *Backpacking Nevada*, and *50 Classic Hikes in Nevada* (University of Nevada Press). Recently, he ventured hundreds of miles around Lake Tahoe and wrote *Top Trails Lake Tahoe* and *Afoot & Afield Reno-Tahoe*. Mike also contributed trip descriptions for *Backpacking California,* and maps and descriptions for updates to the classic Wilderness Press guides, *Sierra North* and *Sierra South*. In addition to his several book titles, Mike has written articles for *Sunset* and *Backpacker* magazines, and for the *Reno-Gazette Journal*.

Mike also instructs hiking, backpacking, and snowshoeing classes at Truckee Meadows Community College and is a frequent speaker for nonprofit groups. In addition, he can be found dispensing trail information while working part time at REI in Reno, where he lives with his wife, Robin, and their youngest son, Stephen, along with their two labs, Barkley and Griffin. David, his oldest son, resides in the area with his wife, Candace.

More Northern California Resources

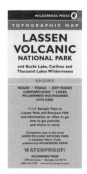

Lassen Volcanic National Park & Vicinity Map
Wilderness Press
Covering the 106,372-acre park, as well as thousands of acres of surrounding land in the Lassen National Forest, Caribou, Thousand Lakes, and Ishi wilderness areas, Hat Creek Valley, and McArthur-Burney Falls Memorial State Park—this map has been completely updated for easier use. It shows more than 450 miles of trails, as well as trailheads, points of interest, campgrounds, picnic areas, ranger stations, access roads, scenic turnouts, and parking areas.
ISBN 978-0-89997-477-4

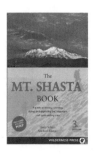

The Mt. Shasta Book
Guide to Hiking, Climbing, Skiing, and Exploring the Mountain and Surrounding Area
Andy Selters & Michael Zanger
This third edition covers dozens of trips both on the 14,162-foot mountain and in its surroundings, with authoritative coverage of hiking and backpacking trails and climbing, snowboarding, and ski routes. A large, folded topographic map shows all the mountain routes and variations.
ISBN 0-89997-404-X

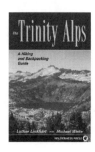

The Trinity Alps
A Hiking and Backpacking Guide
Luther Linkhart & Mike White
With descriptions of over 500 miles of trail and cross-country routes, this guide reveals some of the finest backcountry destinations in an area blessed with a diverse beauty rivaled by few other mountain ranges in the U.S. It includes 34 of the best hiking trips, from dayhikes to weeklong backpacks in the Trinity Alps Wilderness and surrounding area.
ISBN 0-89997-306-X

For ordering information, contact your local bookseller or Wilderness Press, www.wildernesspress.com